Studies in Big Data

Volume 65

The series "Studies in Big Data" (SBD) publishes new developments and advances in the various areas of Big Data- quickly and with a high quality. The intent is to cover the theory, research, development, and applications of Big Data, as embedded in the fields of engineering, computer science, physics, economics and life sciences. The books of the series refer to the analysis and understanding of large, complex, and/or distributed data sets generated from recent digital sources coming from sensors or other physical instruments as well as simulations, crowd sourcing, social networks or other internet transactions, such as emails or video click streams and other. The series contains monographs, lecture notes and edited volumes in Big Data spanning the areas of computational intelligence including neural networks, evolutionary computation, soft computing, fuzzy systems, as well as artificial intelligence, data mining, modern statistics and Operations research, as well as self-organizing systems. Of particular value to both the contributors and the readership are the short publication timeframe and the world-wide distribution, which enable both wide and rapid dissemination of research output.

** Indexing: The books of this series are submitted to ISI Web of Science, DBLP, Ulrichs, MathSciNet, Current Mathematical Publications, Mathematical Reviews, Zentralblatt Math: MetaPress and Springerlink.

More information about this series at http://www.springer.com/series/11970

Reda Alhajj • Mohammad Moshirpour
Behrouz Far
Editors

Data Management and Analysis

Case Studies in Education, Healthcare and Beyond

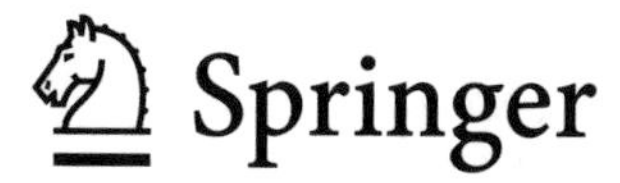

Editors
Reda Alhajj
Department of Computer Science,
University of Calgary
Calgary, AB, Canada

Department of Computer Engineering
Istanbul Medipol University
Istanbul, Turkey

Mohammad Moshirpour
Department of Electrical
and Computer Engineering
University of Calgary
Calgary, AB, Canada

Behrouz Far
Department of Electrical
and Computer Engineering
University of Calgary
Calgary, AB, Canada

ISSN 2197-6503 ISSN 2197-6511 (electronic)
Studies in Big Data
ISBN 978-3-030-32589-3 ISBN 978-3-030-32587-9 (eBook)
https://doi.org/10.1007/978-3-030-32587-9

This Springer imprint is published by the registered company Springer Nature Switzerland AG.
The registered company address is: Gewerbestrasse 11, 6330 Cham, Switzerland

Preface

Research and development in the general area of data science (DS) has grown beyond anticipation in the past few years. The initial wave had focus on modeling and tools drawn from various fields including mathematics, statistics, information science, software engineering, signal processing, probability models, machine learning, data mining, database systems, pattern recognition, visualization, predictive analytics, uncertain modeling, data warehousing, artificial intelligence, and high performance computing. Many projects were defined, developed, and deployed in isolation. In the second wave, general availability of data as well as techniques, tools, libraries, and toolkits, and, more importantly, hardware and software systems to support it collectively contributed to the growth of DS research. Today, we are observing the development and application of complex DS projects in many domains. We can find large-scale projects that require application of DS tools and techniques in each step of the process, from data collection to deployment.

The goal of this volume is to provide application examples of applied DS to solve complex science and engineering problems. In this volume, the contributing authors provide examples and solutions in various engineering, business, bioinformatics, geomatics, education, and environmental science. Through reviewing the contributions in this volume, the professionals and practitioners in each corresponding field can possibly understand the benefits of DS in their domain and understand where a particular theory, technique, or tool would be applied correctly and efficiently.

Calgary, AB, Canada — Reda Alhajj
Istanbul, Turkey
Calgary, AB, Canada — Mohammad Moshirpour
Calgary, AB, Canada — Behrouz Far

Contents

Leveraging Protection and Efficiency of Query Answering in Heterogenous RDF Data Using Blockchain

Sara Hosseinzadeh Kassani, Kevin A. Schneider, and Ralph Deters

Abstract In recent years, the digital world has experienced a massive amount of data being captured in various domains due to improvements in technology. Accordingly, big data management has emerged for storing, managing, and extracting valuable knowledge from collected data. Due to the explosion of the amount of data, developing tools for accurate and timely integration of inherently heterogeneous data has become a critical need. In the first part of this study, we focus on a semantic data integration approach with a case study of a plant ontology to provide a uniform query interface between users and different data sources. In the second part of this study, we propose a distributed Hyperledger-based architecture to ensure data security and privacy preservation in a semantic data integration framework. Data privacy and security can potentially be violated by unauthorized users, or malicious entities. The proposed view layer architecture between heterogeneous data sources and user interface layer using distributed Hyperledger can ensure only authorized users have access to the data sources in order to protect the system against unauthorized violation and determine the degree of users' permission for read and write access.

Keywords Semantic data integration · Blockchain · Security · Query processing

1 Introduction

The World Wide Web (WWW), invented by Tim Berners Lee, is considered as one of the main sources for accessing information and is based primarily on Hypertext Markup Language (HTML), Uniform Resource Locator (URL), and Hypertext Transfer Protocol (HTTP) [1]. Data on the World Wide Web is available in different formats such as structured, semi-structured, and unstructured from various resources

S. Hosseinzadeh Kassani (✉) · K. A. Schneider · R. Deters
Department of Computer Science, University of Saskatchewan, Saskatoon, SK, Canada
e-mail: sara.kassani@usask.ca; kevin.schneider@usask.ca; ralph.deters@usask.ca

R. Alhajj et al. (eds.), *Data Management and Analysis*, Studies in Big Data 65,
https://doi.org/10.1007/978-3-030-32587-9_1

in a decentralized and dynamic environment [2, 3]. The idea behind Semantic Web is about integration and combination of data drawn from diverse sources to have a distributed Web data. URIs (Uniform Resource Identifiers) allow data items to be uniquely identified and avoid unnecessary ambiguities when referring to resources while providing semantics [4, 5]. The idea of a semantic Web, unlike traditional Web, makes data not only human understandable but also machine interpretable [6, 7]. This approach allows sharing and connecting data on the Web from different sources, and is called linked data [8].

RDF is the World Wide Web Consortium (W3C) standard language for representing information on the Web. It provides a flexible data model that facilitates description and exchange of the semantics of Web content. Data in RDF is composed of three parts, namely subject, object, and predicate statements, which is called a triplet. In this manner, RDF provides the tools to construct data integration in Semantic Web. SPARQL Protocol And RDF Query Language (SPARQL) is a W3C standard language for executing complex queries over RDF graphs [9, 10].

The outline of this paper is as follows: Section 2 addresses the main challenges to current semantic data integration systems. A detailed description of the study design and experiment setup for designing and implementing an ontology for *Arabidopsis thaliana* and ontology evaluation is given in Sect. 3. In Sect. 4, we provide a detailed discussion of the proposed architecture of view layer using distributed Hyperledger technology. Finally, Sect. 5 draws the conclusions.

2 Challenges in Semantic Data Integration

2.1 Addressing Data Security Issues

In the current information age, with the increasing number of available data from various sources such as technology, education, healthcare, insurance, finance/banking [11, 12], big data management plays an important role in scientific exploration and knowledge discovery through effective collaboration among researchers [13, 14]. Although scalable big data storage for analyzing and querying large amounts of data exist today, they are not fully capable to adequately meet the needs of collaboration among participants [15].

To overcome the aforementioned challenges, data integration becomes important when building an infrastructure for the query processing across distributed and heterogeneous data sources that may not conform to a single data model. Ontology-based semantic integration approaches are promising to achieve robust and flexible data integration framework [16, 17]. Deficiency of secure methods for sharing vulnerable data may result in unwanted disclosure, security threats, or irreversible losses [18]. Hence, powerful and secure data management framework is a crucial requirement to secure data while being able to query and retrieve RDF data. Security concerns in processing, storing, and transferring of confidential or sensitive data are a serious concern that could cause ethical, intellectual property, and privacy issues [19, 20]. Access control management is another important concern that needs attention while providing a secure environment to prevent data misuse or theft [21]. By providing proper authorization, we can ensure only specific individuals have access to data, making data unavailable to all others [22].

2.2 Addressing Accuracy and Quality of Data Issues

Today large volumes of data are growing exponentially in every domain of science, and valuable knowledge is driven by the capability of collecting and processing of this data. Although data is accumulated and analyzed very quickly in information systems, there is a need to establish approaches that can guarantee a certain degree of data quality [23, 24]. Problems of data quality and trustworthiness must be addressed before preparing the data for subsequent operations. To tackle this challenge, researchers must analyze the quality of data and assure that data is accurate, complete, and consistent in order to decrease operational risk [25, 26].

2.3 Addressing Data Operation and Data Access Issues

The widespread heterogeneous data available in big data systems also have made security critically important. The gap between data processing and security requirements has given rise to many issues and concerns. By compromising fragile defenses, attackers can strike the system not only from outside the system but also from within it [27]. An attacker may attempt to obtain unauthorized read/write permissions against the stored data objects or attempt to reveal or derive the credentials of account owners and try to perform an unauthorized read or write operation on stored data. From data operation perspective, there are four basic operations: write, read, delegate, and revoke [28]. The user needs to be provided with a valid access key to ensure a specific data is being accessed for read or write operation by that authorized user [29]. Also, for a robust auditing system, super-users have privileges to grant delegation and revocation to other users and also customize access rules for extracting queries [30]. Authorization is an even higher priority when private or sensitive data is stored in a multi-user environment, as insufficient authorization and access management system allow attackers to gain access to data and compromise the consistency of the system [31].

3 Study Design and Experiment Setup

3.1 Ontology in Plant Science

The term Ontology is originated from philosophy where it refers to the nature of existence. Particularly, ontology was used to provide a semantic framework for representing knowledge using ontology representation languages. Currently, several ontology representation languages have been proposed including RDF, RDFS, and OWL to capture the semantics of the domain of study [32]. The bio-ontology emerged for enhancing the interoperability within biological knowledge with the best practices on ontology development [33].

The most cited bio-ontology is the Gene Ontology (GO) [34, 35], which is a tool for the unification of biology developed by Gene Ontology Consortium in 2000, present more than 30,000 species-independent control vocabularies for describing gene products including plants. Plant Ontology (PO) focused on developing and sharing unambiguous vocabularies for plant anatomy and morphology. PO consists of two sub-categories: the plant structure ontology and the growth and developmental stages ontology [36]. By defining classes of entities, logical relations, properties, constraints, and range axioms, botany and plant science researchers are able to understand, share, and reuse knowledge in a machine or computer interpretable content, enabling them to detect and reason biologically common concepts in heterogeneous datasets [37].

The Plant Science Ontology's main goal is to design and develop a semantic framework in order to support computerized reasoning. With the help of ontologies, scientists are able to employ PO or GO as a general reference to semantically link large amounts of plant phenotype and genotype data together. However, knowledge engineering requires extensive knowledge of different domains such as biology and engineering, and also standard ontology languages [38, 39].

3.2 *Tools and Implementation of Ontology*

There is no specific method for modeling and building a domain ontology, and the majority of the best methodologies for developing an ontology depends on the purpose of research. For building an ontology, researchers should consider three features. First, identifying the domain and scope of the ontology. Second, choosing the language and logic to construct the ontology. Finally, identifying key concepts of resources (nouns), relationships (verbs), domain, and range axioms.

We study *Arabidopsis thaliana* as a reference plant for building our ontology. *Arabidopsis thaliana* is the best investigated flowering plant species, belonging to the Brassicaceae family. It has been chosen as one of the most widely used model plant organism for studies in plant research in areas such as developmental and molecular genetics analysis, population genetics, and genomics for many years. Its significant properties such as short regeneration time and simple growth requirements make it desirable for model plant studies. Therefore, studying biological processes in this species is important for gaining information about plant science and for utilizing of this knowledge to other relevant plants species.

We have used the Protégé as the principal ontology authoring tool in our ontology-based application. Protégé is an IDE developed at Stanford University by Stanford Medical Informatics team. It is a free and open-source ontology platform that enables users to create and populate ontology and formal knowledge-based

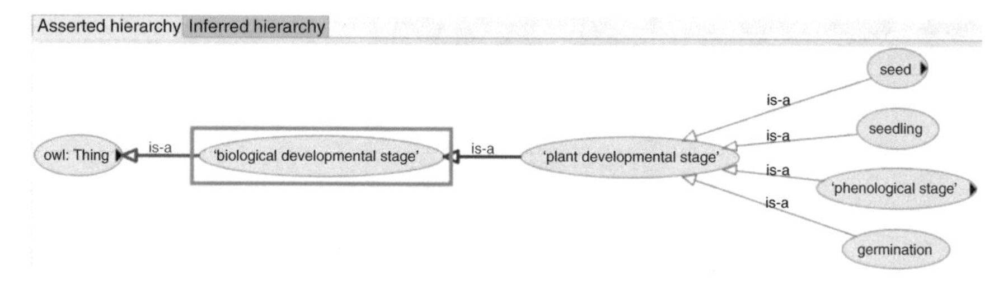

Fig. 1 Class tree of *Arabidopsis thaliana* in Protege

applications more straightforward. There exist many plug-ins for Protégé offering a number of powerful features. We used the OWLViz plug-in to visualize Protégé ontologies. OWLViz is a powerful and highly configurable extension providing a graphical representation of the semantic relationships for helping users to visualize classes in an OWL ontology. OWLViz creates a knowledge-based graph of the classes to different formats such as JPEG and PNG [40].

The process of building ontology for *Arabidopsis thaliana* with the top-down approach is described in detail in this section. This ontology acts as a basis for researchers to conduct queries and reason in a knowledge-based environment. All OWL classes inherit from a single root class called owl:Thing. The class owl:Thing represents the concept of any user-defined class or individuals in order to facilitate reasoning, as illustrated in Fig. 1.

Owl:Thing is developed by W3C located at http://www.w3.org/2002/07/owl as part of OWL vocabulary and is equivalent to rdfs:Resource. The most basic part of the ontology for *Arabidopsis thaliana* ontology is super classes such as biological developmental stage, biological process, and biochemical process as shown in Fig. 2. Each super class consists of subclasses which are arranged in an inheritance hierarchy. The second level in ontology are subclasses which provide more refined and detailed information about superclass, such as germination, life span, seed, and seedling.

OWL properties express association between two entities of a domain. Different types of properties are used to link between concepts. Figure 3 shows the list of declared properties of Arabidopsis thaliana ontology in Protégé for this study. Some of the relations used in this ontology are <growsIn>, <hasPart>, and <hasVariant>.

Domain and range constraints of the properties aid to precisely describe a representation of knowledge. Domain indicates the type of individuals that can be the subject and range specifies the type of individuals that can be the object within the RDF triple. The individuals are the members or instances of a class with certain constraints as illustrated in Fig. 4.

After preparing the ontology, we have used Apache Jena Fuseki server, a HTTP-based query engine, for executing the SPARQL queries over the Web of linked data and extract triple information on the Web page. Apache Jena Fuseki server is a SPARQL server providing hosts for persistent storage or in-memory storage of the datasets and aimed toward supporting developers with building practical semantic

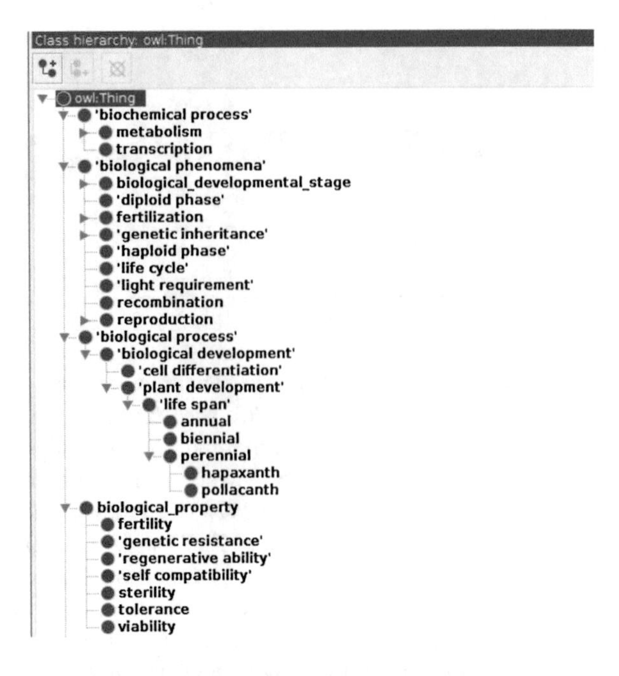

Fig. 2 Class hierarchy of *Arabidopsis thaliana* in Protege

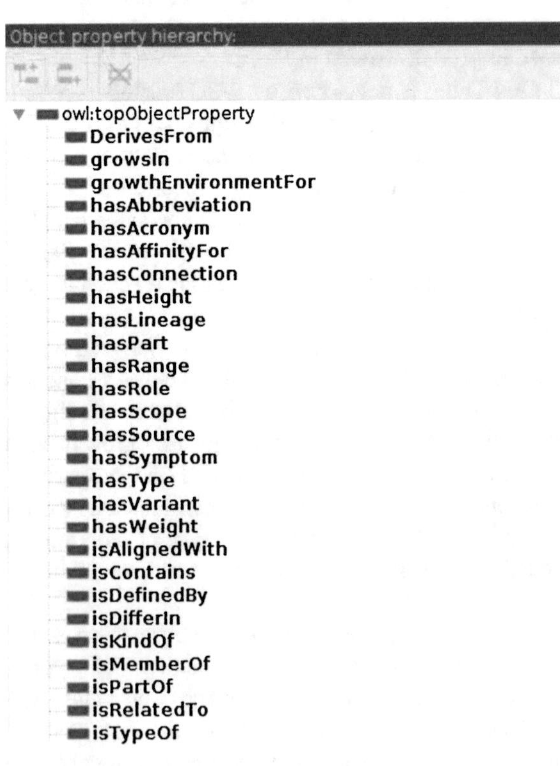

Fig. 3 Object properties of *Arabidopsis thaliana*

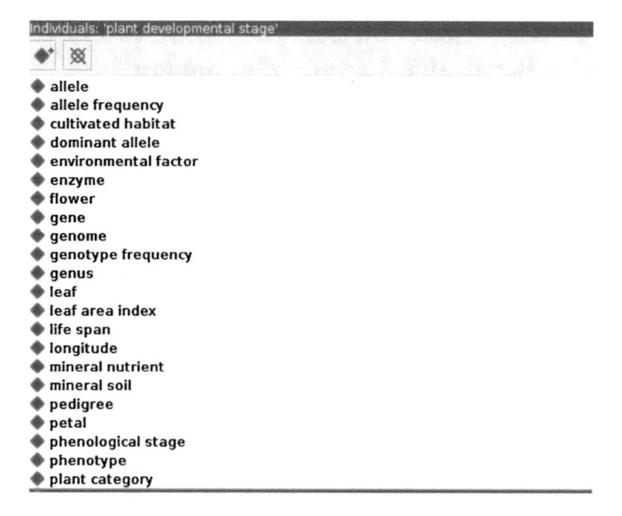

Fig. 4 Individuals of *Arabidopsis thaliana* ontology

Web applications. The class biological property, for example, has several subclasses. Some subclasses of biological property that are used to describe the class are genetic resistance, regenerative ability, seed compatibility, tolerance, and viability. A wide variety of object properties are used to describe relationships between classes and subclasses. The object property growsIn describe the plant-specific requirement for growth and development. The object property maxHeight indicates the plant sample height growth pattern. The ontology of *Arabidopsis thaliana* in this study provides detailed information pertaining to the morphology and developmental stages.

3.3 Ontology Evaluation

After building the Ontology, we should assess the consistency and quality of the ontology using Protégé reasoner. Ontology evaluation and validation ensure the avoidance of excessiveness concepts, terminological ambiguity, and incompatible subclass relationships. Ontologies need to be validated to confirm a standardized OWL profile, the expressivity of ontology, as well as the consistency of structure described in the model with expected semantics to support the exchange of information efficiently. Further consultation with domain experts is needed to examine the scope of the proposed ontology [41, 42]. To evaluate the overall performance of the implementation and ontology syntax, we have used OntoCheck plug-in to evaluate the consistency, conciseness, and correctness of ontology automatically. OntoCheck is an open-source plug-in developed at the University of Freiburg, and it is currently one of the W3C OWL official validating tools [43, 44].

4 View Layer on Semantic Data Integration Using Distributed Ledger Technology

The idea of view-based integration systems presents a single point (the view layer) of a query and data access for a domain of a specific ontology. Users would execute large numbers of expensive queries over the unified view and get back results in order to get the best possible query performance. The main goal of using view layer is to satisfy user-specific requirements while processing data in a timely and secure manner through an integrated framework.

On the other hand, for preventing attackers from exploiting vulnerabilities, a newly initiated approach is needed to verify user's authentication before providing access to the stored data and enhance security. Employing a private blockchain as a secure, decentralized, and distributed corporate ledger system can ensure the correctness and completeness of data in the view layer [45, 46]. The blockchain is a cryptographic technology that has a secure and resilient architecture and is used to track the records of data ownership. Users on a network create a transaction history.

The blocks of data subsequently join together to create chains of blocks, storing a transaction history among users without the need for a centralized control [47, 48]. Once a transaction is published to the blockchain and confirmed as accurate, it cannot be reversed or destroyed and is immutable. We can benefit from this approach to reason about whether an individual is permitted to perform a read/write action.

Each block on the blockchain references to the previous one and contains information regarding the transactions and data about the block. Figure 5 illustrates a blockchain and contents of a block. Usually, the block header contains information about the version of the block and a hash of the data in the block [49].

The significant advantage of blockchain is smart contracts. Smart contracts as a fundamental mechanism in developing access control policies allow users to control access of data by writing a pre-defined set of criteria and condition [50, 51]. The smart contracts will automatically execute the terms of the contract. These contracts increase efficiency by being able to interact with other contracts, storing data, and making decisions. Smart contracts' information is distributed throughout the

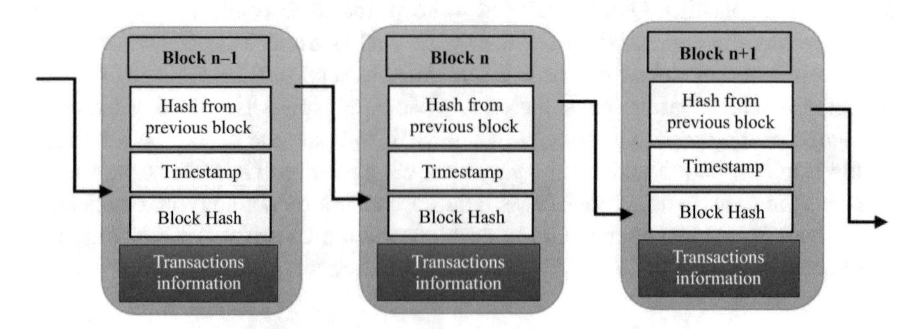

Fig. 5 Structure of blockchain showing chained blocks

blockchain for the cost of a small token and automatically executed upon occurrence of the event [52]. The view layer is transparent to the end users and is able to detect compromised or malicious users; thus, it provides a framework that is able to solve security concerns such as identity management, access control, trust, and authorization. Furthermore, this approach does not allow the user's authentication to be forged or modified and hence remains highly resilient against intrusion [53].

4.1 The Architecture of the View Layer

The idea of our representation model for storing and retrieving views of queries calls for a layer of abstraction over the RDF data sources [54]. This layer of abstraction is called a "view layer" as illustrated in Fig. 6. View layer is dedicated for managing views including storing and retrieving views of queries and also keeping the views updated from the data sources in order to support real-time semantic query processing of the ontology. The views are generated and maintained at the back-end, and each view may be used by several users as a shared view.

View layer also prevents improper access of unauthorized users to sensitive or confidential information based on users corresponding credential levels. In view layer architecture, users are only allowed to have access to data by querying a view of the data, they do not have permission to directly query or access over the original data sources. In this scenario, users with different level of authorization are allowed to have access to the same queries, but not the same results in order to prevent information leakage and security breach.

Figure 7 illustrates an overview to view layer architecture: data flows from a user that sends a query to the view layer. The users' request will be sent to a module called a blockchain access control. The blockchain access control module will examine the users' privileges and make a decision on what kind of access should be granted to users' request. After verifying the level of permission and authorization role of the user, the coordinator module translates or reformulates

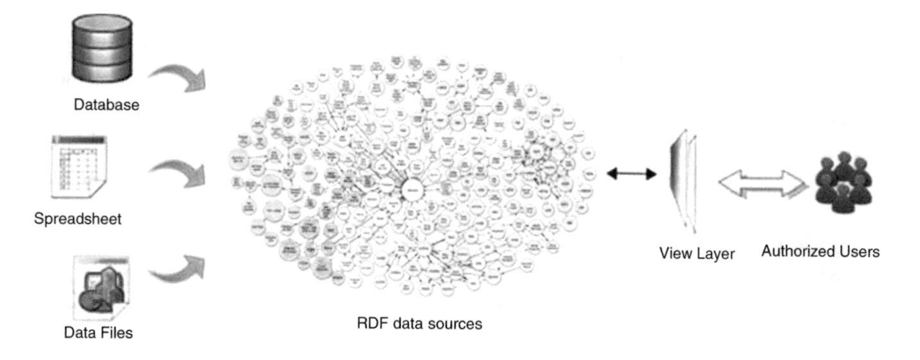

Fig. 6 Data integration system and view layer

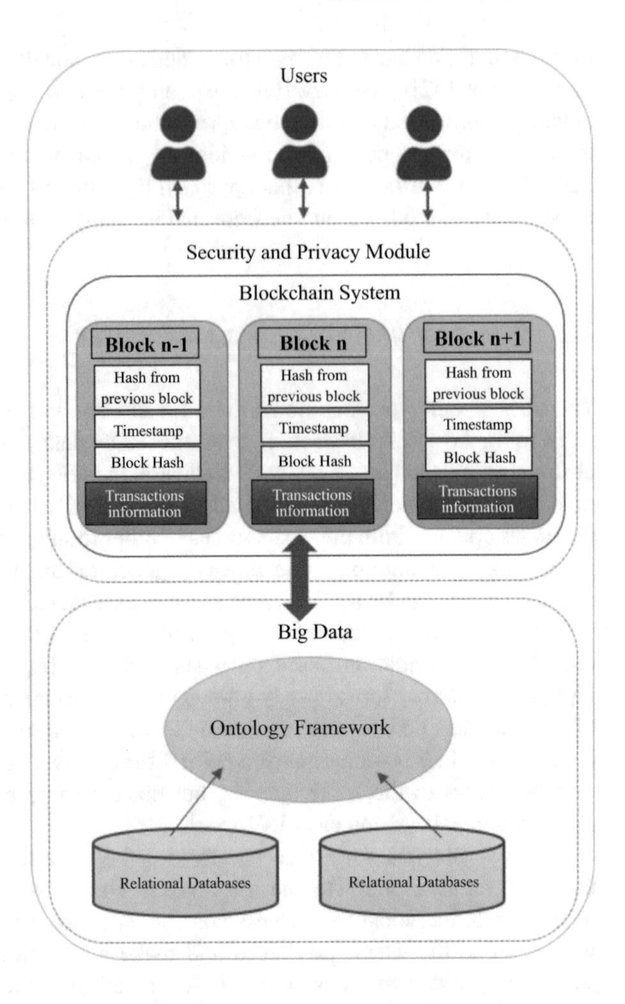

Fig. 7 An overview of view layer architecture

queries into equivalent queries with respect to the data integration schema and user credential. Query processor creates the query result in a database for views in the view manager module and then return the answers to the users while satisfying all security requirements. When a user sends a read or write request to have access to the RDF data store, based on system smart contract rules, the access level will be analyzed and if the user is eligible to have access to data, the requested query will be executed. When a request to the database is accepted, user information and transaction information will be added to the block in order to keep track of all transactions in a distributed ledger.

Blockchain model in the proposed semantic data integration architecture avoids compromising unauthorized data access and protects transactional privacy [22] using a Role-Based Access Control (RBAC) approach. In RBAC, roles are assigned to users and privileges are assigned to roles in order to determine if a user is eligible to have access to data [26, 27]. As demonstrated in Fig. 8, a participant in the system

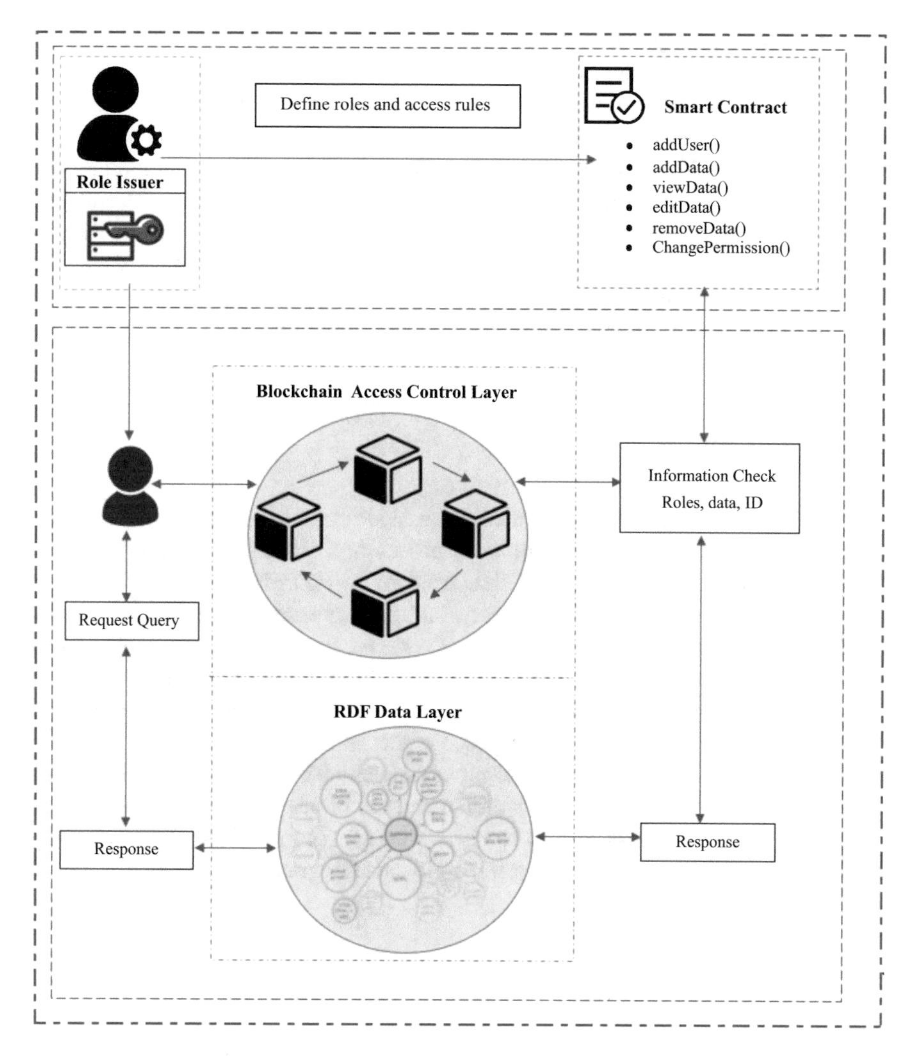

Fig. 8 Blockchain Role-Based Access Control (BRBAC) system

based on the type of role is allowed to have access to a specific data. Roles are issued by the appropriate authority in order to determine whether or not a user (or group of users working together) should be trusted to have access to a specific data. The role-based access control using smart contracts on data verifies the access role of a user. In this architecture, when a user sends requests to have access to data, a rule in smart contract is triggered to check the user assigned role to that data. If the user has a role that has access to privileges then, the user is allowed to view the data.

In the Blockchain Role-Based Access Control (BRBAC) system, the smart contract file contains rules for data and transactions including request, grant, revoke, verify, and also view. The assumption is that access privileges based on defined roles are granted to system users by role issuer to a subset of the RDF data [55]. When a user attempts to access a data, smart contract verifies that the user has a role with appropriate access rights to that data and based on the response from smart contract, the user is allowed or denied having access to a subset or view of data. Using Blockchain Role-Based Access Control approach, a system administrator can assign IDs to data and enable blockchain to control access between users and data store by verifying user data access level using assigned ID. The IDs can be defined to represent a specific data or a query that allows access to a view of data. The blockchain access control module is separated from the data store and hence can be used as an access control layer to the existing infrastructure.

5 Conclusion

Large volumes of data are generated by a wide variety of sources. However, security challenges and complications in processing, storing, and transferring of confidential or sensitive data exist that need to be addressed. These challenges could cause ethical, intellectual property, and privacy issues. There is therefore a need for efficient secure privacy preserving systems. In this study, we implemented a semantic data integration framework with a case study of plant ontology to ensure data quality and trustworthiness in extracting and processing queries over the RDF triples stores. Also, we proposed a secure view-based layer architecture using distributed ledger technology to prevent unauthorized read/write permissions against stored data. The goal of this architecture is to provide a secure and private method in allowing access to data to users with specific privileges by integrating blockchain technology with existing semantic data integration framework.

References

1. Abbate, J. (1999). The electrical century: Inventing the Web. *Proceedings of the IEEE, 87*(11), 1999–2002.
2. Chandarana, P., & Vijayalakshmi, M. (2014). Big data analytics frameworks. In *Circuits, Systems, Communication and Information Technology Applications (CSCITA), 2014 International Conference on* (pp. 430–434). Piscataway, NJ: IEEE.
3. Strawn, G. (2014). Masterminds of the world wide web. *IT Professional, 16*(4), 58–59.
4. Janev, V., & Vranes, S. (2009). Semantic web technologies: Ready for adoption? *IT Professional, 11*(5), 8–16.
5. Howell, S., Rezgui, Y., & Beach, T. (2018). Water utility decision support through the semantic web of things. *Environmental Modelling & Software, 102*, 94–114.
6. Kassani, P. H., Teoh, A. B. J., & Kim, E. (2017). Evolutionary-modified fuzzy nearest-neighbor rule for pattern classification. *Expert Systems with Applications, 88*, 258–269.
7. Ostrowski, D. (2018). Building linked data agents for mobility applications. In *Proceedings - 12th IEEE International Conference on Semantic Computing, ICSC 2018*. Piscataway, NJ: IEEE.

8. Miao, Q., Meng, Y., Fang, L., Nishino, F., & Igata, N. (2015). Link scientific publications using linked data. In *Semantic Computing (ICSC), 2015 IEEE International Conference on* (pp. 268–271). Piscataway, NJ: IEEE.
9. Costanzo, A., Faro, A., Giordano, D., & Spampinato, C. (2012). Implementing Ubiquitous Information services with ontologies: Methodology and case study. In *Computer Science and Information Systems (FedCSIS), 2012 Federated Conference on* (pp. 911–914). Piscataway, NJ: IEEE.
10. Chakraborty, A., Munshi, S., & Mukhopadhyay, D. (2013). Searching and establishment of S-P-O relationships for linked RDF Graphs: An adaptive approach. In *Proceedings - 2013 International Conference on Cloud and Ubiquitous Computing and Emerging Technologies, CUBE 2013*. Washington, DC: IEEE Computer Society.
11. Sara Hosseinzadeh Kassani, S. E. N., & Kassani, P. H. (2015). Introducing a hybrid model of DEA and data mining in evaluating efficiency. Case study: Bank branches. *Academic Journal of Research in Economics and Management, 3*(2), 72–80.
12. Pathak, J., Kiefer, R. C., & Chute, C. G. (2013). Mining drug-drug interaction patterns from linked data: A case study for Warfarin, Clopidogrel, and Simvastatin. In *Proceedings - 2013 IEEE International Conference on Bioinformatics and Biomedicine, IEEE BIBM 2013* (pp. 23–30). Piscataway, NJ: IEEE.
13. Wang, S., Man, Y., Zhang, T., Wong, T. J., & King, I. (2013). Data management with flexible and extensible data schema in clans. *Procedia Computer Science, 24*, 268–273.
14. Kanchi, S., Sandilya, S., Ramkrishna, S., Manjrekar, S., & Vhadgar, A. (2015). Challenges and solutions in big data management-An overview. In *Proceedings - 2015 International Conference on Future Internet of Things and Cloud, FiCloud 2015 and 2015 International Conference on Open and Big Data, OBD 2015* (pp. 418–426). IEEE.
15. Kassani, P. H., & Kim, E. (2016). Pseudoinverse Matrix Decomposition Based Incremental Extreme Learning Machine with Growth of Hidden Nodes. *International Journal of Fuzzy Logic and Intelligent Systems, 16*(2), 125–130.
16. Moujane, A., Chiadmi, D., Benhlima, L., & Wadjinny, F. (2009). A study in the P2P data integration process. In *Computer Systems and Applications, 2009. AICCSA 2009. IEEE/ACS International Conference on* (pp. 57–58). Piscataway, NJ: IEEE.
17. Kassani, P. H., & Teoh, A. B. J. (2017). A new sparse model for traffic sign classification using soft histogram of oriented gradients. *Applied Soft Computing Journal, 52*, 231–246.
18. Al Nuaimi, N., AlShamsi, A., Mohamed, N., & Al-Jaroodi, J. (2015). e-Health cloud implementation issues and efforts. In *Industrial Engineering and Operations Management (IEOM), 2015 International Conference on* (pp. 1–10). IEEE.
19. Treiblmaier, H., Madlberger, M., Knotzer, N., & Pollach, I. (2004). Evaluating personalization and customization from an ethical point of view: An empirical study. In *System Sciences, 2004. Proceedings of the 37th Annual Hawaii International Conference on* (p. 10). IEEE.
20. Sugumaran, M., Murugan, B. B., & Kamalraj, D. (2014). An architecture for data security in cloud computing. In *2014 World Congress on Computing and Communication Technologies* (pp. 252–255). IEEE.
21. Paul, R., et al. (2008). An ontology-based integrated assessment framework for high-assurance systems. In *Semantic Computing, 2008 IEEE International Conference on* (pp. 386–393). IEEE.
22. Park, H.-A., Lee, D. H., & Zhan, J. (2008). Attribute-based access control using combined authentication technologies. In *Granular Computing, 2008. GrC 2008. IEEE International Conference on* (pp. 518–523). IEEE.
23. Lv, Z., Song, H., Basanta-Val, P., Steed, A., & Jo, M. (2017). Next-generation big data analytics: State of the art, challenges, and future research topics. *IEEE Transactions on Industrial Informatics, 13*(4), 1891–1899.
24. Taleb, I., El Kassabi, H. T., Serhani, M. A., Dssouli, R., & Bouhaddioui, C. (2016). Big data quality: A quality dimensions evaluation. In *2016 Intl IEEE Conferences on Ubiquitous Intelligence & Computing, Advanced and Trusted Computing, Scalable Computing and Communications, Cloud and Big Data Computing, Internet of People, and Smart World Congress (UIC/ATC/ScalCom/CBDCom/IoP/SmartWorld)* (pp. 759–765). IEEE.

25. Karkouch, A., Al Moatassime, H., Mousannif, H., & Noel, T. (2015). Data quality enhancement in Internet of Things environment. In *Computer Systems and Applications (AICCSA), 2015 IEEE/ACS 12th International Conference of* (pp. 1–8). IEEE.
26. Botha, M., Botha, A., & Herselman, M. (2014). Data quality challenges: A content analysis in the e-health domain. In *2014 4th World Congress on Information and Communication Technologies, WICT 2014* (pp. 107–112). IEEE.
27. Kayem, A. V. D. M., Martin, P., & Akl, S. G. (2011). Efficient enforcement of dynamic cryptographic access control policies for outsourced data. In *Information Security South Africa (ISSA), 2011* (pp. 1–8). IEEE.
28. Balani, R., Wanner, L. F., Friedman, J., Srivastava, M. B., Lin, K., & Gupta, R. K. (2011). Programming support for distributed optimization and control in cyber-physical systems. In *Proceedings - 2011 IEEE/ACM 2nd International Conference on Cyber-Physical Systems, ICCPS 2011* (pp. 109–118). IEEE Computer Society.
29. Farroha, B., Essman, K., Farroha, D., & Cohen, A. (2011). Development of an integrated security framework to enable the control and security of a heterogeneous enterprise. In *Systems Conference (SysCon), 2011 IEEE International* (pp. 103–108). IEEE.
30. Ferrara, A. L., Fachsbauer, G., Liu, B., & Warinschi, B. (2015). Policy privacy in cryptographic access control. In *Computer Security Foundations Symposium (CSF), 2015 IEEE 28th* (pp. 46–60). IEEE.
31. Upadhyaya, A., & Bansal, M. (2015). Deployment of secure sharing: Authenticity and authorization using cryptography in cloud environment. In *Conference Proceeding - 2015 International Conference on Advances in Computer Engineering and Applications, ICACEA 2015* (pp. 852–855). IEEE.
32. Yang, K.-A., Yang, H.-J., Yang, J.-D., & Kim, K.-H. (2005). Bio-ontology construction using object-oriented paradigm. In *12th Asia-Pacific Software Engineering Conference (APSEC'05)* (p. 6). IEEE.
33. Kim, K.-H., Yang, J.-D., Choi, J.-H., Yang, K.-A., & Ha, Y.-G. (2007). A semantic inheritance/inverse-inheritance mechanism for systematic bio-ontology construction. In *2007 29th Annual International Conference of the IEEE Engineering in Medicine and Biology Society* (pp. 398–401). IEEE.
34. Gan, M., Dou, X., Wang, D., & Jiang, R. (2011). DOPCA: A new method for calculating ontology-based semantic similarity. In *Proceedings - 2011 10th IEEE/ACIS International Conference on Computer and Information Science, ICIS 2011* (pp. 110–115). IEEE.
35. Bandyopadhyay, S., & Mallick, K. (2014). A new path based hybrid measure for gene ontology similarity. *IEEE/ACM Transactions on Computational Biology and Bioinformatics, 11*(1), 116–127.
36. Silalahi, M., Cahyani, D. E., Sensuse, D. I., & Budi, I. (2015). Developing indonesian medicinal plant ontology using socio-technical approach. In *2015 International Conference on Computer, Communications, and Control Technology (I4CT)* (pp. 39–43). IEEE.
37. Li, X., Zhang, Y., Wang, J., & Pu, Q. (2016). A preliminary study of plant domain ontology. In *Proceedings - 2016 IEEE 14th International Conference on Dependable, Autonomic and Secure Computing, DASC 2016, 2016 IEEE 14th International Conference on Pervasive Intelligence and Computing, PICom 2016, 2016 IEEE 2nd International Conference on Big Data*. IEEE.
38. Qi, H., Zhang, L., & Gao, Y. (2010). Semantic retrieval system based on corn ontology. In *Proceedings - 5th International Conference on Frontier of Computer Science and Technology, FCST 2010* (pp. 116–121). IEEE.
39. Mizoguchi, R., Sano, T., & Kitamura, Y. (1999). An ontology-based human friendly message generation in a multiagent human media system for oil refinery plant operation. In *Proceedings of the IEEE International Conference on Systems, Man, and Cybernetics, 1999* (pp. 648–653). IEEE.
40. Kassani, S. H., & Kassani, P. H. (2018). Building an ontology for the domain of plant science using prot\'eg\'e. *arXiv.org*. arXiv:1810.04606.

41. Bezerra, C., Freitas, F., & Santana, F. (2013). Evaluating ontologies with competency questions. In *2013 IEEE/WIC/ACM International Joint Conferences on Web Intelligence (WI) and Intelligent Agent Technologies (IAT)* (pp. 284–285). IEEE.
42. Khan, S., Qamar, U., & Muzaffar, A. W. (2015). A framework for evaluation of owl biomedical ontologies based on properties coverage. In *2015 13th International Conference on Frontiers of Information Technology (FIT)* (pp. 59–64). IEEE.
43. OntoCheck. [Online]. Retrieved from https://protegewiki.stanford.edu/wiki/OntoCheck
44. Schober, D., Tudose, I., Svatek, V., & Boeker, M. (2012). OntoCheck: Verifying ontology naming conventions and metadata completeness in Protégé 4. *Journal of Biomedical Semantics, 3*(2), S4.
45. Samaniego, M., & Deters, R. Supporting IoT multi-tenancy on edge devices. In *Proceedings - 2016 IEEE International Conference on Internet of Things; IEEE Green Computing and Communications; IEEE Cyber, Physical, and Social Computing; IEEE Smart Data, iThings-GreenCom-CPSCom-Smart Data 2016* (pp. 2017, 66–2073). IEEE.
46. Chen, J., & Xue, Y. (2017). Bootstrapping a blockchain based ecosystem for big data exchange. In *Big Data (BigData Congress), 2017 IEEE International Congress on* (pp. 460–463). IEEE.
47. Patel, D., Bothra, J., & Patel, V. (2017). Blockchain exhumed. In *Asia Security and Privacy (ISEASP), 2017 ISEA* (pp. 1–12). IEEE.
48. Guo, H., Meamari, E., & Shen, C.-C. (2018). Blockchain-inspired event recording system for autonomous vehicles. In *2018 1st IEEE International Conference on Hot Information-Centric Networking (HotICN)* (pp. 218–222). IEEE.
49. Lewis, A. (2015). Blockchain technology explained. *Blockchain Technology*, 1–27.
50. Wright, C., & Serguieva, A. (2018). Sustainable blockchain-enabled services: Smart contracts. In *Proceedings - 2017 IEEE International Conference on Big Data, Big Data 2017* (pp. 4255–4264). IEEE.
51. Jämthagen, C., & Hell, M. (2017). Blockchain-based publishing layer for the keyless signing infrastructure. In *2016 Intl IEEE Conferences on Ubiquitous Intelligence & Computing, Advanced and Trusted Computing, Scalable Computing and Communications, Cloud and Big Data Computing, Internet of People, and Smart World Congress (UIC/ATC/ScalCom/CBDCom/IoP/SmartWorld)* (pp. 374–381). IEEE.
52. Aste, T., Tasca, P., & Di Matteo, T. (2017). Blockchain technologies: The foreseeable impact on society and industry. *Computer, 50*(9), 18–28.
53. Cheng, J.-C., Lee, N.-Y., Chi, C., & Chen, Y.-H. (2018). Blockchain and smart contract for digital certificate. In *2018 IEEE International Conference on Applied System Invention (ICASI)* (pp. 1046–1051). IEEE.
54. Samaniego, M., & Deters, R. (2017). Virtual resources & blockchain for configuration management in IoT. *Journal of Ubiquitous Systems & Pervasive Networks, 9*(2), 1–13.
55. Uchibeke, U. U., Kassani, S. H., Schneider, K. A., & Deters, R. (2018). Blockchain access control ecosystem for big data security. In *2018 IEEE International Conference on Internet of Things (iThings) and IEEE Green Computing and Communications (GreenCom) and IEEE Cyber, Physical and Social Computing (CPSCom) and IEEE Smart Data (SmartData)* (pp. 1373–1378). IEEE.

Big Data Analytics of Twitter Data and Its Application for Physician Assistants: Who Is Talking About Your Profession in Twitter?

Monica Mai, Carson K. Leung, Justin M. C. Choi, and Long Kei Ronnie Kwan

Abstract In the current era of big data, huge volumes of a wide variety of valuable data—which may be of different veracity—are easily generated or collected at a high velocity in various real-life applications. A rich source of complex big data is social networking sites (e.g., Twitter, Facebook, LinkedIn), in which many people are connected with each other. For many of these creators of social network data (i.e., users on the social networking sites), it is not unusual for them to have hundreds or even thousands of friends or connections. Among these friends or connections, some of them care about you as an individual user or friend, while some others care or talk about your profession. It is interesting to know how many of your friends or connections know about your profession, understand it, and talk about it. This chapter presents a system for big data analytics of Twitter data. In particular, we design a system to allow non-computer experts to extract interesting information from the social network (especially, Twitter) data. To demonstrate the practicality of the system, we also conduct a case study to demonstrate how the system helps physician assistants (PAs) to find interesting pattern from tweets about their profession.

1 Introduction

In the current era of big data, huge volumes of a wide variety of valuable data—which may be of different veracity—are easily generated or collected at a high velocity in various real-life applications. As big data are new oil, embedded in these big data are implicit, previously unknown, and potentially useful information and

M. Mai
Max Rady College of Medicine – Master of Physician Assistant Studies, University of Manitoba, Winnipeg, MB, Canada

C. K. Leung (✉) · J. M. C. Choi · L. K. R. Kwan
Department of Computer Science, University of Manitoba, Winnipeg, MB, Canada
e-mail: kleung@cs.umanitoba.ca

R. Alhajj et al. (eds.), *Data Management and Analysis*, Studies in Big Data 65,
https://doi.org/10.1007/978-3-030-32587-9_2

valuable knowledge. With the following characteristics of big data, data science solutions are in demand:

- Volume, which focuses on the quantity of big data;
- Variety, which focuses on types, contents, or forms of big data;
- Value, which focuses on the usefulness of data;
- Veracity, which focuses on the quality of data (e.g., precise data, imprecise and uncertain data);
- Velocity, which focuses on the speed at which data are collected or generated;
- Validity, which focuses on interpretation of data and discovered knowledge from the data; and
- Visibility, which focuses on visualization of data and discovered knowledge from the data.

In general, data science solutions apply techniques like data mining, machine learning, as well as mathematical and statistical modelling to discovery knowledge and useful information from these big data. Rich sources of complex big data include social networking sites (e.g., Twitter, Facebook, LinkedIn), in which many people are connected with each other.

The beginning of the twenty-first century saw an explosion of online social networking activity with the advent of social media sites such as Twitter [1]. Twitter is an online social networking and blogging service that allows users to read the tweets of other users by "following" them. As such, a Twitter user A may be interested in knowing the popular followees. In other words, for any Twitter user A, if many of his friends follow some individual users or groups of users, then user A might also be interested in following the same individual users or groups of users. Note that, relationships between social entities are mostly defined by following (or subscribing) each other. Each user (social entity) can be following multiple users and be followed by the same or different followers. Note that the follow/subscribe relationship between follower and followee is not the same as the mutual friendship because a user A can follow another user B while user B may not know user A. This creates a relationship with direction in a social network. We use A→B to represent the follow/subscribe (i.e., "following") relationship that user A is following user B.

Social networks have an enormous number of users. As of the end of 2018, there were more than 321 million monthly active Twitter users. With user numbers in the millions, inevitably, massive amounts of data are generated through short messages called "tweets" which are sent in real time using any digital devices such as a cell phone or computer. Tweets were originally restricted to only 140 characters, but this limit was doubled (to a maximum of 280 characters for tweets in most languages) in November 2017. When composing a new tweet, in addition to text of a maximum of 280 characters, users can add photos, video, and/or GIF (i.e., a bitmap image in Graphics Interchange Format). Since 2015, users have had ability to add poll questions. Moreover, users can also enable location so as to share their precise latitudinal and longitudinal locations. Furthermore, one of the main features of Twitter is the use of the hashtag symbol (#) followed by a keyword related to the subject topic [2], i.e., "#keyword." The ability to search Twitter by topics that are mentioned within the tweets allows us to access and interpret large amounts of data. Another key feature is the use of the "@" sign followed by a username, i.e., "@username" for mentioning other Twitter users or replying to other Twitter users. Moreover, the users can reply, retweet (i.e., repost), like, and view activity of a tweet [3]. The process of data mining involves the extraction and analysis of large amounts of data to discover and summarize information into meaningful results [4]. This process involves a variety of computationally intensive techniques which find and analyze patterns that have the potential to create predictive models and bring changes to the political and social landscape of the world [5].

Facebook is another social networking site, in which users can create a personal profile, add other Facebook users as friends, and exchange messages. In addition, Facebook users can also join common-interest user groups and categorize their friends into different customized lists (e.g., classmates, co-workers). The number of (mutual) friends may vary from one Facebook user to another. It is not uncommon for a user C to have hundreds or thousands of friends. Note that, although many of the Facebook users are mostly linked to some other Facebook users via the mutual friendship (i.e., if a user C is a friend of another user D, then user D is also a friend of user C), there are situations in which such a relationship is no longer mutual. To handle these situations, Facebook added in 2011 the functionality of "subscribe," which was relabeled as "follow" in 2012. Specifically, a user can subscribe or follow public postings of some other Facebook users without the need of adding them as friends. So, for any Facebook user C, if many of his friends followed some individual users or groups of users, then user C might also be interested in following the same individual users or groups of users. Furthermore, the "like" button allows users to express their appreciation of content such as status updates, comments, photos, and advertisements.

Social networking analysis enables discovery of interesting knowledge or information from social networks or social network data by applying techniques like data mining. Data mining aims to extract implicit, previously unknown and potentially useful information from data (say, social network data). Over the past few years, many algorithms have been developed to mine social networks. Most of these algorithms were designed for the use by data scientists or data analysts, but not necessary for non-computer scientists.

Due to explosive growth of social networks, the amount of big data grows rapidly. In addition to data scientists or data analysts, many users of social networks (including non-computer scientists) would like to find some interesting information or discover some knowledge from the social networks. However, as many of the developed social network analytic algorithms were not designed for non-computer scientists, these people may face some challenges when attempting to use some of these existing systems. In this chapter, we present a data science system to help non-computer scientists to perform data analytics on social network data. This is a *key contribution of this chapter*.

In BIDMA 2016, we [6] presented a data science solution for big data analytics of social network data. In particular, the solution helps users to discover who cares most about the users on Facebook. While the solution is useful, there are situations in which users would like to find out not only who cares about the users as individuals but also about their profession. These situations occur frequently, especially when the profession is relatively new or uncommon. To deal with these situations, we present a data science system that helps users to discover who cares about their profession (cf. individuals) on another social networking site—namely, Twitter.

Key contributions of this book chapter include the design and development of a data science system that helps non-computer scientists to perform data analytics on social network data to discover knowledge about who cares about their profession on Twitter.

The remainder of this chapter is organized as follows. We first provide some background information and related works. Then, we describe our data science solution for data analytics of social network data—specifically, Twitter's tweets. We illustrate an application of this data science solution on helping users to discover who cares about an emerging profession—namely, physician assistants (PAs). Finally, we draw conclusions:

2 Background and Related Works

2.1 Data Analytics on Facebook for Discovery of Most Interactive Friends of Users

In BIDMA 2016, we [6] presented a data science solution for big data analytics of social network data. Such a data science solution helps answer the questions "who cares most about you on Facebook?" In particular, the solution finds those friends who are most interactive toward the primary user. To distinguish these interactive friends from lurkers, we measure the number of "like" or comments of these friends made to the post by the primary user. We also measure the number of tags and posts of these friends in the primary users' timeline. Our data science solution automatically extracts relevant data from Facebook using Facepager, Facebook's Graph API, and Rfacebook package. The solution then cleans the extracted social data and includes relevant contents in the discovery of most interactive friends. The use of the arules package helps discover frequent interactions among the users and their most interactive friends. The discovered association rules—which reveal these interactions and friendships—are then visualized by the same package.

The aforementioned data science solution finds the most interactive friends of the primary Facebook users. This reveals who cares most about the primary users. However, there are situations in which the primary users also want to find out who cares most about their occupations or professions. These situations occur especially when the professions are relatively young. Physician Assistant (PA) is one of these relatively young occupations.

2.2 Background on Physician Assistants

Physician Assistants (*PAs*) are academically prepared and highly skilled health care professionals who provide a broad range of medical services. Specifically, they are accelerated medically educated clinicians who practice within a formalized relationship with physicians. The PA practice of medicine includes the following:

- Perform diagnoses,
- Obtain medical histories,
- Perform physical exams,
- Order and interpret diagnostic studies,
- Provide therapeutic procedures,
- Prescribe medications, as well as
- Educate and counsel patients.

Although educated and qualified as medical generalists, PAs receive additional education and experience on the job and may work in a wide variety of practice settings.

Historically, the PA profession evolved in the USA during the mid-1960s, in response to a shortage and uneven geographical distribution of physicians. The PA profession alleviated physicians from performing routine technical tasks in hospitals allowing the following:

- More patients to be served, and
- Physicians to focus where their skills would be better utilized.

This rapidly evolved to include utilizing PAs in primary care settings. The first trainees were highly skilled military medics who had no equivalent medical role in civilian life. So, programs were developed to build on their qualifications and experience, leading to the establishment of the PA profession. As of 2017, the PA profession has grown over 40 countries [7].

In Canada, advanced care professionals performing as primary care clinicians and medical assistants have served the Canadian Armed Forces since the 1900s as Sick Berth Attendants or Military Medics. In 1984, the Canadian Armed Forces adopted "Physician Assistant" as the role for senior medics. In 1991, the Canadian Armed Forces officially changed the name of the Senior Medical Technician (aka 6B medic) to Physician Assistant. The Canadian Military PA graduates are the first formally trained Canadian PAs. In October 1999, the Canadian Academy of Physician Assistants—now the Canadian Association of Physician Assistants (CAPA)—was formed with support of the Canadian Armed Forces.

The CAPA is a nationally incorporated bilingual professional association that advocates on behalf of its members at the direction of a volunteer Board of Directors which represents Physician Assistants (PAs), PA students, and other members across Canada and internationally. CAPA has members in all national regions as well as the Canadian Forces sharing a desire to help develop Canadian health care, and to advocate for the professions' model of cooperative, collaborative, patient centered quality health care.

Currently, there are only four programs that train PAs in Canada, and they are listed below:

- Both (1) Physician Assistant program and (2) Physician Assistant Baccalaureate in an allied health program, offered through Canadian Forces Health Services Training Centre Program by the Canadian Forces;
- Bachelor of Health Sciences (BHSc) degree in Physician Assistant offered by McMaster University;
- Bachelor of Science Physician Assistant (BScPA) Degree offered by the Consortium of PA Education—which comprise of University of Toronto, Northern Ontario School of Medicine, and the Michener Institute for Education at University Health Network (UHN); and
- Master of Physician Assistant Studies (MPAS) offered by University of Manitoba.

In Manitoba, PAs are Associate Regulated Members of the College of Physicians and Surgeons of Manitoba requiring an approved Practice Description and Contract of Supervision before being allowed to practice medicine. The Contract of Supervision identifies the primary and any alternative physician who is allowed to supervise the PA. The PAs Scope-of-Practice mirrors that of their physicians with permission to perform restricted acts, provide prescription, or write medical orders established by regulations and provincial law.

The advancement of the physician assistant profession greatly depends on current PAs and how their value is interpreted by other health care professionals, politicians, and the public. Although well established in the USA, Canada's PA profession is relatively young and remains unfamiliar to the majority of Canadians [8]. Only four provinces have formal statutes that allow the practice at this time:

- Manitoba,
- Ontario,
- New Brunswick, and
- Alberta.

According to the CAPA, there are over 800 nationally certified PAs across Canada with an addition of about 85 newly trained PAs practicing each year. As the number of PAs entering the work force continues to grow, the level of discussions regarding the PA profession is occurring on multiple levels. Politicians, civilians, and other health care professionals have begun to see the value and positive impact PAs have on the health care system.

As described above, a role of PAs is to advocate their professions. "What people think" has always been an important piece of information for decision-making. The success of the PA profession is dependent on the belief that PAs are beneficial to the healthcare system and that the introduction of the new profession has had a positive outcome. To elaborate, if belief or opinions are negative, the initial review from the social media might be enough to discourage future provinces in legislation for provincial acceptance of PAs to practice and stop further funding of current PAs. Conversely, Twitter can be an avenue for promoting the career with positive opinions of the profession, which can increase public acceptance and advocates for further passing of legislature for the practice of PAs. Hence, PAs may be interested in discovering not only who cares about them but also who cares about their profession. Please note that, although we use PA as a profession for our illustrative example and case study of our data science solution, our solution can be easily adapted to many other professions.

2.3 Data Analytics on Twitter

Traditional methods on analyzing big social media site Twitter are to use surveys, focus groups, and interviews, which are all limited to smaller samples. Due to the sampling nature of these methods, the results may be less accurate as they may be biased. In addition, these methods can be time-consuming, costly, and inaccurate due to low response rates that are typically below 50% [9]. Social media have several advantages when used to analyze data. The vast number of users provides access to a broader range of opinions. The findings can bring to light new issues that would otherwise be overlooked. Social media can be used to gauge public opinion and even to help develop it [5].

With a new method of gathering information by data mining the social networking sites, we can ask more questions and draw more conclusions on a much larger scale. Furthermore, gathering information through data mining allows for faster insight, better decision-making, reduced cost, and overall higher throughput and output.

In BIDMA 2017, Sorvisto et al. [10] designed and implemented a micro-batch streaming application that streams live data from Twitter's public streaming application programming interface (API) and predicts sentiment in near real time. Their results demonstrate that proprietary/closed-source tools can give comparable performance to open-source sentiment analysis tools for targeted sentiment analysis with live Twitter data. Such an API could be adapted for data analytics of Twitter tweets about physician assistants.

3 Our Data Science Solution

In the past, PAs conducted manual analysis on small samples of Twitter data. Unfortunately, such a traditional approach can be time-consuming and impractical in the current era of big data. Hence, a computerized Twitter data analytic tool that is capable of handling and analyzing big data is desirable.

In this section, we describe our data science solution for big data analytics of Twitter. Please note that, although we analyze Twitter data, our solution can be easily adapted for analyzing other social network data such as Facebook or LinkedIn data. Moreover, we design and develop the solution in such a way that it is easy for computer scientists and non-computer scientists to use.

3.1 Data Extraction

In general, one can use a standard-tier Twitter Search API platform to search for tweets published in past 7 days. By applying this platform regularly (say, every 7 days), one would be able to collect tweets over a certain period. Alternatively, one can use premium-tier or enterprise-tier Twitter search API platform to collect tweets published in past 30 days and tweets from as early as 2006.

Moreover, one can use the following to sample, filter, and collect real-time tweets from Twitter Streaming API:

- Amazon Web Services (AWS), which is an online server that provides cloud computing with various CPU's memory, storage, and networking capacity; and
- RStudio, which is an open-source programming software for statistical computing and graphics.

By using the streamR package in the Comprehensive R Archive Network (CRAN), one can access Twitter Streaming API via the R programming language. Specifically, we can access Twitter's filter, sample, and user streams. We can also parse the output into data frames. Consequently, real-time tweets are then saved in a continuous loop after each hour in JavaScript Object Notation (JSON) format. When using a standard-tier Twitter Streaming API, 400 keywords, 5000 user IDs, and 25 location boxes can be used in the filters.

In addition to the text in the tweets, we also capture the following information in the metadata associated with the tweets:

- Status information (e.g., posted date/time, tagged place); and
- User information (e.g., name and location in the user bio; location information such as sub-region, region, and country in the user profile);

3.2 Data Filtering

We filter Twitter data based on user preference. Specifically, we apply user-specified keywords and hashtags to filter the data. To reduce the workload of users, our data science solution provides the following features:

- Generating acronyms or short forms: For example, our solution generates "PA" for "physician assistant," "Dr" for "doctor"
- Enumerating variants: For example, our solution enumerates "Doctors" as a variant (or a plural form) of "Doctor"

- Generating synonyms: For example, our solution generates "GP" (general practitioner), "MD" (doctor of medicine), and "FamDr" (family doctor) for "doctor"
- Enumerating similar keywords or hashtags: For example, after learning from a hashtag "#BCNeedsPAs," our solution enumerates similar hashtags for other provinces and territories (e.g., "#ABNeedsPAs," "#SKNeedsPAs," "#MBNeedsPAs," "#ONNeedsPAs," "#QCNeedsPAs," "#NBNeedsPAs," "#NSNeedsPAs" "#NLNeedsPAs," "#PENeedsPAs," "#YTNeedsPAs," "#NTNeedsPAs," and "#NUNeedsPAs"). This feature would be very useful when the number of similar keywords or hashtags is high (e.g., for all 50 states in the USA)

3.3 Data Analysis

Once the Twitter data are collected and filtered, we analyze the filtered data to discover interesting knowledge and/or valuable information that is implicit, previously unknown, and potentially useful, but embedded in the data. In particular, we apply the following techniques:

- Data mining—especially, frequent pattern mining
- Sentiment analysis
- Data and result visualization

Frequent pattern mining aims to discover implicit, previously unknown, and potentially useful information and knowledge—presented in the form of sets of frequently co-occurring items (aka frequent itemsets)—from data. In this case, applying frequent pattern mining to Twitter tweets enables users (e.g., data analysts, physician assistants (PA)) to understand the distributions of tweets about a certain topic or occupation (e.g., PA) such as:

- Popular (or frequently used) tags,
- Relationships between certain tags and date,
- Relationships between certain tags and the day of the week, as well as
- Relationships between certain tags and the location (e.g., profile location, twitting location). Note that the twitting location may not necessarily be the same as the profile location. For instance, a Manitoban may have twitted during his vacation in BC. Similarly, a Canadian may have twitted during his business trip to Germany.

Besides frequent pattern mining (which focus on the counts or frequency of patterns), we also conduct sentiment analysis (which focuses on the semantics of tweets). This analysis would give users (e.g., data analysts, PA) an idea of the general feelings (e.g., positive, negative, or neutral) about a certain topic or occupation (e.g., PA) from the people who tweets about it.

As "a picture is worth a thousand words," a visual representation of the mined information and discovered knowledge (e.g., frequent patterns, sentiment) is more comprehensive to users (e.g., data analysts)—especially, those non-computer scientists (e.g., PA, policy makers)—than its equivalent textual form. Hence, we display these mined information and discovered knowledge visually.

4 Evaluation on Real-Life Twitter Data About Physician Assistants

To evaluate our data science solution for big data analytics of Twitter and to demonstrate its practicality, we applied the solution to Twitter data—namely, tweets—about a specific real occupation of physician assistant (PA). To elaborate, our solution first extracts data by using a standard-tier Twitter Search API platform. As such a platform searches for tweets published only in the past 7 days, our solution uses this API platform on a weekly basis. For the demonstration purpose, we extract 1,867 Canadian tweets—out of a total of 64,120 relevant tweets—for about 90 days (from September 26 to December 18 inclusive) about PA. Here, we extract both the text in the tweets, as well as their metadata (e.g., status information like posted date/time and tagged place; user information like name and location in the user profile) from a set of users who tweeted about PA. The tweets were filtered based on relevant hashtags—i.e., hashtags about PA such as "#PA" and "BCNeedsPAs."

Our data science solution then applies different data analyses on the filtered tweets. For instance, the solution counts the daily frequency of tweets and displays the results in a textual form in Table 1. An equivalent visualized or graphical form is as shown in Fig. 1. Both the figure and the table show an average of about 30 tweets per day, with exception two spikes. Upon deeper analysis, it was revealed that spikes occurred when two special events were held:

- October 26–29 when the annual CAPA conference was held, and
- November 27 when the PA day was held.

During these two intervals, more people tweeted about the two respective events related to PA. Moreover, one can easily observe the spikes from Fig. 1 than from Table 1, which implies that graphical representation can be more comprehensible to readers than its equivalent textual representation.

In addition, our data science solution also analyzes and visualizes the frequency of tweets based on the day of the week as shown in Fig. 2. The figure shows that, among the seven days, people mostly tweet on Monday. The number of tweets on the remaining four workdays is quite stable, whereas the number of tweets drops over the weekend. This figure reveals the weekly pattern of PAs. Unlike doctors (especially those in emergency rooms who need to be on shift), PA's working hours are more stable. They only work on regular hours during the weekday and off work during the weekend. Hence, they spend time relaxing on weekend than tweeting. They have more topics to tweet on Monday when they come back from weekend. This could be an attractive point for recruiting students to study for PA instead of medical doctors (MD).

Table 1 The daily frequency of tweets during September 26–December 18 (in textual form)

Date	#tweets	Date	#tweets
2017-09-26	8	2017-11-07	48
2017-09-27	13	2017-11-08	34
2017-09-28	21	2017-11-09	28
2017-09-29	33	2017-11-10	15
2017-09-30	9	2017-11-11	6
2017-10-01	3	2017-11-12	7
2017-10-02	13	2017-11-13	19
2017-10-03	8	2017-11-14	12
2017-10-04	21	2017-11-15	32
2017-10-05	23	2017-11-16	34
2017-10-06	19	2017-11-17	32
2017-10-07	15	2017-11-18	9
2017-10-08	6	2017-11-19	10
2017-10-09	18	2017-11-20	11
2017-10-10	9	2017-11-21	16
2017-10-11	25	2017-11-22	31
2017-10-12	16	2017-11-23	44
2017-10-13	17	2017-11-24	53
2017-10-14	5	2017-11-25	14
2017-10-15	4	2017-11-26	29
2017-10-16	18	2017-11-27	181
2017-10-17	6	2017-11-28	45
2017-10-18	15	2017-11-29	22
2017-10-19	4	2017-11-30	31
2017-10-20	10	2017-12-01	27
2017-10-21	10	2017-12-02	16
2017-10-22	0	2017-12-03	3
2017-10-23	23	2017-12-04	11
2017-10-24	24	2017-12-05	27
2017-10-25	20	2017-12-06	19
2017-10-26	29	2017-12-07	12
2017-10-27	90	2017-12-08	20
2017-10-28	100	2017-12-09	6
2017-10-29	53	2017-12-10	13
2017-10-30	44	2017-12-11	11
2017-10-31	15	2017-12-12	13
2017-11-01	16	2017-12-13	3
2017-11-02	26	2017-12-14	22
2017-11-03	13	2017-12-15	13
2017-11-04	6	2017-12-16	9
2017-11-05	20	2017-12-17	8
2017-11-06	28	2017-12-18	14

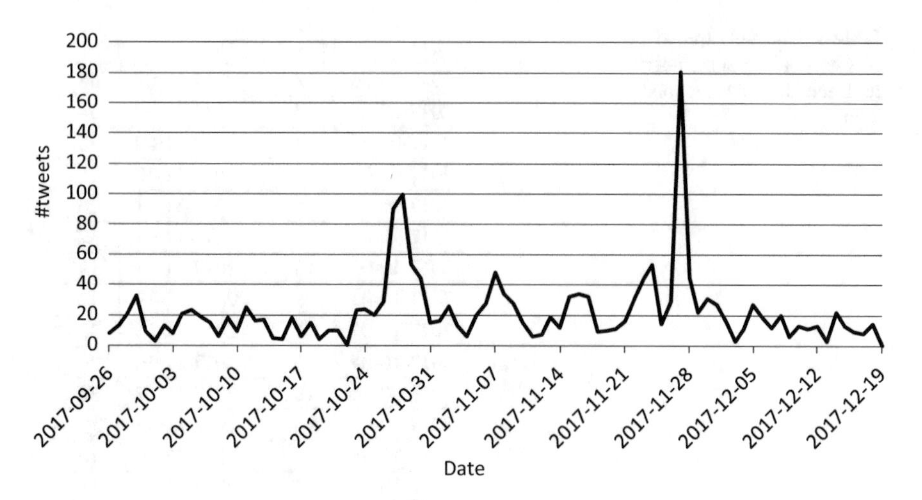

Fig. 1 The daily frequency of tweets during September 26–December 18

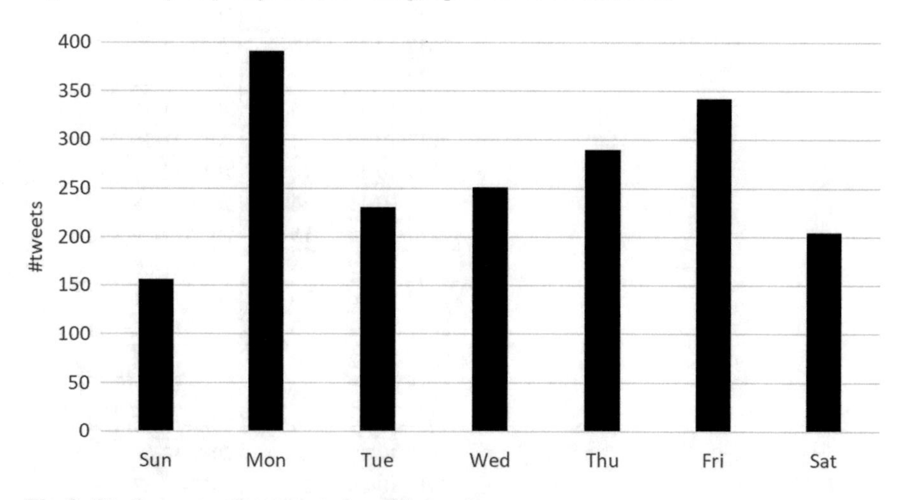

Fig. 2 The frequency of tweets vs. day of the week

Recall that, in addition to time, our data science solution also collects another piece of metadata about users—namely, profile location. Figure 3 shows the frequency or percentage of tweets among all regions (i.e., ten provinces and three territories of Canada). The figure reveals that 30% of the tweets were from users who declared the profile location at the coarse-grained level as Canada without identifying the location at a finer-grained level (e.g., provincial level). 45% of the tweets were from Ontario where the following PA-offering institutes are located:

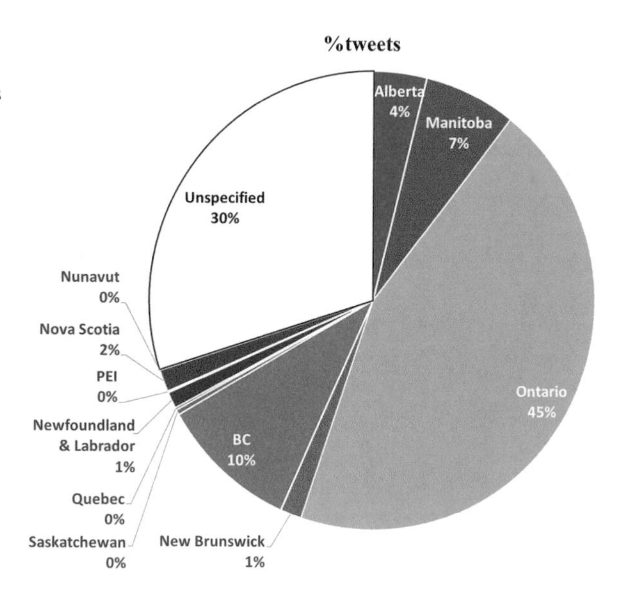

Fig. 3 The percentage of tweets among all ten provinces and three territories (plus unspecified Canadian profile locations) in Canada

- McMaster University, and
- Consortium of PA Education—which comprise of University of Toronto, Northern Ontario School of Medicine, and the Michener Institute for Education at University Health Network (UHN).

By ignoring the "unspecified" course-grained region in Fig. 3 to get Fig. 4, it becomes much clearer about the distribution of tweets based on their specified provinces and territories. The figure reveals that 64% of the tweets were from Ontarians. This is followed by 14% British Columbians, 10% Manitobans, 5% Albertans, and only 2% in New Brunswick, Nova Scotia, as well as Newfoundland and Labrador. Recall that only four provinces—namely, Ontario, Manitoba, Alberta, and New Brunswick—have formal statutes that allow the practice at this time. It is interesting to note that, despite the absence of formal statutes from both BC or Nova Scotia, there were still 14% of British Columbians tweeted. Detailed analysis reveals that most of the tweets from BC discuss about whether or not to establish formal statutes at British Columbia.

Moreover, among all users who tweeted in our evaluation data, we also compare the number of PA vs. non-PA. We found 26 identified PA out of 534 users who were captured in our study, i.e., <5% of the 534 users. However, these 5% of users (PAs) posted 48% of the tweets. Out of the top-ten users who tweeted, eight were PAs. In other words, although only a small percentage of the users in our evaluation were PAs, those PAs tweeted a high volume of tweets. This shows they care about their profession.

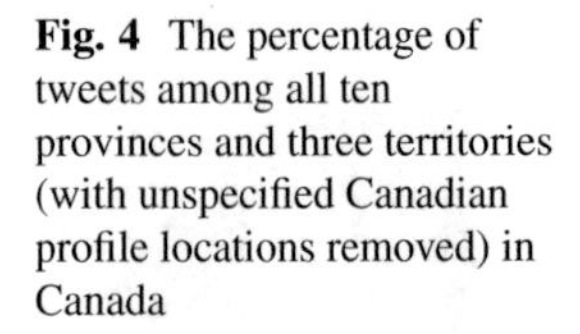

Fig. 4 The percentage of tweets among all ten provinces and three territories (with unspecified Canadian profile locations removed) in Canada

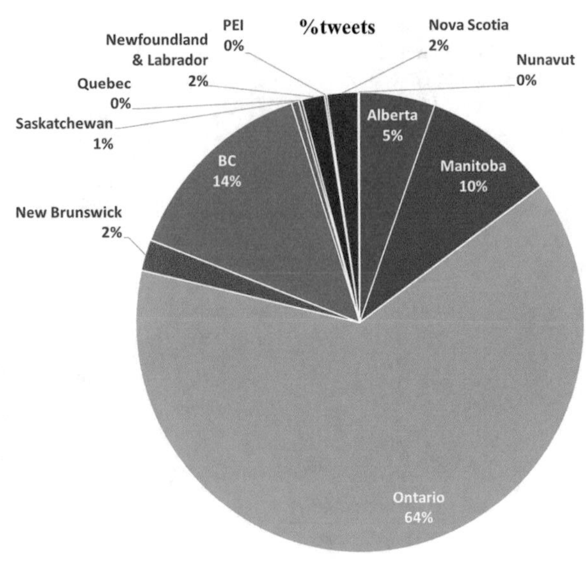

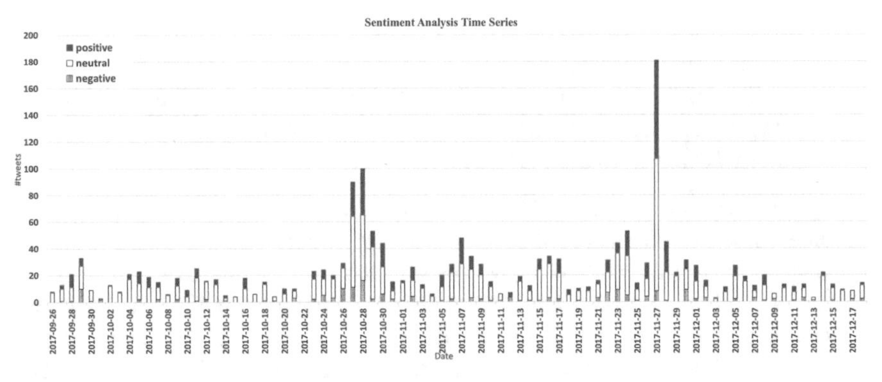

Fig. 5 Trends in the sentiment of tweets over time

In addition to finding frequency of tweets, we also conduct sentiment analysis. The results show

- 29.7% of the tweets are positive,
- 60.3% of the tweets are neutral, and
- Only 9.9% of the tweets are negative.

In order to find the trend in the sentiment of tweets over time, we plot changes in the sentiment of tweets in Fig. 5. It shows that, when the absolute number of tweets increases, the number of negative tweets also increases. The good news is the number of negative tweets increases disproportionally.

Consistent with Fig. 5, Table 2 shows that there are more positive tweets in November than the other 3 months. To have a fair comparison and to observe the

Table 2 The number of monthly sentiments of tweets

	Sept	Oct	Nov	Dec
Positive	20	187	283	65
Neutral	51	402	514	159
Negative	13	74	75	23

Table 3 The percentage of monthly sentiments of tweets

	Sept (%)	Oct (%)	Nov (%)	Dec (%)
Positive	23.8	28.2	32.5	26.3
Neutral	60.7	60.6	58.9	64.4
Negative	15.5	11.1	8.6	9.3

Table 4 The number of different sentiment of tweets between groups of PA ad non-PA

	PA	Non-PA
Positive	218	337
Neutral	398	728
Negative	85	100

Table 5 The number of different sentiment of tweets among different provinces in mo

	Ontario	BC	Manitoba	Alberta	New Brunswick
Positive	245	54	41	17	9
Neutral	511	116	85	25	14
Negative	84	17	8	3	7

trend, we normalize the number of tweets to get Table 3. A good news observed from this table is that the percentage of negative tweets decreased over time (from 15.5% of the tweets are negative in September to only 9.3% in December).

We also analyzed our earlier results in a similar fashion by drilling into more details. Table 4 shows that there is no scientific difference between the PA and non-PA in terms of positive, neutral, or negative tweets.

Table 5 shows that there are scientific differences among tweets from users living in different regions. Specifically, there are more positive tweets from Ontarians than (the 121 positive tweets) from the other four provinces combined.

5 Conclusions

In this chapter, we presented a data science solution that conducts big data analytics of social media data (especially, Twitter data). The solution routinely extracts tweet contents and metadata from social networking sites, filters the extracted data, and analyzes the filtered data. The analysis includes frequent pattern mining and sentiment analysis. To enable users (e.g., data analysts) to easily comprehend the mined information and discovered knowledge, our data science solution represents the mined information and discovered knowledge in visual or graphical representation than its equivalent textual representation. To demonstrate the feasibility and practicality of our solution, we apply it for physician assistants (PAs) so as to help asking the question: Who is talking about your profession in Twitter? In particular, who is talking or tagging PAs?

Acknowledgements This project is partially supported by (1) Natural Sciences and Engineering Research Council of Canada (NSERC), and (2) University of Manitoba. The first author also thanks K. Bairos-Novak, D.L. DeKezel, and T.S. DeKezel for their assistance and support during this project.

References

1. Jones, I., & Liu, H. (2013). Mining social media: Challenges and opportunities. In *Proceedings of the 2013 International Conference on Social Intelligence and Technology* (pp. 90–99). IEEE.
2. Maruyama, M., Robertson, S. P., Douglas, S., Semaan, B., & Faucett, H. (2014). Hybrid media consumption: How tweeting during a televised political debate influences the vote decision. In *Proceedings of the 17th ACM Conference on Computer Supported Cooperative Work & Social Computing* (pp. 1422–1432). ACM.
3. Mohammad, S. M., & Kiritchenko, S. (2015). Using hashtags to capture fine emotion categories from tweets. *Computational Intelligence, 31*(2), 301–326.
4. Attewell, P., Monaghan, D. P., & Kwong, D. (2015). *Data mining for the social sciences: An introduction*. Oakland, CA: University of California Press.
5. June, P., Choi, H., & Park, S. (2011). Social media's impact on policy making. *SERI Quarterly, 4*(4), 125.
6. Leung, C. K., Jiang, F., Poon, T. W., & Crevier, P. (2018). Big data analytics of social network data: Who cares most about you on Facebook? In *Highlighting the importance of big data management and analysis for various applications* (pp. 1–15). Cham: Springer.
7. Journal of the American Academy of Physician Assistants (JAAPA), & Journal of Physician Assistant Education (JPAE). (2017). *The PA profession: 50 years and counting*. Philadelphia, PA: Wolters Kluwer.
8. Bowen, S. (2016). Potential of physician assistants to support primary care: Evaluating their introduction at 6 primary care and family medicine sites. *Can Fam Physician, 62*(5), e268–e277.
9. Cobanoglu, C., Warde, B., & Moreo, P. (2001). A comparison of mail, fax, and web-based survey methods. *International Journal of Market Research, 43*(4), 1–15.
10. Sorvisto, D., Cloutier, P., Magnusson, K., Al-Sarraj, T., Dyskin, K., & Berenstein, G. (2018). Live Twitter sentiment analysis: Big data mining with Twitter's public streaming API. In *Applications of data management and analysis* (pp. 29–41). Cham: Springer.

An Introductory Multidisciplinary Data Science Course Incorporating Experiential Learning

Nelson Wong and Jalal Kawash

Abstract This paper describes a novel data science course at the University of Calgary. The course is for non-major students, who have a limited technical background. It incorporates experiential learning aspects such as team work and working with real-world data.

1 Introduction

Large amounts of data are being constantly generated by existing applications, such as social media, business services, and scientific applications. Many such datasets are also readily available at the fingertips of users. Dealing with such large amounts of data magnifies existing challenges and poses new challenges. Empowering future scientists, engineers, or even graduates from outside these disciplines with data analysis techniques is becoming more desirable.

In this paper, we present an introductory course, SCIE/DATA 201—*Thinking with Data* at the University of Calgary. The target audience is first-year multidisciplinary students. The course has no prerequisites. It is designed to incorporate and promote experiential learning [1].

The course was run two times: Once in Summer 2017 (with 20 students) and once in Fall 2017 (with 139 students). Student feedback indicated that the incorporated hands-on activities during tutorials enhanced the students' learning experience.

Teaching data science has been slowly finding its way to university programs. For example, Marttila-Kontio et al. discuss advanced data analytics in business management [2]. Radchenko and Maksimenkova address the questions about teaching data science and the areas that borrow the techniques from data science [3]. Others suggest "datathons" as a mean of data science education, proposing to host data hackathons to augment teaching [4]. Teaching data science in a flipped

N. Wong (✉) · J. Kawash
Department of Computer Science, University of Calgary, Calgary, AB, Canada
e-mail: nelson@cpsc.ucalgary.ca; kawash@cpsc.ucalgary.ca

R. Alhajj et al. (eds.), *Data Management and Analysis*, Studies in Big Data 65,
https://doi.org/10.1007/978-3-030-32587-9_3

classroom environment is discussed by Cassel et al. [5]. Similar to our work, their students are with limited technical background.

In the next section, we will provide the course details. Student feedback is discussed in Sect. 3. Section 4 concludes the paper.

2 The Course

The course we are describing is SCIE/DATA 201—*Thinking with Data*. It is an introduction to tools and techniques for managing, visualizing, and making sense of data. Students build a fundamental understanding of and an experience with the complete data analysis lifecycle: obtaining data, cleaning and transforming it, performing exploratory analysis, and presenting data using interactive visuals. The course also introduces a range of tools and techniques for data cleaning, exploratory visualization, and sensemaking.

SCIE/DATA 201 is a three-unit course that focuses on experiential learning. Weekly, the course consists of 100 min of lectures for delivering course concepts and 150 min of tutorials for hands-on activities. The grading in the course consists of five group-based assignments (30%), two projects (50%), and a final exam (20%). Assignments and projects are included in the appendices. Course outcomes are as follows. By the end of the course, students should be able to:

1. Obtain data using different data collection methods such as observation and surveys.
2. Remove and correct inconsistencies in datasets using tools such as OpenRefine (www.openrefine.org).
3. Perform basic data analysis with tools such as Excel and Tableau (www.tableau.com).
4. Show data through digital and physical representations.
5. Present analytic results effectively.
6. Entertain ethical implications of collecting, analysing, and using data.

During lectures, the instructor introduces a broad range of fundamental concepts and techniques for interpreting, managing, and visualizing data. The topics include:

- Data literacy
- Data collection
- Data cleaning and
- Basic statistics
- Exploratory data analysis
- Qualitative analysis
- Data visualization
- Presentations
- Ethics considerations

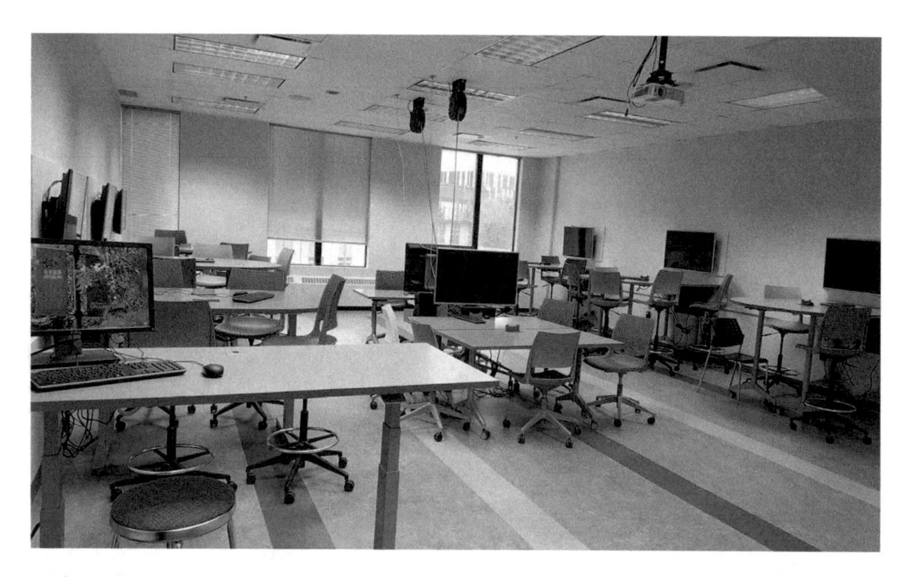

Fig. 1 Tutorial room

During tutorials, students can apply what they learn in lectures using practical activities. Most activities are performed in groups of four or five; each tutorial session has five groups of students. There are two tutorials (75 min each) per week and tutorials are structured in blocks. Each block is a 2-week period that focuses on a specific concept matching the lecture topics taught in the same period. A typical block is organized as follows.

- First week, first tutorial: Teaching assistants demonstrate how to use software applications such as OpenRefine, Excel, and Tableau. Students do small in-class exercises.
- First week, second tutorial: Teaching assistants provide some more examples and exercises to the students. An assignment related to the concept of the block will be given to the students. Students work on the assignment.
- Second week, first tutorial: Students continue to work on the assignment in groups.
- Teaching assistants provide guidance to each group.
- Second week, second tutorial: Each group performs a presentation between 5 and 10 min about their assignment.

Since many activities are done in teams during tutorials, the tutorial room is specifically designed to facilitate group work. Figure 1 shows the layout of the room. One desk is in the front for teaching assistants. A podium computer is connected from the desk to a projector screen (out of view in Fig. 1). There are eight workstations for students: two in the centre and three on each side of the room. Each workstation can fit four to six students and is equipped with a desktop computer

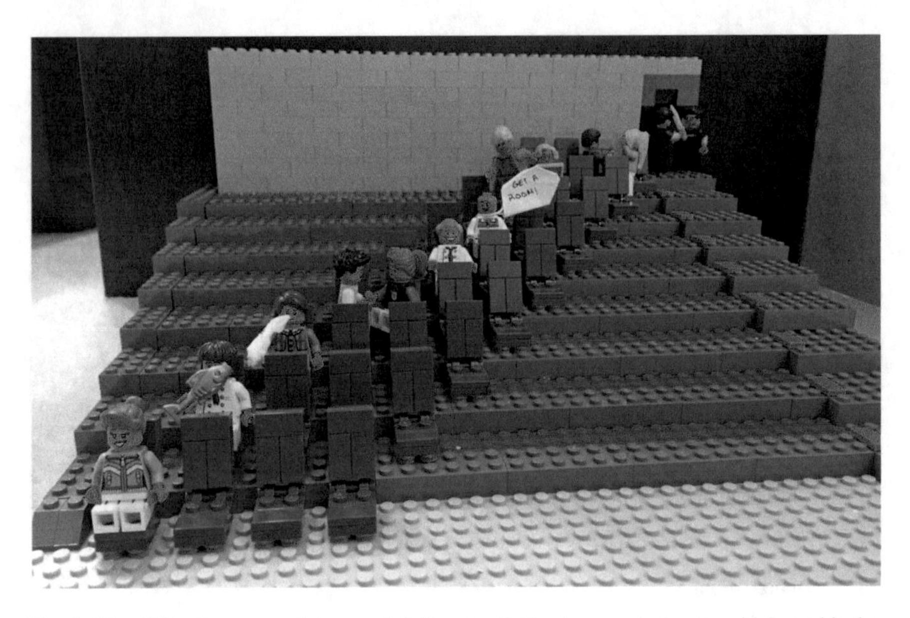

Fig. 2 Visualizing the appropriateness of different activities in a movie theatre with Lego blocks

connected to a large monitor. Plenty of space is available among workstations to promote activities between groups.

The activities given during tutorials provide students with hands-on experiences working with real-world datasets. The datasets are either collected by students or provided by the teaching assistants. Here we list five activities that pertain to each biweekly assignment:

- Each group constructs sketches with colour pencil and physical visualizations with tokens, such as Lego pieces, jelly beans, and coins, to represent some datasets. Groups present their work to each other and critique other groups' work in a round-robin fashion. Figures 2, 3, and 4 show some sample work from one of the activities.
- Each group picks a topic and creates a survey using SurveyMonkey or Google Forms to collect data about the topic. The surveys are then completed and critiqued by other groups.
- Each group receives a dataset. The datasets are then cleaned and transformed using Excel and OpenRefine. Groups then present their cleaned dataset and describe the cleaning process to all other groups.
- Each group creates interview questions related to a chosen topic and conducts interviews with students from other groups.
- Each group creates digital visualizations using tools such as Excel and Tableau to answer some questions from a dataset. The visualizations are then presented to and critiqued by other groups.

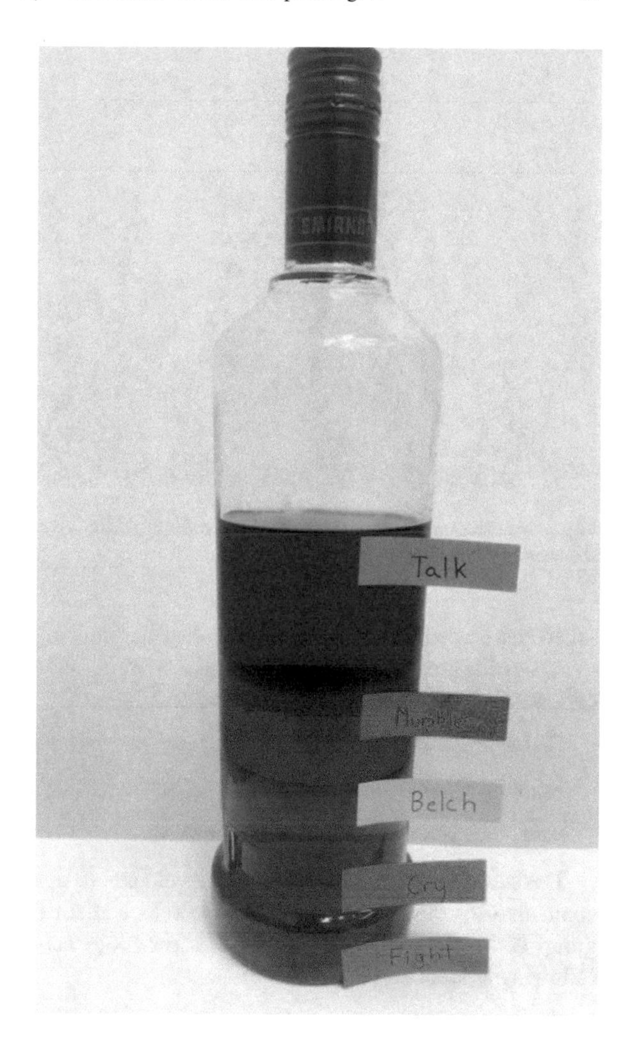

Fig. 3 Visualizing the appropriateness of different activities in a bar with a liquor bottle

In addition, students can reflect on their experience in tutorials, and apply what they learn to two projects. One is an individual project and the second is a group project. Students need to collect, clean, analyse, and present data relevant to a topic of their interests.

3 Student Feedback

The university requires student feedback about the course and their learning to be collected near the end of the term. There is an overarching theme across the comments that we received—*hands-on activities* during tutorials are important. We

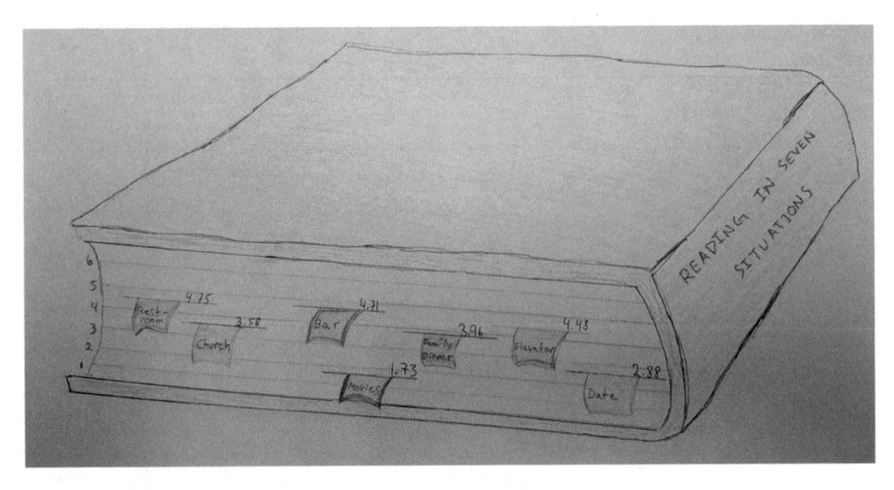

Fig. 4 Visualizing the appropriateness of reading indifferent situations and locations with hand sketched visualization

asked the students to name one aspect of the course that was especially effective in supporting their learning. The responses were overwhelmingly pointing towards tutorials and activities, as one student puts it:

> The tutorials help out a lot because we actually get to apply what we learn in class.

Another states

> Hands-on experience helped me learn the most.

The survey instruments also ask the students to discuss the things the instructor could modify that would have further helped them learn. Realizing the value of group activities students typically ask for more activities as represented by the following student comment:

> The instructor can include more group activities or activities in general [during lecture]

Some comments specifically requested the use of a Classroom Response System (CRS) to replace the open discussion, as is clearly indicated by the following comment specifically naming the Top Hat CRS (www.tophat.com):

> Instead of open discussion, use Top Hat.

Based on student feedback, the interactivity nature of tutorials was a success. Students engage with the exercises and believe the exercises substantially enhance their learning experiences. Students would also like to see more activities during lectures. Due to the physical constraints of the lecture theatre we used, most activities were conducted during tutorials. However, as suggested by the feedback, we are planning to use Top Hat during lectures in the next offering of the course to increase engagement [6] and improve content retention [7].

4 Conclusion

SCIE/DATA 201—*Thinking with Data* is an introductory course in data science for first-year multidisciplinary students. It incorporates experiential learning and allows students to have hands-on experience in a complete data analysis pipeline. Student feedback shows that practical hands-on activities improved their learning experience.

Appendix 1

Assignment 1: Non-digital Data Visualizations

This assignment helps you learn about *physical visualizations* and *sketches*. Non-digital visualizations allow you to communicate visually without being limited by what software tools can create. This is a group-based assignment. Your group needs to submit written answers (physical copy) and do a presentation during your tutorial. All group members must attend the presentation.

Contributions

Everyone in the same group will receive the same mark by default. However, if certain members of a group do not contribute as much as they should have, their marks will be adjusted according to how much contributions they have to the assignment.

Deliverables

You need to submit both *Parts A and B.*

A. Written Answers

You need to create five questions regarding the dataset provided. You should then submit *one printed document* that clearly answers the five questions. The file should be organized so that it is easy to read. For each question, you need:

- A snapshot of the physical visualization *or* sketch.
- A description of your physical visualization or sketch to help us understand your work

You must use *physical visualizations for at least two questions and sketches for at least two questions*. For physical visualization, you can pick physical tokens such as Legos, coins, jelly beans, etc. For sketches, you should use (colour) *pens/pencils/markers and paper only* (i.e., do NOT use electronic devices for sketching). Be *creative*!

B. Oral Presentation

Your presentation must be 5–10 min, followed by 1 or 2 min of question period. Present one physical visualization and one sketch that you think are the most interesting.

Assignment 2: Data Collection

This assignment helps you learn about *data collection* and *surveys*. This is a group-based assignment. Your group needs to submit written answers (physical copy) and do a presentation during your tutorial. All group members must attend the presentation.

Contributions

Everyone in the same group will receive the same mark by default. However, if certain members of a group do not contribute as much as they should have, their marks will be adjusted according to how much contributions they have to the assignment.

Deliverables

You need to submit both *Parts A and B.*

A. Written Answers

Each team should submit *one printed document* that clearly answers the following questions about your dataset that you collected via a survey using Google Forms or SurveyMonkey (If you use SurveyMonkey, you may need to pay for the software in order to download your data). All survey questions should be coherent with each other and should help you achieve the goal of the survey. The dataset needs to have *at least ten rows and five attributes.*

- What did you hope to understand from this dataset? What was your goal for collecting this dataset?
- What is your dataset? Provide a clear description of the chosen dataset including a description of all the attributes.
- Indicate the levels of measurement (nominal, ordinal, interval, or ratio) for each attribute. You can provide the reasonings of your answers if needed.
- Show screenshots of your whole survey. All contents must be legible (this question will be marked based on the quality of your survey)

- Include a table of your dataset. If you have more than ten rows of data, you only need to print the first ten rows. Similarly, if you have more than five attributes, you only need to print the five most relevant attributes. Make sure all contents are legible.

B. Oral Presentation

Your presentation must be 5–10 min, followed by 1 or 2 min of question period. The presentation should be about your survey and dataset. You should use visual aids (e.g., pictures or screenshots) to help you deliver your contents.

Assignment 3: Data Cleaning

This assignment helps you learn about *data cleaning*. This is a group-based assignment. Your group needs to submit written answers (physical copy) and do a presentation during your lab. All group members must attend the presentation.

Contributions

Everyone in the same group will receive the same mark by default. However, if certain members of a group do not contribute as much as they should have, their marks will be adjusted according to how much contributions they have to the assignment.

Deliverables

You need to submit both *Parts A and B.*

A. Written Answers

Use the dataset provided for this assignment. The dataset contains inconsistent formatted data entries, missing values, etc.

Your task is to clean this dataset. You need to show us the processes of cleaning five sets of "dirty" entities (e.g., all empty spaces at the beginning of a certain column would be considered as one set, and duplicated rows would be considered as another set). The processes should be substantially different from each other (e.g., removing excess spaces from column 1 and removing excess spaces from column 2 are considered as one single process). For each cleaning process, you need to clearly show us:

- A before cleaning screenshot of the dataset—highlighting the "dirty" parts
- The steps (e.g., formula, technique, manual work, etc.) that you have used to clean that abnormality

- An after screenshot of the cleaned data—highlighting the parts that were "cleaned"
- An explanation of why you thought these entities were needed to be cleaned

The dataset does not need to be completely cleaned. Make sure all five processes are *clearly explained* and all screenshots are *legible*. You *must use Excel in at least one of the processes and OpenRefine in at least one of the processes.*

B. Oral Presentation
Your presentation must be 5–10 min, followed by 1 or 2 min of question period. The presentation should clearly show the processes of cleaning all five sets of "dirty" entities. You can use visual aids (e.g., pictures or screenshots) to help you deliver your contents.

Assignment 4: Qualitative Data Analysis

This assignment helps you learn about *qualitative data analysis*. This is a group-based assignment. Your group needs to submit a written report (physical copy) and do a presentation during your tutorial. All group members must attend the presentation.

Contributions

Everyone in the same group will receive the same mark by default. However, if certain members of a group do not contribute as much as they should have, their marks will be adjusted according to how much contributions they have to the assignment.

Deliverables

You need to submit both *Parts A and B.*

A. Written Answers
Your task is to conduct an interview that consists of *five main interview questions* and analyse the interview data. In the written report, you should do the following (five marks per point):

- Explain the topic of your interview and why you were interested to know about the topic.
- List the five main interview questions and their corresponding follow-up questions.

- Create an affinity diagram—attach legible photo(s) of the diagram, and explain the diagram (e.g., what the groups/categories are and why they are formed the way they are, etc.)
- Discuss your findings (e.g., Are there unexpected findings? Did you find what you are looking for? How do you interpret your results? etc.)
- Reflect on the process (e.g., What can be improved? Did you miss any questions? Will you rephrase any of your questions? Why? etc.)

B. Oral Presentation

Your presentation must be 5–10 min, followed by 1 or 2 min of question period. Present the *key elements* from your report. You should decide what to include in the presentation. You can use visual aids (e.g., pictures or screenshots) to help you deliver your contents.

Assignment 5: Digital Data Visualizations

This assignment helps you learn about *digital data visualizations* using *Excel* and *Tableau*. This is a group-based assignment. Your group needs to submit a written report (physical copy) and do a presentation during your lab. All group members must attend the presentation.

Contributions

Everyone in the same group will receive the same mark by default. However, if certain members of a group do not contribute as much as they should have, their marks will be adjusted according to how much contributions they have to the assignment.

Deliverables

You need to submit both *Parts A and B*.

A. Written Answers

Use the dataset provided for this assignment.

For each point listed below, clearly state the question, show the process, and include a screenshot of the visualization (it needs to have legend, title, axis, etc.). All interesting facts must be different from each other. Try to use different charts for the points below.

1. Find an interesting fact on this dataset and visualize your finding with Excel.
2. Find an interesting fact on this dataset and visualize your finding with Excel.

3. Find an interesting fact on this dataset and visualize your finding with Tableau.
4. Find an interesting fact on this dataset and visualize your finding with Tableau.
5. Find an interesting fact on this dataset and visualize your finding with Excel or Tableau.

B. Oral Presentation

Your presentation must be 5–10 min, followed by 1 or 2 min of question period. Your presentation should clearly show your questions, processes, and visualizations. You can use visual aids to help you deliver your contents.

Appendix 2

Individual Project

This *individual* project helps you strengthen what you learned from Assignment 1, 2, and 3—*obtaining*, *cleaning*, and *visualizing* data.

Deliverables

You need to submit a written report that includes *Part A, B, C, and D* in *one PDF* file via *D2L*.

A. Introduction

Write an introduction of your project. Tell us what your *main goal/problem/-topic* is and *explain* why you picked that. Provide any *background information* we need to know in order to understand your project.

B. Obtaining Data

Obtain a dataset that can help you solve the main problem or gain understanding of the specific topic (from Part A). You can use any methods introduced in lectures to obtain your data. Your dataset must have *at least 20 rows and eight attributes*. In addition, your dataset (the source if downloaded, and the actual data) must be different from other datasets you used in any other submissions in the course (including your group project).

You must include:

- The *reasons* of using the particular dataset
- *Where* and *how* you obtain the dataset
- If you use a survey, include
  - Screenshots of your whole survey (all contents must be legible)
  - Descriptions of your target participants

- If you download your dataset, include
  - A link where you downloaded the data
- A table of your dataset. If you have more than 20 rows of data, you only need to print the first 20 rows. If you have more than 8 attributes, you only need to print the eight most *relevant* attributes. All contents must be legible.

Make sure you use your dataset *ethically* and *do not violate any copyright laws*.

C. Cleaning Data

Perform any data cleaning necessary—reformatting data, removing duplicates, removing erroneous data points, etc. You can use any programs of your choice to clean the dataset.

You should indicate which attributes are dirty. For each dirty attribute, you must include:

- An explanation why you think the data needs to be cleaned
- A screenshot showing the dirty data (before cleaning)
- A screenshot showing the clean data (after cleaning)

The screenshots must be *legible* and clearly show the differences between dirty and clean data.

If you think your data is clean to start off with and do not need any cleaning, you must:

- Clearly explain why you think the data is clean
- Include any procedures that you do to make sure you have obtained clean data

D. Visualizing Data

Keeping the *overall problem/goal* (from Part A) in mind, create *at least three visualizations* that help you solve the problem or achieve your goal. The visualizations must be either *physical or sketches*. For physical visualization, you can pick physical tokens such as Legos, coins, jelly beans, etc. For sketches, you should use (colour) *pens/pencils/markers and paper only*.

Note: *Digital visualizations are not allowed in this project*. By not using digital tools to create visualizations, you can think out of the box—creating visualizations that are not limited by what digital tools can do. (You will need to use digital tools in your group project; not here.) You may receive *bonus marks* for creative visualizations.

For each visualization, you must:

- Include a photo of the visualization (must be legible)
- Explain what information you want to convey
- Explain why you think the visualization is a good way to convey the information (e.g., how the visualization helps solve the overall problem?)

Group Project

This *group* project helps you learn about the whole *data analysis pipeline*. There are *three parts* in the project. It may become necessary to amend this specification at some point. If that is the case, you will be notified via D2L.

Contributions

Everyone in the same group will receive the same mark by default. However, if certain members of a group do not contribute as much as they should have, their marks will be *adjusted* according to how much contributions they have to the project.

Part 1: Topic Approval

As a group, you need to decide the main goal/topic of your project. It should be something that interests you, so you will have fun working on the project and learn something about the area. For example, a main goal can be "find out more about climate change." You should plan ahead and think about how to gather data and the size of your dataset. Public data including government records, health data, census data, environmental data, etc. are good candidates. You are also encouraged to collect your own data via surveys. Data from your other courses could also be a good fit. Do *NOT* begin gathering data before receiving approval from your TA.

Deliverables

Submit a *physical copy* that succinctly states the following points (*one or two sentences* would be enough):

- Project goal/main problem you want to solve/a topic that interests you
- Data collection method(s) (e.g., survey, download, etc.)
- Size of the dataset (*at least 50 rows and ten attributes*) that you are aiming for

Your TA will let you know whether your topic is approved. Note that you can change your topic after the due date. However, you will need TA's approval again.

Part 2: Written Report

You will need to *obtain data* and *transform/clean* the data so that the dataset will be ready for analysis; create a set of *analysis questions* that help you solve the main problem; and answer the analysis questions with appropriate *visualizations*.

Deliverables

You need to submit a written report that includes *Sections A, B, C, D, and E* in *one PDF* file via *D2L*. There is no hard limit for how long your report should be, but you should provide a clear and comprehensive discussion of your analysis and findings. You should present your analysis succinctly, in a way that an outsider can understand. *Your job is to convince us that you know how to work with the dataset and have a clear understanding of each steps in the data analysis pipeline.*

- *Section A: Introduction*
  Write an introduction of your project. Tell us what your *main goal/problem/-topic* is and *explain* why you pick that. Provide any *background information* we need to know in order to understand your project.
- *Section B: Obtaining Data*
  Obtain a dataset that can help you solve the main problem or gain understanding of the specific topic (from Part 1). You can use any methods introduced in lectures to obtain your data. Your dataset must have *at least 50 rows and ten attributes*. In addition, your dataset (the source if downloaded, and the actual data) must be different from other datasets you used in any other submissions in the course. You must include:

  - The *reasons* of using the particular dataset
  - Where and how you obtain the dataset
  - If you use a survey, include

    Screenshots of your whole survey (all contents must be legible)
    Descriptions of your target participants

  - If you download your dataset, include

    A link where you downloaded the data

  - A table of your dataset. If you have more than 50 rows of data, you only need to print the first 50 rows. If you have more than ten attributes, you only need to print the ten most *relevant* attributes. Make sure all contents are legible.

  Make sure you use your dataset *ethically* and *do not violate any copyright laws*.
- *Section C: Cleaning Data*
  Perform any data cleaning necessary—reformatting data, removing duplicates, removing erroneous data points, etc. You can use any programs of your choice to clean the dataset. You should indicate which attributes are dirty. For *each* dirty attribute, you must include:

  - An explanation why you think the data needs to be cleaned
  - A screenshot showing the dirty data (before cleaning)
  - A screenshot showing the clean data (after cleaning)

The screenshots must be *legible* and clearly show the differences between dirty and clean data.

If you think your data is clean to start off with and do not need any cleaning, you must:

- Clearly explain why you think the data is clean
- Include any procedures that you do to make sure you have obtained clean data

- *Section D: Analysis Questions*

  Create *five analysis questions* that you will address. By answering these questions, you should have a better understanding of your overall topic.
- *Section E: Visualizations and Findings*

  You need to analyse your dataset with the help of *digital visualizations*. For *each* question in Section D, you must provide:

  - A proper visualization created by some software tools (e.g., Excel or Tableau)
  - A discussion of your findings based on the visualization (You can use extra images, diagrams, and annotations to help you explain your answer.)
  - The reasons why you choose the specific visualization to help you answer the question

Part 3: Presentation

Your group will need to conduct a presentation *during lecture*. You can use your own laptop (you may need a VGA connector) or use the computer (Windows) at the podium. Your presentation must be between 5 and 10 min, including question period (this is different from the timing of your assignment presentations).

Note that you may not have finished all sections of your project at the time of presentation and that is fine. The presentation can be about the parts that you have done and what you are planning to do. *The goal of the presentation is to let your classmates know what your project is about and to show the instructor your progress*. You will need to decide what to be included in your presentation. It will be marked based on the contents and how well it is conducted.

References

1. Kolb, A., & Kolb, D. (2005). Learning styles and learning spaces: Enhancing experiential learning in higher education. *Academy of Management Learning and Education, 4*(2), 193–212.
2. Marttila-Kontio, M., Kontio, M., & Hotti, V. (2014). Advanced data analytics education for students and companies. In *Proceedings of the 2014 Conference on Innovation & Technology In Computer Science Education (ITiCSE '14)* (pp. 249–254). New York: ACM.
3. Radchenko, I., & Maksimenkova, O. (2016). Principles of citizen science in open educational projects based on open data. In *Proceedings of the 12th Central and Eastern European Software Engineering Conference in Russia (CEE-SECR '16)*. New York: ACM.

4. Anslow, J. B., Brosz, J., Maurer, F., & Boyes, M. (2016). Datathons: An experience report of data hackathons for data science education. In *Proceedings of the 47th ACM Technical Symposium on Computing Science Education (SIGCSE '16)* (pp. 615–620). New York: ACM.
5. Cassel, L., Dicheva, D., Dichev, C., Goelman, D., & Posner, M. (2016). Data science for all: An introductory course for non-majors; in flipped format (abstract only). In *Proceedings of the 47th ACM Technical Symposium on Computing Science Education (SIGCSE '16)* (pp. 691–691). New York: ACM.
6. Collier, R., & Kawash, J. (2018). Effectively using classroom response systems for improving student content retention. In *Computers Supported Education, Communications in Computer and Information Science* (Vol. 865, pp. 3–21). Basel: Springer.
7. Kawash, J., & Collier, R. (2018). On the use of classroom response system as an integral part of the classroom. In *Proceedings of the 10th International Conference on Computer-Supported Education (CSEDU'18)* (pp. 38–46). Setúbal: SciTePress.

Homogeneous Vs. Heterogeneous Distributed Data Clustering: A Taxonomy

Rasha Kashef and Marium Warraich

Abstract Recent advances in computer architecture and networking allow for the opportunity to parallelize the data clustering process. By dividing the problem into smaller partitions, tackling each one in parallel, and then combining the partial solutions, the parallel algorithms can cluster large amounts of data much more efficiently. In specific scenarios, the dataset is inherently distributed over multiple nodes, making it impossible and even infeasible to apply centralized clustering, which has created a need for performing clustering in distributed environments. Distributed clustering solves two problems: infeasibility of collecting data at a central node, due to either technical and/or privacy limitations, and intractability of traditional clustering algorithms on large datasets. In this paper, we provide a novel taxonomy of distributed data clustering algorithms and provide insight into their distributed modeling strategies. The taxonomy classifies the distributed clustering processes as either a homogeneous or heterogeneous process. Various distributed performance and quality measures are also addressed.

Keywords Data clustering · Distributed processing · Performance · Quality measures

1 Introduction

The clustering task can be defined as partitioning a dataset into meaningful groups (clusters) such that, under a particular definition of similarity, objects within a cluster are similar to one another (high intra-cluster similarity) but

R. Kashef (✉)
Electrical, Computer, and Biomedical Engineering Department, Ryerson University, London, ON, Canada
e-mail: rkashef@ryerson.ca

M. Warraich
Department of Management Science, Ivey Business School, London, ON, Canada
e-mail: mwarraich.msc2018@ivey.ca

R. Alhajj et al. (eds.), *Data Management and Analysis*, Studies in Big Data 65,
https://doi.org/10.1007/978-3-030-32587-9_4

differ from objects in other clusters (low inter-cluster similarity). This subject has been explored extensively under various disciplines over the past three decades. A large number of clustering algorithms [1–8] have been devised in statistics, data mining, pattern recognition, information retrieval, and other related fields. Traditionally, data clustering has been studied as a centralized process, characterized by a dataset that is located at a central node to which a clustering process is applied. In certain scenarios, the dataset is inherently distributed over multiple nodes, making it impossible and even infeasible to apply centralized clustering. The attributes ascribed to the distributed clustering system can be identified in terms of the local models, a global model for the clustering process, and the clustering strategy itself. In this paper, we used the clustering strategy attribute to classify the distributed clustering process into two main categories as either homogeneous or heterogeneous, depending on whether the nodes all share the same clustering strategy or invoke different clustering strategies, respectively. In each of the two categories, the local models and the global model are generated based on the architecture of the network. The remainder of this paper is organized as follows: in Sect. 2, an overview of clustering analysis is provided. Classical types of data and clustering process distributions, distributed clustering architectures, and local and global models are defined and discussed in Sect. 3. Section 4 provides our taxonomy of distributed clustering based on the adopted clustering strategies. Section 5 discusses different distributed clustering performance measures. Finally, we conclude the paper in Sect. 6.

2 Clustering Analysis

Clustering analysis is an unsupervised machine learning approach that partitions data points into groups such that data points within the same cluster are of high similarity to each other than those in different groups defined by a given similarity measure. It aims at identifying groups of customers or products with similar behaviors that eventually support firms and organizations to further smoothen their business model and process. Clustering analysis is used to predict the association/correlation in data and has broad application including market/customer segmentation, pattern recognition, biological studies, and Web document classification [1–8].

2.1 Properties of Clustering Methods

Clustering methods can be classified into different categories based on their clustering properties.

2.1.1 Partitional Vs. Hierarchical

A partitional-based clustering method obtains disjoint partitions of the data instead of a structure of clusters, such as the dendrogram generated by a hierarchical-based clustering approach. Partitional-based algorithms have been efficiently applied in applications involving large-scale data for which the process of building a dendrogram is computationally expensive. One main drawback of the partitional algorithms is the need to decide on the number of clusters a priori.

2.1.2 Hard Vs. Fuzzy

A hard-clustering algorithm assigns each data point to exactly one cluster by allocating a binary membership value either 0 or 1. Fuzzy clustering allocates degrees of membership for each data point to each cluster. Fuzzy clustering can be converted to hard clustering by allocating each data point to the cluster with the maximum degree of membership.

2.1.3 Distance Vs. Density

A distance-based clustering method assigns a data point to a particular cluster based on its distance from the cluster or its representative(s), while a density-based clustering approach expands a cluster as long as the density (or the number of data points) in the neighborhood satisfies some density threshold. Distance-based clustering methods can typically find only spherical-shaped clusters and encounter difficulty at discovering clusters of arbitrary shape, while density-based clustering algorithms are capable of finding clusters of different shapes and distributions.

2.1.4 Deterministic Vs. Stochastic

Deterministic-based clustering algorithms use deterministic optimization which can find clusters in a number of deterministic steps. Most of the partitional-based clustering techniques are deterministic which are designed to optimize a squared error function. Stochastic-based clustering algorithms adopt probabilistic optimization which randomly searches the entire state space consisting of all possible solutions.

2.2 Similarity Measures

In general, a critical step in clustering analysis and recommendation systems is the computation of the similarity between items and the selection of items with the highest similarity. The Pearson Correlation, cosine similarity, and Jaccard similarity are common similarity measures that are widely used in different clustering applications [1, 2].

2.3 *The Clustering Performance Measures*

Cluster validation is the process of estimating how well a partition fits the structure underlying the data. Evaluating clustering is more challenging than evaluating classification, as labels are available in supervised learning and performance statistics, such as accuracy, can be computed. Clustering validation measures can be categorized into two main groups, external clustering validation and internal clustering validation. External measures evaluate the result based on available supervised information, while internal measures evaluate the result based on the information intrinsic to the data alone [9]. External quality measures can be classified into F-measures based and Entropy-based measures. Different scalar validity indices have been proposed in [10, 11] as internal quality measures, none of which is perfect as standalones, and therefore several indices should be used to evaluate the quality of the clustering algorithm. Some indices are used to assess the quality of un-nested clusters produced by hard-clustering algorithms, and others are employed to evaluate the quality of fuzzy clusters generated by fuzzy clustering approaches. Another family of indices is applicable to hierarchical clustering algorithms. In addition, we can use one index to assess two different partitions produced by two different clustering algorithms.

3 Distributed Data Clustering

Distributed clustering assumes that the objects to be clustered reside at different nodes. Table 1 shows the different types of data and clustering process distribution.

- *Centralized Data–Centralized Clustering (CD-CC)*: This is the standard approach where the clustering process and data both reside on the same node.
- *Distributed Data–Centralized Clustering (DD-CC)*: Data might be dispersed across different nodes, a typical case in the Web domain, while the clustering process runs on a single node.

Table 1 Different types of data and clustering process distribution

	Centralized data	Distributed data
Centralized Clustering	CD-CC	DD-CC
Distributed Clustering	CD-DC	DD-DC

- *Centralized Data–Distributed Clustering (CD-DC)*: Data is stored in one node, with clustering processes running on different nodes accessing the same data; a typical case of parallel processing.
- *Distributed Data–Distributed Clustering (DD-DC)*: The highest level of distribution, in which both the data and the clustering processes are distributed over multiple nodes.

3.1 Distributed Networks

Two traditional approaches for performing distributed data clustering are either performing local clustering at each node to generate a local model which can be transmitted to a central node that aggregates them together into one global model *or* each node selects a small set of representative objects and transmits them to a central node, which combines the local representatives into one global representative of the whole dataset to carry out data clustering. The two approaches involve one central node to facilitate the distributed clustering process. A more departing approach does not involve a centralized operation, this fits to the peer-to-peer (P2P) class of algorithms. P2P networks can be unstructured and structured. In P2P networks, nodes communicate directly with each other to perform the clustering task. Communication in P2P networks can be very costly due to network traffic leading to flooding of messages [12–14].

3.2 Local and Global Clustering Models

Distributed clustering is carried out on two different levels: the local level and the global level. On the local level, all of the nodes independently carry out clustering, and local models are generated at each node. After clustering is completed on the local nodes, a global model is determined which can be accessed by all nodes to update their local models. The quality of the global model derived from the data should be either equal to or comparable to a model derived using a centralized method. Each node is required to build and maintain a local model of the problem space that it is responsible for. In terms of data clustering, this model is the cluster prototype (i.e., representatives). The global model is a representation of the entire cluster set produced by all nodes, it is constructed based on the local models generated at each node, and it is considered as a common repository of knowledge that is accessible to all nodes. The global model is what makes individual nodes aware of the big picture and serves as a catalog for nodes to consult with and determine whether the desired clustering quality has been achieved. The nodes then update their local models based on the global model generated.

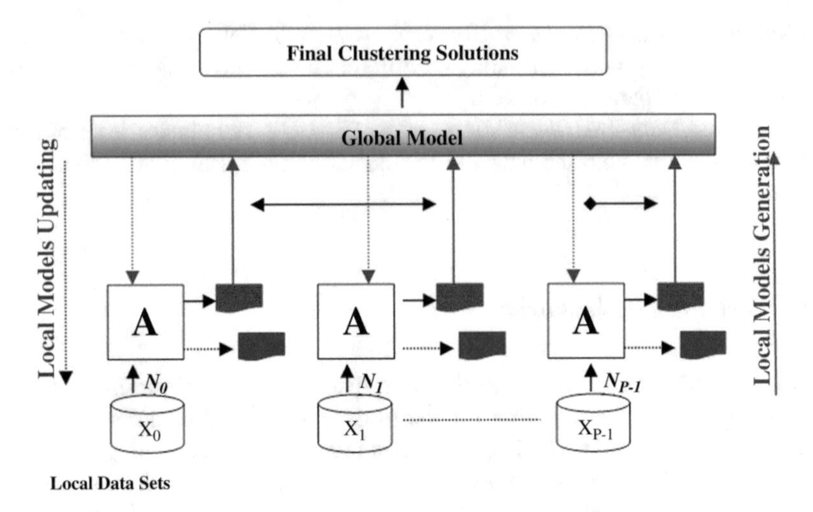

Fig. 1 General distributed clustering architecture

3.3 *Distributed Clustering Architectures*

Let N_0, N_1, ..., N_{P-1} be the set of nodes in the system, each node performs a clustering strategy A. Let $Z_0, Z_1, \ldots, Z_{P-1}$ be the corresponding set of local models, each local model Z_p, $p = 0, 1, \ldots, P - 1$ consists of the prototype representation of the collection of local objects X_p, the node N_p owns. Z_A is the final global model of the whole cluster set generated by all nodes. The general distributed clustering architecture is shown in Fig. 1.

The architecture shown in Fig. 1 is based on the fact that all nodes contribute to building one global model. A different architecture can be designed based on the existence of a facilitator node, which collects the local models from all nodes and builds one global model with an overall clustering.

4 Taxonomy of Distributed Clustering

Defining a distributed clustering system involves three main attributes: the structure of the local model, the final global model, and the clustering strategy itself. The lattermost attribute classifies the distributed clustering system as homogeneous or heterogeneous, depending on whether one or multiple different clustering strategies are adopted across all nodes, respectively.

Definition: Clustering Strategy
Clustering a set of n objects into a number of groups follows a certain clustering strategy A that involves several parameters including the similarity measure, a clustering algorithm, and initializations. Different combinations of these parameters define different clustering strategies for the clustering process.

Definition: Homogeneous Nodes
The nodes, $N_0^A, N_1^A \ldots, N_{P-1}^A$ that communicate with each other and run the same clustering strategy A, such that each node has its local dataset, are called homogeneous nodes.

Definition: Heterogeneous Nodes
Let $N_0^{A0}, N_1^{A1} \ldots, N_{P-1}^{AP-1}$ be any set of P nodes (each node has its own local dataset) in the system, such that each node N_i follows a clustering strategy A_i. These nodes are called *heterogeneous nodes*.

In homogeneous distributed clustering, each node follows a similar clustering strategy to its neighbors and similar local models are generated at each node. On the other hand, distributed heterogeneous clustering assumes that the adopted algorithms use different clustering strategies at each node; the nodes cooperate to achieve better overall clustering performance. Both homogeneous and heterogeneous distributed clustering can be classified into two main sub-categories, All-nodes-Global model or Facilitator-Global model, based on the communication protocol executed between nodes when collecting the local models and generating the global model. In the All-nodes-Global model, all nodes communicate with each other to either generate the global model (the clustering goal), or to enhance each other's performance by broadcasting messages (e.g., local objects) or exchanging local models. In the Facilitator-Global model, a facilitator node collects the local models from all nodes, constructs the global model, and sends this global model back to the other nodes to update their local models. Based on the above classification of distributed data clustering, taxonomies of the distributed data clustering schemes are illustrated in Tables 2 and 3.

Table 2 Taxonomy of distributed homogeneous clustering

All-nodes-global model		Facilitator-global model	
Distributed program	Distributed task	Single-local model	Multiple-local model

Table 3 Taxonomy of distributed heterogeneous clustering

All-nodes-global model		Facilitator global model	
Intermediate cooperation	End-results cooperation	Intermediate cooperation	End-Results cooperation

4.1 Homogeneous Distributed Clustering

In homogeneous distributed clustering, each node invokes the same clustering strategy, and homogeneous local models (i.e., prototypes) are generated at each node.

4.1.1 All-Nodes-Global Model: Distributed-Program

In the Distributed-Program model, a complete version of the clustering algorithm is distributed and executed over all nodes simultaneously, and all nodes contribute in the generation of the global model. The PKM [15], PFCM [16], DCC [17], PDDP [18], PBKM [19], MKmeans [20], and PAutoClass [21] are examples of the Distributed-Program model. Some of these distributed clustering algorithms are described next.

The Parallel k-Means (PKM)

The centralized k-means algorithm is an iterative procedure and requires the number of clusters k to be given a priori. The initial partitioning is randomly generated and the dataset is partitioned into k non-overlapping regions identified by their centroids that minimize the objective function criterion as shown in Eq. (1).

$$\sum_{i=1}^{k} \sum_{x \in S_i} \|x - c_i\| \tag{1}$$

where $\|x - c_i\|$ is Euclidian distance between the data vector x and the centroid c_i. In the parallel k-means algorithm (PKM) [15] the node N_0 as the "root node" computes the initial centroids and then broadcasts these k initial centroids to all other nodes. Each node is responsible for *n/P* vectors rather than the entire set. As a result, each node will compute the distances between its local vectors to each of the centroids. A series of assignments are generated mapping vectors to the closest centroid. Each node then gathers the sum of all vectors allocated to a given cluster and computes the mean of the vectors assigned to a particular cluster. Thus, the k-means program is distributed over the entire set of P nodes.

The Parallel Fuzzy c-Means (PFCM)

The Parallel Fuzzy c-means algorithm (PFCM) [16] requires the dataset to be divided into an equal number of data points, so that each node computes with its *n*/*P* data points loaded into its own local memory. The overall fuzzy membership function u_{ij} is divided up between the nodes with a local representation My_u_{ij} storing the membership of the local data points only. Global centroids are produced by global reduction of local centroids; these global centroids are used to update the local membership matrix My_u_{ij} at each node. The PFCM belongs to the family of distributed-program homogenous clustering, as the centralized FCM is applied at each node and the root node is responsible for collecting the global solution.

Distributed Collaborative Clustering (DCC)

The DCC algorithm [17] belongs to the family of distributed homogeneous collaborative clustering. In this model the goal is not to achieve one global clustering solution, but rather maximizing the quality of the local clustering solution at each node through collaboration. This is achieved through augmenting the local clustering solutions with recommendations from peer nodes after exchanging cluster prototypes. The Distributed Collaborative Clustering (DCC) algorithm assumes a set of P nodes, where the data at each node is clustered independently to form an "initial local clustering." The goal is to enhance each individual local clustering by gaining access to summarized cluster information from other nodes. Each node broadcasts its cluster prototypes to all other nodes. Every other node collects this information from its peers, calculates similarity values between local data and the peer cluster prototypes, and then sends a list of recommended local objects to be merged with the peer clusters. The original node receives recommendations from all of its peers, and based upon its own judgment it either merges the recommended objects or rejects them. This process results in an expanded local clustering that is both of higher quality and of more coverage than the initial local clustering.

4.1.2 All-Nodes-Global Model: Distributed-Task

The Distributed-Task model assumes that only a part, the most computationally intensive task, of the clustering algorithm is distributed over the nodes. Parallel k-windows [22] and DENCLUE-IM [23] algorithms follow this category of distributed clustering. The Parallel k-windows is described next.

Parallel k-Windows (PK-windows) Clustering

The idea behind the k-windows algorithm [22] is the use of windows to determine clusters. A window is defined as an orthogonal range in d-dimensional Euclidian space, where d is the number of numerical features of each data vector. Therefore, each window is a d-range of initial fixed area a. Each object that lies within a window is considered to belong to the corresponding cluster. The main idea is to construct a tree-like data structure with the properties that give the ability to perform a fast search of the set of objects. An orthogonal range search is based on this pre-processing where the tree is constructed. Thus, objects that lie within a d-range can be found by traversing the tree. Iteratively, the k-windows algorithm moves each window in the Euclidian space by centering them on the mean of the data vectors included. This iterative process continues until no further movement results in an increase in the number of vectors that lie within each window. Subsequently the algorithm enlarges every window in order to contain as many vectors as possible from the corresponding cluster. When trying to parallelize the k-windows algorithm, it is obvious that the step that requires the most computational effort is the range search. For this task, a parallel algorithmic scheme that uses Multi-Dimensional Binary Tree for a range search is presented.

4.1.3 Facilitator-Global Model: Single-Local Model

On the facilitator node, a global clustering model based on the representatives is constructed and sent back to the local nodes. The local nodes update their clustering solution based on the global model. The algorithms belonging to this model construct a single structure of homogeneous local models at each node; the facilitator collects these models to build one global model. The DCPCA [24], CHC [25], KDEC [13], DMBC [26], and Dk-windows [27] belong to this family of homogeneous distributed clustering. The DCPCA algorithm is described next.

Distributed Clustering Using Principal Component Analysis (DCPCA)

Principal Component Analysis (PCA) [24] is a popular technique to construct a representation of the data that captures maximally variant dimensions of the data. It computes a representation with a set of basis vectors that are the dominant eigenvectors of the covariance matrix generated by the data. PCA involves linear transformation of a collection of (statistically) related variables into a set of transformed variables, usually referred to as principal components. In a distributed environment, it would be advantageous to perform the computations for PCA locally, thereby minimizing the amount of data communication and the computation at one central node. The entire data matrix X is comprised of different smaller portions stored at different nodes. A facilitator node performs the PCA on this collected data and broadcasts the global PCs to each node.

4.1.4 Facilitator-Global Model: Multiple-Local Models

In this model, multiple-local models are generated, and the facilitator node generates one global model from any of the multiple-local models. The Distributed Density-based Clustering (DDBD) [28] algorithm follows this family of multiple-local models.

The Distributed Density-Based Clustering (DDBD)

The DDBD generates two different local models. It first clusters the data locally and extracts suitable representatives out of these clusters, which are sent to a facilitator node where the complete clustering is stored based on the local clustering. Two suitable local models called REPscor and REPk-means [28] are designed to create the local model based on the definition of the complete set of specific core points.

4.2 *Heterogeneous Distributed Clustering*

The distributed clustering algorithms that have been discussed thus far are homogeneous algorithms. In the case of different clustering algorithms with different clustering strategies, the clustering process is called heterogeneous clustering process. Using different clustering methods that cooperate in the clustering process helps in obtaining better clustering results at the global model. Heterogeneous distributed clustering algorithms can cooperate either on the intermediate level or the end-result level.

4.2.1 Intermediate Cooperation

In an intermediate-based cooperation, the heterogeneous clustering algorithms cooperate, negotiate, and obtain the best results at either each step or following a specified number of steps. Using this strategy, various cooperation methods can be used to implicitly enhance the quality of each individual clustering methods at the intermediate stages. Enhanced Bisecting k-means is an example of intermediate-based cooperative model [19].

Enhanced Bisecting k-Means Using Intermediate Cooperation (CBKM)

In some scenarios when a fraction of the dataset is left behind with no other way to re-cluster it again at each level of the binary tree, a "refinement" is needed to re-cluster the resulting clustering. Current techniques to refine the clustering results produced by the BKM (Bisecting K-means) uses end-result enhancement as k-means (KM) clustering. In this hybrid model, KM waits for the former BKM to finish its clustering and then it takes the final set of centroids as initial seeds for a better refinement. On the other hand, the CBKM concurrently combines the results of the BKM and KM at each level of the binary hierarchical tree using cooperative and merging matrices. Experimental analysis show that the CBKM achieves better clustering quality than that of KM and BKM.

4.2.2 End-Result Cooperation

In heterogeneous distributed clustering, algorithms cooperate at the final step; this model of cooperation is always used to refine the clustering quality produced by a former algorithm(s). An example of the distributed heterogeneous End-result clustering is distributed hybrid clustering, which assumes multiple clustering algorithms are used in cascade (i.e., the clustering algorithms cooperate at the end-result level) to cluster the dataset. Distributed hybrid clustering is carried out by either communication between all the different nodes or through the interaction between only facilitator nodes. The Parallel Hybrid Principal Direction Divisive Partitioning (PDDP) and k-means algorithm fit under the family of hybrid distributed clustering [18].

Parallel Hybrid Principal Direction Divisive Partitioning (PDDP) and k-Means

The Principal Direction Divisive Partitioning (PDDP) [18] is an unsupervised document-clustering algorithm based on the principal component analysis. The quality of the clustering solutions obtained, and the cost of the computations are shown to be good. The PDDP algorithm starts with a root cluster comprising the entire set of documents. Then it splits the set into two parts using the principal direction, this process runs recursively and results in a binary tree. To avoid generating clusters of unbalanced sizes, PDDP selects the next cluster with the largest scatter value to be split. The scatter value measures the cohesiveness of the documents within a cluster. The set of documents are represented by a term-document matrix M, in which each column corresponds to a document and each row corresponds to a particular word. For the parallel PDDP, the matrix M is stored in the Compressed Sparse Row (CSR) format. Each of the P nodes has a data structure consisting of the following three arrays. MM, a real number array containing the real values of the nonzero elements of M stored on each node row by row. CM matrix, an integer array for the column indices corresponding to the array MM. RM matrix, an integer number array containing the pointers to the beginning of each row in the arrays MM and CM. The parallel PDDP algorithm is fast in clustering Web documents datasets. However, the quality of its clustering for some cases may not be as good as that produced by the PKM clustering algorithm. Thus, the PKM is used to refine the clustering solutions that results from the parallel PDDP algorithm. This hybrid combination is based on *end-result* cooperation between both the parallel PDDP and PKM, this strategy of cooperation is mainly to enhance the clusters produced by the PDDP algorithm and to give the k-means algorithm a good initial point.

5 Distributed Clustering Performance Measures

Several distributed algorithms have been discussed, showcasing the different distribution schemes and strategies used. The performance of distributed algorithms compared to the corresponding centralized ones is evaluated through various metrics, some of these measures are illustrated next.

5.1 Execution Time

The time taken by a clustering algorithm to execute on a single node is called the centralized execution time and is denoted by T_c. The execution time of the corresponding parallel clustering algorithm on P identical nodes is called the parallel execution time and is denoted by T_p. A parallel clustering algorithm incurs several overheads during execution, including overheads due to idling, communication, and contention over shared data structures. The total sum of time spent by all nodes doing work, which is not done by the centralized clustering algorithm, is termed as the total overhead T_o. Since the total time spent by all nodes is $P * T_p$, and the total overhead is T_o, we can see that,

$$T_p = (T_c + T_o) / P \tag{2}$$

5.2 Speedup

The speedup performance measure is defined as the ratio of the execution time for clustering a dataset into k clusters on one central node to the execution time for identically clustering the same dataset on P nodes. Speedup is a summary of the efficiency of the distributed/parallel clustering algorithm.

$$\text{Speedup} = T_c / T_p \tag{3}$$

5.3 The Efficiency

The *Efficiency* of a distributed clustering algorithm is defined as the ratio of the speedup obtained to the number of nodes used. Therefore,

$$\text{Efficiency} = \frac{\text{Speedup}}{P} \text{ or Efficiency} = \frac{T_c}{T_c + T_o}\% \tag{4}$$

5.4 Isoefficiency Function

The efficiency of a parallel clustering algorithm is defined as the ratio of the speedup obtained to the number of nodes used. Therefore,

$$\text{Efficiency} = T_c / \left(T_c + T_o\right) \tag{5}$$

The isoefficiency function [29] connects the size of the problem to the number of nodes necessary to preserve a reasonable efficiency, thus showing the scalability of the parallel clustering algorithm. For a problem of size SZ (not the size of the input, but the number of operations the centralized clustering algorithm executes to solve the clustering problem; $T_c = \text{SZ} \times \text{Cost of executing one operation}$), assuming that the cost of executing one operation is one unit of time, the efficiency is defined as:

$$\text{Efficiency} = \left(\text{SZ} / \left(\text{SZ} + T_o\left(\text{SZ}, P\right)\right) \tag{6}$$

To achieve constant efficiency, $T_o(\text{SZ},P)/\text{SZ}$ must be maintained as a constant. If efficiency is fixed, SZ can be expressed as:

$$\text{SZ} = \text{Efficiency} / \left(1 - \text{Efficiency}\right) * T_o\left(\text{SZ}, P\right) \tag{7}$$

From that, for a specific $T_o(\text{SZ},P)$, SZ can be usually obtained as a function of P. This is the isoefficiency function for the given parallel clustering problem. This function indicates that the rate of growth of SZ requires keeping the efficiency of the parallel clustering algorithm fixed as P increases. Most of the distributed clustering algorithms use the *Speedup* and *Efficiency* measures in conjunction with the *isoefficiency* function to test their performance in comparison with the corresponding centralized clustering algorithms.

5.5 Distributed Messaging Cost

The total time spent by all nodes doing work, which is not done by the centralized clustering algorithm, is proposed as the total messaging cost M_c. The total messaging cost M_c is the sum of the idling time T_I, the messaging time T_M, and the communication time T_u.

$$M_c = T_I + T_M + T_u \tag{8}$$

The total distributed execution time T_d is the maximum running time from all nodes defined as:

$$T_d = \max_{p=0}^{P-1}\left(M_c^P + C_c^P\right) \quad (9)$$

where M_c^P and C_c^P are the messaging cost and computational cost of each node, respectively.

6 Conclusion

It is desirable to develop distributed clustering approaches that have low communication complexity. Quality and complexity of the global model derived from the data should be either equal to or comparable to a model derived using a centralized method. Handling inherently distributed datasets has become an important issue due to the emergence of different distributed applications. We provided a taxonomy that summarizes the current research trends in distributed data clustering based on the clustering strategy. Measuring the performance of distributed clustering algorithms is addressed through a discussion of some of the well-known performance and speedup measures.

References

1. Xu, R., & Wunsch, D. (2005). Survey of clustering algorithms. *IEEE Transactions on Neural Networks, 16*(3), 645–678.
2. Steinbach, M., Karypis, G., & Kumar, V. (2000). A comparison of document clustering techniques. In *Proc. KDD Workshop on Text Mining* (pp. 109–110). Setúbal: SciTePress.
3. Duda, R. O., Hart, P. E., & Stork, D. G. (2001). *Pattern classification*. New York: Wiley.
4. Vrahatis, M. N., Boutsinas, B., Alevizos, P., & Pavlides, G. (2002). The new k-windows algorithm for improving the k-means clustering algorithm. *Journal of Complexity, 18*, 375–391.
5. Hammouda, K. M., & Kamel, M. S. (2003). Incremental document clustering using cluster similarity histograms. In *Proc. IEEE/WIC International Conference on Web Intelligence* (pp. 597–601). Washington, DC: IEEE Computer Society.
6. Hammouda, K. M., & Kamel, M. S. (2004). Efficient phrase-based document indexing for web document clustering. *IEEE Transactions on Knowledge and Data Engineering, 16*(10), 1279–1296.
7. Savaresi, S. M., & Boley, D. L. (2001). On the performance of bisecting K-means and PDDP. In *Proc. 2001 SIAM International Conference on Data Mining* (pp. 1–14). Philadelphia: SIAM.
8. Karray, F. O., & Desilva, C. W. (2004). *Soft computing and intelligent systems design: Theory, tools and applications*. London: Pearson Education.
9. Rezaei, M., & Fränti, P. (2016). Set matching measures for external cluster validity. *IEEE Transactions on Knowledge and Data Engineering, 28*(8), 2173–2186.

10. Rendón, E., Abundez, I., Arizmendi, A., Quiroz, E. M., & M, E. (2011). Internal versus external cluster validation indexes. *International Journal of computers and communications, 5*(1), 27–34.
11. Reichart, R., & Rappoport, A. (2009). The NVI clustering evaluation measure. In *Proc. Thirteenth Conference on Computational Natural Language Learning* (pp. 165–173). Stroudsburg, PA: Association for Computational Linguistics.
12. Datta, S., Bhaduri, K., Giannella, C., Wolff, R., & Kargupta, H. (2006). Distributed Data Mining in Peer-to-Peer Networks, in *IEEE Internet Computing, 10*(4), 18–26.
13. Klusch, M., Lodi, S., & Moro, G. (2003). Agent-based distributed data mining: the KDEC scheme. In *Intelligent information systems* (Lecture notes in computer science) (Vol. 2586, pp. 104–122). Berlin: Springer.
14. Kashef, R., & Kamel, M. S. (2006). Distributed cooperative hard-fuzzy document clustering. In *Proc. 3rd Annual Scientific Conference of the LORNET Research Network (I2LOR06).* Montreal: ARIES Publications.
15. Stoffel, K., & Belkoniene, A. (1999). Parallel k/h-means clustering for large data sets. In *Euro-Par '99 parallel processing* (Lecture notes in computer science) (Vol. 1685, pp. 1451–1454). Berlin: Springer.
16. Kwok, T., Smith, K., Lozano, S., & Taniar, D. (2002). Parallel fuzzy c-means clustering for large data sets. In *Euro Par '02 parallel processing* (Lecture notes in computer science) (Vol. 2400, pp. 365–374). Berlin: Springer.
17. Hammouda, K. M., & Kamel, M. S. (2006). Collaborative document clustering. In *Proc. SIAM Conference on Data Mining (SDM06)* (pp. 453–463). Philadelphia: SIAM.
18. Xu, S., & Zhang, J. (2004). A hybrid parallel web document clustering algorithm and its performance study. *Journal of Supercomputing, 30*(2), 117–131.
19. Kashef, R. F., & Kamel, M. S. (2009). Enhanced Bisecting K-means Clustering Using Intermediate Cooperation. *Journal of Pattern Recognition, 42*(11), 2557–2569.
20. Rehioui, H., Idrissi, A., Abourezq, M., & Zegrari, F. (2016). DENCLUE-IM: A new approach for big data clustering. *Procedia Computer Science, 83*, 560–567.
21. Pizzuti, C., & Talia, D. (2003). P-AutoClass: Scalable parallel clustering for mining large data sets. *IEEE Transactions on Knowledge and Data Engineering, 15*(3), 629–641.
22. Alevizos, P. D., Tasoulis, D. K., & Vrahatis, M. (2003). Parallelizing the unsupervised k-windows clustering algorithm. In *Parallel processing and applied mathematics* (Lecture notes in computer science) (Vol. 3019, pp. 225–232). Berlin: Springer.
23. Zhang, J., Wu, G., Hu, X., Li, S., & Hao, S. (2013). A parallel clustering algorithm with MPI–MKmeans. *Journal of Computers, 8*(1), 10–17.
24. Kargupta, H., Huang, W., Sivakumar, K., & Johnson, E. (2001). Distributed clustering using collective principal component analysis. *Knowledge and Information Systems, 3*, 422–448.
25. Johnson, E. L., & Kargupta, H. (1999). Collective, hierarchical clustering from distributed, heterogeneous data. In *Large-scale parallel data mining* (Lecture notes in computer science) (Vol. 1759, pp. 221–244). Berlin: Springer.
26. Kriegel, H. P., Kröger, P., Pryakhin, A., & Schubert, M. (2005). Effective and efficient distributed model-based clustering. In *Proc. Fifth IEEE International Conference on Data Mining (ICDM05)* (pp. 258–265). IEEE.
27. Tasoulis, D. K., & Vrahatis, M. N. (2004). Unsupervised distributed clustering. In *Proc. International Conference on Parallel and Distributed Computing and Networks* (pp. 347–351). IEEE.
28. Januzaj, E., Kriegel, H. P., & Pfeifle, M. (2003). Towards effective and efficient distributed clustering. In *Proc. Workshop on Clustering Large Data Sets (ICDM03)* (pp. 49–58). IEEE.
29. Gupta, A., & Kumar, V. (1993). Isoefficiency function: a scalability metric for parallel algorithms and architectures. *IEEE Transaction, Parallel and Distributed Technology, 1*, 12–21.

Order Acceptance Policy for Make-To-Order Supply Chain

Jun Ma, Yiliu Tu, and Ding Feng

Abstract This paper explores a dynamic order acceptance policy of firms in a decentralized supply chain (SC) to improve the profits of an SC by using the machine learning method. The dynamic arrival and due date orders in SC were divided into three types according to the profit that the SC can obtain. Two echelons of the SC, in which a supplier that cooperate with other firms in SC will receive orders in and out of the SC, are employed in this study. Capturing four order characteristics in make-to-order SC, we examine whether this model can make a higher profit by using a simulation model of Support Vector Machines (SVMs) rather than First Come First Serve (FCFS) and Artificial Neural Network (ANN). The experimental results indicate that SVMs is an efficient tool for firms in a dynamic SC to improve the performance of the SC. A numerical example is used to validate the results.

Keywords Supply chain · Simulation · SVMs · Order acceptance strategy

J. Ma
School of Management, Shenyang University of Technology, Shenyang, Liaoning, People's Republic of China

Department of Mechanical and Manufacturing Engineering, University of Calgary, Calgary, AB, Canada
e-mail: jun.ma2@ucalgary.ca

Y. Tu (✉)
Department of Mechanical and Manufacturing Engineering, University of Calgary, Calgary, AB, Canada
e-mail: paultu@ucalgary.ca

D. Feng
School of Mechanical Engineering, Yangtze University, Jingzhou, Hubei, People's Republic of China

R. Alhajj et al. (eds.), *Data Management and Analysis*, Studies in Big Data 65,
https://doi.org/10.1007/978-3-030-32587-9_5

1 Introduction

Make-to-order supply chain often faces the uncertainty of orders practice. Order acceptance policy is one of the important managerial issues in the supply chain (SC) management, which will affect the profits of the SC to some extent. Guerrero and Kern [1] argue that the order acceptance policy of a firm in the SC affects the profits of the SC. Especially, the order arrivals are uncertain and their due date is dynamic in SCs in which firms cooperate and compete for each other. Although some significant progress has been made by using simulation, optimization, and heuristic methods, some high-profit orders are still rejected, and negative-profit orders are accepted in SC. Each of these order acceptance methods has both its advantages and disadvantages. Optimization algorithms, such as mixed integer linear programming (MILP), are simple, but lack sensitivity to dynamic orders and competitive SC. On the other hand, most acceptance order management methodologies in SC ignore this problem or handle it in terms of past experience. Some methods, even very popular in practice, such as FCFS (first come, first serve), balancing between a big order and many small orders, and FCLS (first come, last serve) are often incomplete. Some high-profit orders often were rejected by using these methods under production capacity limitation [2, 3]. These problems have seriously affected the performance of an SC.

It has been widely recognized in practice that the order acceptance policy of a firm in an SC affects the profits of the make-to-order SC under the firm's capacity limitation. Thus, the following questions naturally arise. How does the dynamic order acceptance policy of a firm in competitive make-to-order SC affect the performance (e.g., profits) of an SC? In which way is the performance of the SC evaluated? How does a firm select an order under its capacity limitation? How much more profits will the whole SC obtain? How much profit will the firm lose and gain? To answer these questions, this paper proposes a modeling initiative to formalize an order acceptance policy for the suppliers in the SC. Considering the order in and out of the SC, the order acceptance policy can be perceived as a tool and indicator to identify what kind of orders will contribute more to the profits of the SC. Although in the past few decades some research papers have been found which aim to improve the performance of SCs. As to our best knowledge, a meaningful report or paper that explicitly answers these questions has not been found in the literature.

Order acceptance problems in a single firm can be classified into four dimensions: the characteristics of order stream, the structure of products to be manufactured, the level of planning decision, and the flexibility of order acceptance [4]. The order acceptance problem in a make-to-order SC is sometimes different from the order acceptance problem in a single firm. All orders are placed by various customers and the components and finished goods inventories are generated to buffer or store these orders according to their due dates. More often the firm in a make-to-order SC sacrifices the profit of its own to obtain the optimal profit of the whole SC. How to further optimize the profits of an SC based on order acceptance policy is an intriguing, strategic decision that has been facing SC management.

Our study builds upon earlier order acceptance policy research and order rejection research and makes some new ideas. In this paper, we consider an order acceptance problem of a supplier in the SC with different order characteristics and different demands. Two kinds of orders with distinctive characteristics were considered. Both their arrival time and due date are dynamic. One is from downstream of this SC which is regular and stable relatively, and others are from out of this SC which is uncertain and unstable. If a supplier accepts a vast number of orders out of the SC, it will have a negative effect on its cooperation and reputation in SC. On the contrary, if the supplier rejects the order, it will affect profits and lead to idle manufacturing resources. Different orders have distinctive characteristics including the size, due date, and distribution of the orders, whether the production capacity is available to satisfy the customers and so on. In our paper, we explore an SVM model to balance and select these dynamic orders according to the characteristics of an order to improve the performance of the SC. Additionally, the orders faced by a supplier every day in our study are separated into three types, including (1) high-profit order. Both the SC and the supplier get more profits from it. If the order is rejected, the supplier and SC will lose the profits directly; (2) low-profit order. Rejecting it, the whole SC will get more profits. But the supplier will lose a part of the profits. Because if the supplier accepts this order, his/her production capacity will be not enough for the order in SC during the lead-time. Next step will be the profit sharing of the SC; (3) negative-profit order. Rejecting it. Both the whole SC and suppliers get more profits.

In this paper, (1) In order to investigate how the order acceptance policy of a supplier affects the SC profits, we capture four order characteristics in make-to-order SC, i.e., order's size, due date, residual production capacity in the supplier, and order probability in make-to-order SC. (2) For the sake of verifying how the order acceptance policy of a supplier affects the SC profits, we simulate the problems for suppliers in an SC by using FCFS, ANN, and SVMs to filter the orders that will benefit for a whole SC. (3) For the sake of explaining machine learning method in detail, we check the performance of the SC under FCFS and SVMs. (4) We study the free competition in an SC with complete demand information sharing. Every firm in SC is a decentralized decision-maker. There are lots of elements affecting the profits of an SC, which are either discrete or continuous. Another key difference in this paper is that we have used simulation to identify the profits of an SC based on the SVMs method considering both discrete-event and continuous simulation. To the best of our knowledge, it is the first study that SVMs were used to analyze dynamic order acceptance and rejection policy in competitive make-to-order SCs.

The rest of this paper is organized as follows. In Sect. 3, the SVMs are discussed. In Sect. 4, we present an SC simulation model by using SVMs for make-to-order SC according to SC utility maximization. We illustrate our results with a numerical example in Sect. 5. Conclusion and future work are given in Sect. 6.

2 Literature Review

Early in 1969, order acceptance was attended by scholars. Miller [5] considers an n-server queueing system with m customer classes distinguished by the reward associated with serving customers of that class and formulated this problem as an infinite horizon continuous time Markov decision problem. Over the last decades, several methods have been applied to solve the order acceptance problems to improve the profit of SC, e.g., simulation, heuristic method, regression method, mixed integer linear programming (MILP), and Machine learning method. (1) *Simulation*: To date, simulation is an effective way to solve the order acceptance problems with different models. There are several relevant literature reviews in this field. Holweg and Bicheno [6] describe how a participative simulation model is used to demonstrate SC dynamics and to model possible improvements to an entire SC. The Lean Leap Logistics Game' was developed primarily to foster collaboration. Lee et al. [7] propose an architecture of combined modeling for SC simulation, which includes the equation of continuous portion in the SC and how these equations can be used in the SC simulation models. Petrovic [8] develops for analyzing SC behavior and performance in the presence of uncertainty by using a special purpose simulation tool, SCSIM (Supply Chain SImulation Model). Simulation has been widely adopted in order acceptance since early 1970 [9–11]. (2) *Heuristic method*: In the early 1990s, Heuristic methods were adopted by Stern and Avivi [12] to solve the order acceptance problems of a textile firm. Slotnick and Morton [13] develop the optimal branch-and-bound procedure that uses a linear (integer) relaxation for bounding and performs the sequencing and job acceptance decisions jointly. They then developed a variety of fast and high-quality heuristics based on this approach. Barut and Sridharan [14] investigate the effectiveness of a tactical demand-capacity management policy to guide operational decisions in order-driven production systems. The policy is implemented via a heuristic that attempts to maximize revenue by selectively accepting or rejecting customer orders for multiple product classes when demand exceeds capacity constantly over the short term. (3) *Regression method*: Regression models show good performance when used to support customer order acceptance decisions in complex plants with dynamic order arrivals and either deterministic or stochastic processing times [15, 16]. (4) *Mixed integer linear programming (MILP)*: MILP, a popular method, is used in order acceptance research. Lei and Guo [17] formulate the order acceptance and scheduling problem in a flow shop as a mixed integer linear programming model and develop an effective parallel neighborhood search algorithm. Nobibon and Leus [18] present two MILP procedures and two branch-and-bound algorithms to the problem with up to 50 jobs within reasonable CPU times. Charnsirisakskul et al. [19, 20] develop a MIP formulation and use numerical analysis to examine simultaneous order acceptance with a two-level due date structure as in Og et al. [21]. (5) *Machine learning method*: In recent years, several machine learning methods were used to differentiate the higher-profit order from the lower-profit order. A genetic algorithm (GA) was adopted in some of these papers. Rom and Slotnick [22] use a genetic algorithm to solve the order acceptance problem with tardiness penalties. Rahman et al. [23] develop a Genetic Algorithm based approach that is applied repeatedly for re-optimization as each new order arrives. Chen et al. [24] propose a diversity controlling genetic algorithm (DCGA) for selection and scheduling problems in production systems. Park et al. [25] propose two new Particle Swarm Optimization (PSO) approaches to order acceptance problem. Afterward, genetic programming evolved rules are combined with an existing Tabu Search (TS) heuristic and with the proposed PSO algorithms as hybrid approaches to order acceptance problem. In 1994, the neural network approach was considered in order acceptance problem. Wang et al. [4] develop a neural network approach for order acceptance decision support in job shops with machine and manpower capacity constraints. The order acceptance problem was solved as a sequential multiple criteria decision problem by using a neural network approach.

The detailed themes of order acceptance which the scholars focused are different. The relevant literature can be classified into three major categories. (1) The first category is related to *due date and lead-time setting*. Keskinocak and Tayur provided a survey of due date management (DDM) research. Three basic approaches were explored by Wester et al. [26]. One is the monolithic approach; the acceptance decision is based on detailed information on a current production schedule for all formerly accepted orders. The second is the hierarchic approach, the acceptance strategy is based on global capacity load profiles only, while the detailed scheduling of accepted orders takes place at a lower level (possibly later in time). The third one is the myopic approach, which the acceptance decision is similar to the one in the hierarchic approach, but scheduling is myopic, i.e., once the machine becomes idle only the next order to be produced is actually scheduled. (2) *Time-related penalty*: The penalty is a major tool that controls the delivery date timely in SC practice. Some literature studied profit optimization under a penalty for delay delivery. Nobibon and Leus [18] study a generalization of the order acceptance and scheduling problem in a single machine environment where a pool consisting of firm planned orders, as well as potential orders, is available from which an over-demanded company can select. Og et al. [21] examine simultaneous order acceptance and scheduling decisions where the orders are defined by their release dates, due dates, deadlines, processing times, sequence dependent setup times, and revenues in a single machine environment. The penalty is a traditional way of revenue management [22, 27–29]. (3) *Uncertain demand*: uncertain demand is a crucial factor which affects the profit of SC. In recent years, a number of authors have increasingly focused their attention on uncertain demands in an SC. Yang and Fung [30] consider that demands in different periods are random variables and are independent of one another, and replenishment of inventory deviates from the scheduled quantities. Aouam and Brahimi [31] formulate a model that integrates production planning and order acceptance decisions while taking demand uncertainty into account. Kilic et al. [32] consider a food production system that processes a single perishable raw material into several products having stochastic demands.

3 Support Vector Machines

3.1 Definition of Support Vector Machines

Support vector machines (SVMs), also known as support vector networks [33–35], were initially proposed by Vapnik and his coworkers in 1995. SVMs are supervised learning models with associated learning algorithms that analyze data

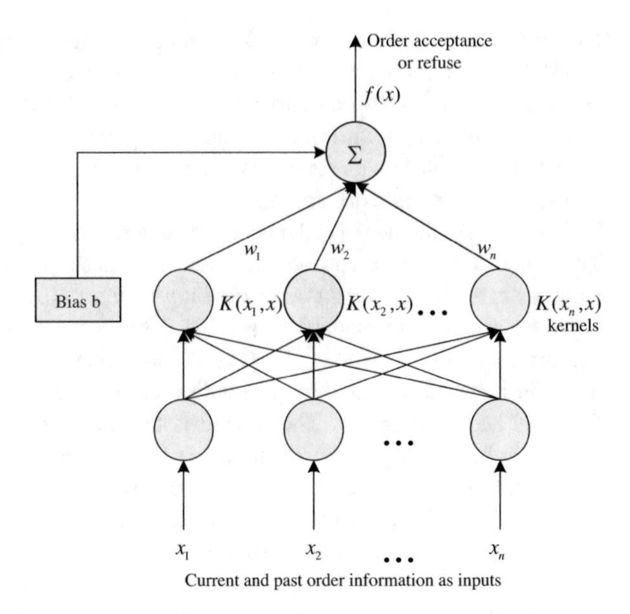

Fig. 1 Schematic view of an SVM for order acceptance

used for classification and regression analysis. SVMs are a newer type of universal function approximators that are based on the structural risk minimization principle from statistical learning theory [34]. SVMs aim at minimizing an upper bound of the generalization error through maximizing the margin between the separating hyperplane and the data. This is an approximate implementation of the Structure Risk Minimization principle [36]. SVMs have been proved to have mostly good performances in the analysis of pattern classification and nonlinear regression [37–39]. Figure 1 shows the schematically view of an SVM for order acceptance problems.

3.2 Support Vector Machines for Classification

In this section, we briefly discuss the basic features of support vector machines (SVMs) model for classification. At the outset, given training dataset $\{(x_i, y_i), x_i \in \mathbb{R}^d, y_i \in (+1, -1), i = 1, \cdots, n\}$. x_i is a vector in the input space $\mathbb{R}^d$. And y_i is the class index. Then, constructing the optimal separating hyperplane to give the maximum separation between the decision classes. Classification linear inseparable problem can be transferred into formula (1).

$$\min\ f = \frac{1}{2}\|w\|^2 + C\sum_{i=1}^{N}\varepsilon_i \tag{1}$$

$$s.t. \quad y\left[w^T \varnothing(x_i) + b\right] \geq 1 - \varepsilon_i, \quad i = 1, \cdots, N.$$

$$\varepsilon_i \geq 0, \quad i = 1, \cdots, N.$$

Nonlinear classification problem can be mapped into a linear classification problem in the high-dimensional feature space by mapping the input vectors x into the high-dimensional feature space. A linear classification problem built in the new space can represent a nonlinear classification problem in an original space. The maximum margin hyperplane will be given in the high-dimensional feature space.

The optimal hyperplane classification problem can be transformed into a Lagrangian dual problem by using Lagrange optimization. It is an optimization problem of a quadratic function under the constraints of inequality. The classification function is shown in formula (2).

$$f(x) = \text{sign}\left\{\sum_{i=1}^{N} a_i^* y_i k(x_i, y_i) + b^*\right\} \tag{2}$$

Where a_i^* are the nonnegative Lagrange multipliers.

3.3 *The Kernel Function and Model Parameters of SVMs*

The function $k(x_i, y_i)$ is the kernel function. Common kernel functions are the linear kernel $k(x_i, y_i) = \langle x_i, y_i \rangle$, the polynomial kernel $k(x_i, y_i) = (\langle x_i, y_i \rangle + R)^d$ and the Gaussian radial basis function $k(x_i, y_i) = \exp\left\{\frac{\|x_i - x_j\|^2}{2\sigma^2}\right\}$. We choose Gaussian radial basis function as a kernel function in this paper. g, C, important coefficients, which will affect the accuracy of the result will be given using n-fold cross validation method.

4 Simulation Models

4.1 *Basic Assumptions*

In this section, we propose an SC model with components supplier, components manufacturers, and demand market. The SC includes the production, transportation, marketing, and store of the product associated with the different costs. The decision-makers on the SC network are the suppliers and the manufacturers, who aim at obtaining the maximum profits under time and capacity constraints. Suppliers make a decision under their profit maximization goal. We focus on an SC in which a

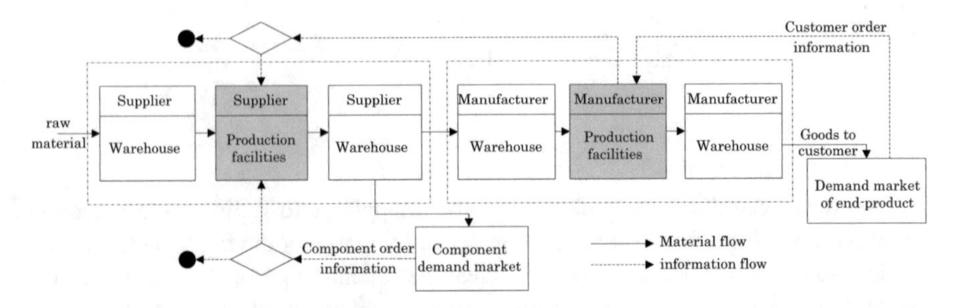

Fig. 2 Schematic view of an SC

supplier will balance between demands in/out of SC, and at the same time we also assume that this SC is in completion with other SCs in the same market. The SC also includes a raw material inventory, production facilities, and an end-product inventory as illustrated in Fig. 2.

Assumptions about SC operations and processes are as follows:

ASSUMPTION 1: The manufacturers in the SC employ a make-to-order (MTO) market strategy, and they can accept or reject a particular order according to order's size, their production capacity, the due date of order, the occurrence probability of the order in SC.

ASSUMPTION 2: The total demand excesses the production capacity of a firm in the SC over the given period.

ASSUMPTION 3: The demand distribution of end-product can be obtained from the historical data.

ASSUMPTION 4: The information on the order's size, due date, and demand distribution of orders as well as the residual production capacity are observable.

ASSUMPTION 5: The firms employ FCFS (first come, first serve) rule to process its accepted orders. The succeeding order will be immediately processed once the preceding order is completed.

4.2 Defining Variables

The SC as perceived in this paper consists of suppliers and manufacturers. It produces l types of end-products. Orders in the SC arrive stochastically and follow a certain distribution. Orders out of the SC arrive randomly. The size of orders in SC also follows a certain distribution. The size of orders out of the SC is randomly distributed. For clarity, the notation was listed in Table 1.

We use *ordertype* (OS, DD, PCS, PD) to represent the order information that supplier receives out of the SC. *OS* : *The order′s size* denotes the order's size out of the SC the supply receives; *DD* : *Due date* denotes the order's due date that supplier receives the order out of the SC; *PCS* : *production capacity surplus* denotes the residual production capacity of the firm in the SC when the order is placed by

Table 1 Notation for order acceptance policy

T	The year of order loading horizon
i	i Order index $i = (1, 2, \cdots, N)$
q	The size of order i, $i = (1, 2, \cdots, N)$
$\mathrm{TP}_{\mathrm{sc}}$	Total profit of SC
TP_M	Total profit of the manufacturer in SC
TP_S	Total profit of supplier in SC
P_l	Selling price of type l product
RV	Revenue
D_l	Demand of type l product
HC	Holding cost
IC_M	Inventory cost of manufacturer
IC_S	Inventory cost of supplier
DD_i	The due date of order i, $i = (1, 2, \cdots, N)$
MP_i	The total time of manpower required for order i
PT_i	The total production time for order i on firm
P_{ns}	The fee of a normal shift
WH	The working hours of normal shift
α	The fee of overtime shift is α times of normal shift
OC_i	The production capacity for order i
MC_i	The open machine production capacity for order i
PC_i	The open manpower production capacity for order i
FC_M	The fixed cost of manufacturer in SC
FC_S	The fixed cost of supplier in SC

a customer; *PD* : *Probability of demand distribution* denotes the probability of an order arrives in SC when the supplier receives an order out of the SC. The product ordering process in SC is shown in Fig. 3.

4.3 Simulation Logics

We aim to maximize the profits of SC considering order acceptance policy of supplier in the SC. The simulation process is described as follows:

1. The initialization phase: the number of working days in a year is m days/per year. The number of order occurred in the SC in a year is N. The number of order occurred out of the SC in a year is K.
2. Generally, we assume an elastic demand function, sensitive to the dominant firm's price, which is a monotone decreasing function of the price. l denotes the number of end-products' type of SC that will compete with other SC in the same markets.

$$D_k = f\left(p_1, p_2, \cdots, p_l\right), \forall k, l. \tag{3}$$

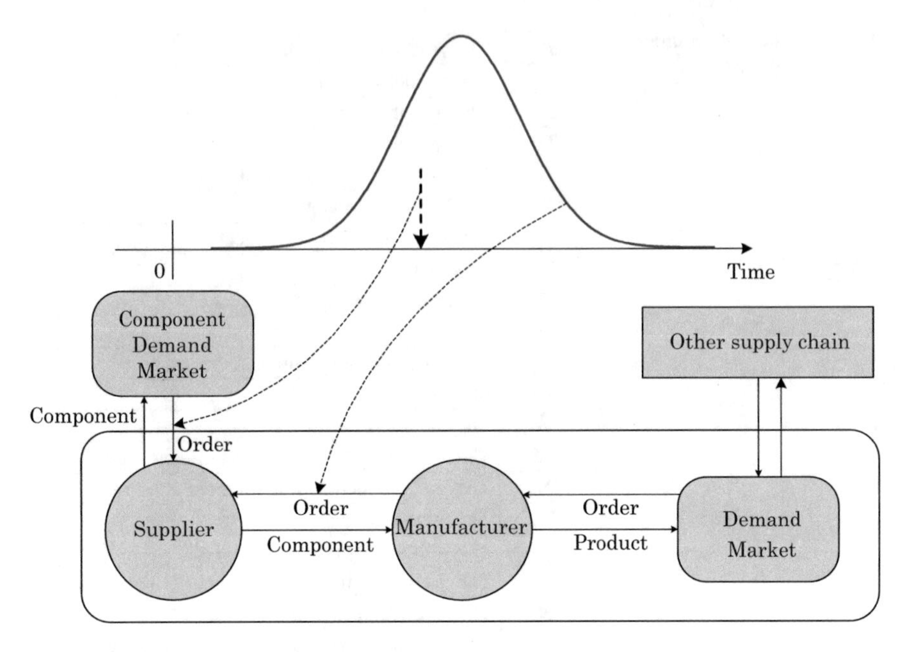

Fig. 3 Chain of product ordering

3. The order's size and arrival time in the SC are a certain distribution. The order received out of the SC is stochastic. The information of orders received out of the SC includes order's size, due date, the residual production capacity, and the occurrence probability of the order. The demand is the sum of the total order's quantity.

$$D_k = \sum_{i=1}^{N} q_i, \tag{4}$$

4. If an order arrives from out of the SC, an MTO (make-to-order) supplier can decide whether accept the order according to the order's size, due date, residual production capacity, and the occurrence probability of order. Figure 4 shows the supplier trade-off model.
5. If one of the MTO suppliers and MTO manufacturers rejects the orders, the SC will reject these orders directly. If the MTO manufacturer's capacity is available for this order, he/she needs further to know whether the necessary MTO suppliers are available to fulfill this order.
6. If suppliers and the manufacturer in the SC decide to accept this order, the suppliers and the manufacturer will schedule the order following the FCFS rule. It is assumed that the accepted orders cannot be canceled or changed by the customers lately.

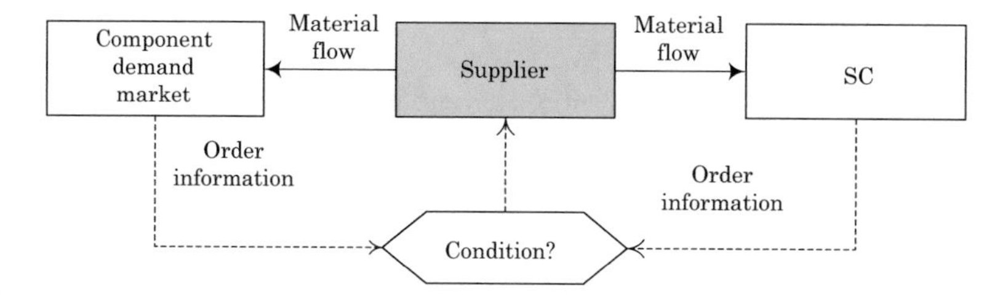

Fig. 4 Supplier's trade-off model

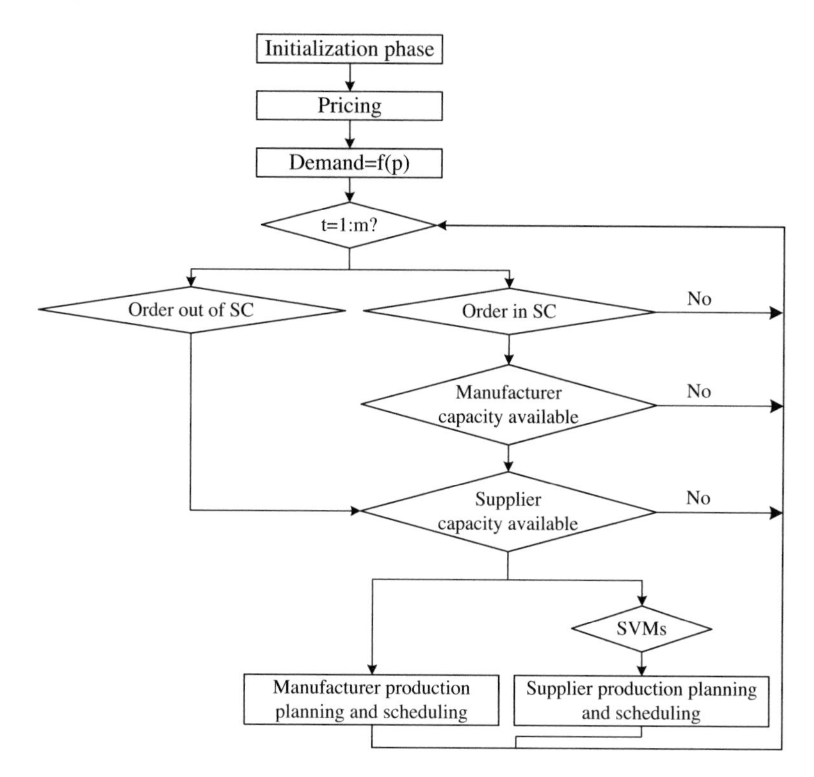

Fig. 5 Schematic view of SC simulation logic with SVMs

7. If $t > m$, calculate the profit of the suppliers, the manufacturer, and the whole SC. Figure 5 is the schematic view of the SC operation logic.

4.4 Simulation Model Descriptions

The model was built to simulate the MTO process in SC practice. The simulation model and relevant assumptions are described as follows:

4.4.1 The Manufacturer

A manufacturer in an SC normally prices the end-product and accepts orders from a customer directly. As well studied [40–42], a customer demand is the function of the end-product's price from this SC and other SCs' end-product's prices. The order's sizes in 1 year are normally distributed.

$$D_k = f\left(p_1, p_2, \cdots, p_l\right), \forall k, l. \tag{5}$$

Accepting the order from the customer demand, the manufacturer often decomposes the order into parts according to the end-product BOM (Bill of Material). If the residual production capacity allows the manufacturer to fulfill this order before its due date, the manufacturer will further seek for the necessary suppliers for fulfilling the order. In terms of the feedbacks from these suppliers, the manufacturer will decide whether the order is accepted or not. If the order is finally accepted, the manufacturer will schedule the order as according to FCFS (first come, first serve) rule together with other orders. Figure 6 shows the production scheduling principle.

If the normal shift cannot complete the order, an overtime shift will be arranged. The fee of overtime shift is α times of the fee of normal shift (P_{ns}). The end-product in a workshop will be sent to a warehouse, whose inventory is I_j daily and inventory cost is C_I each year. Formula (6) is the annual inventory cost of the manufacturer.

$$\text{IC}_M = \sum_{j=1}^{m} I_j \times C_I / m \tag{6}$$

The variable cost of the manufacturer includes a fee of a normal shift, a fee of overtime shift, material or component cost, and transportation cost. Formula (7) is the annual variable cost of the manufacturer.

$$\text{VC}_M = \sum_{j=1}^{m}\sum_{i=1}^{\text{WH}} q_{ij} \times P_l + \sum_{j=1}^{m}\sum_{i=\text{WH}}^{24} q_{ij} \times P_l \times \alpha + P_S \times Q_S + \text{TC}_M \tag{7}$$

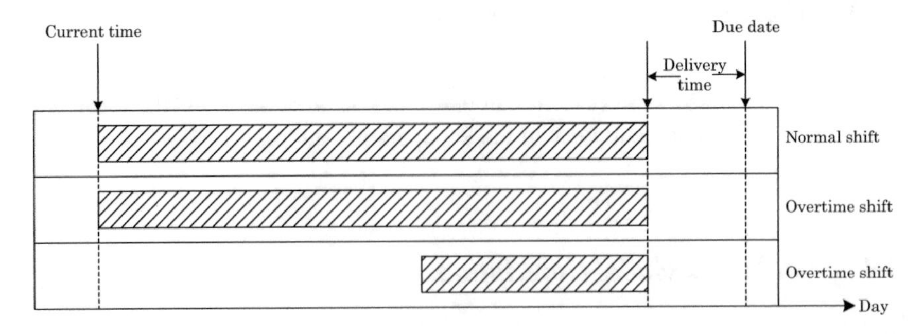

Fig. 6 Production planning and scheduling based on FCFS rule

The fixed cost of the manufacturer is denoted by FC_M. Let RV_M denotes the revenue of the manufacturer. Formula (8) is the profit of the manufacturer.

$$P_M = \mathrm{RV}_M - \mathrm{IC}_M - \mathrm{CV}_M \tag{8}$$

4.4.2 The Supplier

When receiving the order information from the manufacturer, a supplier will make a decision whether he/she would accept the order according to his/her residual production capacity before the due date of the order. Accordingly, the supplier will send a feedback to the manufacturer in due course. The supplier can also accept orders from other SCs. Whether the supplier accepts an order from this SC or other SCs, we assume that the supplier can make this decision based on the profit of an SC by using SVMs (support vector machines) to calculate. Figure 7 shows the order acceptance policy process based on SVMs.

1. According to supplier's history training data, we build a separating hyperplane by using margin maximization.

$$y(x_i) = w^T \varnothing (x_i) + b, \forall i. \tag{9}$$

2. The corresponding classification decision function is

$$f(x_i) = \mathrm{sign}\left(w^T \varnothing (x_i) + b\right), \forall i. \tag{10}$$

3. The optimal separating hyperplane is the farthest one from the training data. So, the objective function and constraint can be followed.

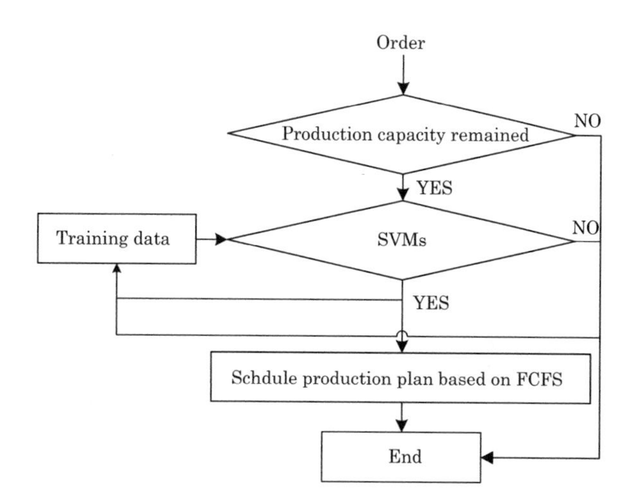

Fig. 7 Order acceptance policy process based on SVMs

$$\arg\max_{w,b}\left\{\frac{1}{\|w\|}\min_{i}\left[y_i\left(w^T\varnothing\left(x_i\right)+b\right)\right]\right\} \tag{11}$$

$$\text{s.t.}\, y_i\left[w^T\varnothing\left(x_i\right)+b\right]\geq 1-\varepsilon_i, i=1,2,\cdots,N.$$

4. Formula (11) can be transferred into a Lagrange function as follows:

$$L\left(w,b,\varepsilon,\alpha,\mu\right)=\frac{1}{2}\|w\|^2+C\sum_{i=1}^{N}\varepsilon_i-\sum_{i=1}^{N}\alpha_i\left(y_i\left(wx_i+b-1+\varepsilon_i\right)\right)-\sum_{i=1}^{N}\mu\varepsilon_i \tag{12}$$

Then, the optimal separating hyperplane function can be obtained by using Karush–Kuhn–Tucker (KKT) condition and SMO algorithm. The optimal separating hyperplane function is the criterion to allow the supplier to discriminate between two classes of orders (one yielding a higher profit contribution than the other), resulting in selective rejection of orders for the class with the lower-profit contribution.

The profit of SC is the sum of the profits of the supplier and the manufacturer in SC. The formulas of profit of the supplier are same as the manufacturer's.

$$P_{\text{SC}}=P_M+P_S \tag{13}$$

4.5 Criteria and Constraints of Order Acceptance Problems

4.5.1 Criteria

We consider three major performance criteria in the order acceptance problems: profit of SC, the average profits of each order, acceptance rate of order.

Profit of SC: the profit of SC is evidently the main goal to be maximized from SC perspective. In this paper, we do not consider profit sharing problems in SC. In fact, some firms will lose part of their profits to some extent. Profit sharing is an important problem that must be considered in the next cooperation.

Average profits of each order: in practice, the average profit of each order is a normal criterion in revenue management. It is especially important to know whether the decision to accept an order is right or not.

Acceptance rate of product order (ARPO): with decreasing of this criterion, the firms in SC maximize the profit of SC in the minimum number of order. However, a lower ARPO may imply customer credit. ARPO criterion should be considered from two sides.

4.5.2 Constraints

Production capacity constraint: the workload of supplier and manufacturer from the accepted orders to the scheduling time cannot exceed the residual production capacity of a firm. The production capacity is determined by the bottle-neck between production facilities and manpower.

$$\mathrm{OC}_i \leq \min\{\mathrm{MC}_i, \mathrm{PC}_i\} \quad (14)$$

MC_i: The machine production capacity for order *i*. It is the sum of machine production time from now to due date subtracting delivery time for order *i*.

PC_i: The manpower production capacity for order *i*. It is the sum of manpower production time from now to due date subtracting delivery time for order *i*.

5 Simulation Results

In this section, we present an example of an SC in two demand markets to illustrate this model. There are two manufacturers competing in two demand markets to sell two types of product. Two suppliers ship the components to these two manufacturers. We focus on one supplier who serves in an SC. See Fig. 8.

5.1 Experimental Environment

Let *ordertype*(OS, DD, RPC, PD) denote supplier' order information. We simulate 10 years' operations of SC in experiment. The parameters of this experiment are showed in Table 2.

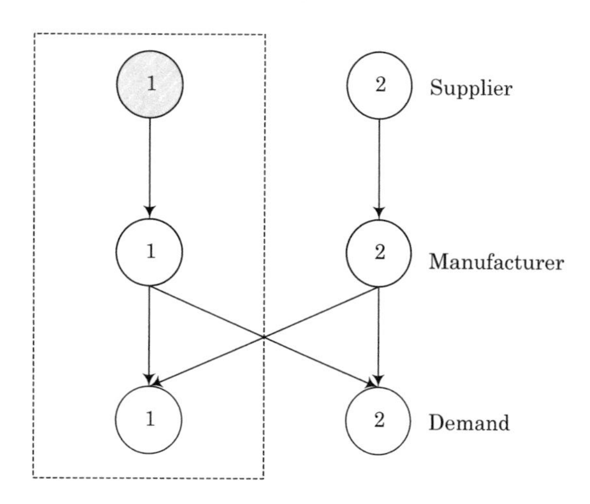

Fig. 8 The supply chain topology

Table 2 the parameters of experiment

Symbol	Value	Explanation
μ_1	1,000,000	Mean value of normal distribution for order quantity in SC
σ_1	50,000	Standard deviation of normal distribution order quantity in SC
μ_2	500,000	Mean value of uniform distribution for order quantity out of SC
σ_2	20,000	Standard deviation of uniform distribution order quantity in SC
σ^2	10	The parameters of SVMs model
C	4	The parameters of SVMs model
g	16	The parameters of SVMs model
DT_{MD}	2	Delivery time from manufacturer to demand market
DT_{SM}	2	Delivery time from supplier to manufacturer
IC_M	0.2	Inventory cost per product of manufacturer each year
IC_S	0.2	Inventory cost per component of supplier each year
DC	1000	Delivery cost per truck
QT	10,000	The quantity of each truck
P	10	Price of finished product
P_{ns}	100	The fee of a normal shift
α	1.5	The fee of overtime shift is α times of normal shift

The demand functions faced by manufacturers given by:

$$d_1 = -7000000 p_{11} + 4000000 p_{21} + 200000000$$
$$d_2 = -7000000 p_{12} + 4000000 p_{22} + 190000000$$

5.2 Experiment Results

This simulation experiment demonstrates the acceptance order policy of the supplier in two SCs and the performances of an SC based on FCFS and SVMs. FCFS implies that the supplier generally accepts and process orders sequentially if the supplier can complete an order by the due date of the order. At this study, we simply ignore other factors which may influence the supplier's decision to accept or reject an order, since these factors can be handled by rule-based decision-making process and it will not affect the results of current model. In this simulation experiment, the supplier makes order acceptance decision based on the profits of the whole SC it joined in. Average profits of the order and acceptance rate of product order (ARPO) are used to compare the results between FCFS and SVMs.

As shown by the simulation experiment results, the residual production capacity before the latest time of delivery is the key to affect the profits of SC. Table 3 shows the effects of SVMs and FCFS. The profits of SC increase in 7 out of

Table 3 Experimental results by comparison of FCFS and SVMs

	FCFS		SVMs	
Year	Profits of each order	ARPO (%)	Profits of each order	ARPO (%)
1	7373225.10	65.28	7521597.82	61.11
2	5960299.61	81.94	6357002.13	79.17
3	10030365.06	56.94	11371533.38	54.17
4	8929871.99	61.11	8929871.99	61.11
5	8523504.92	72.22	8523504.92	72.22
6	7638737.75	68.06	7817884.20	66.67
7	9456588.78	66.67	10008879.15	65.28
8	7075919.77	69.44	8627833.86	68.06
9	8349738.63	66.67	8475064.98	50.00
10	10605066.51	65.28	10605066.51	65.28

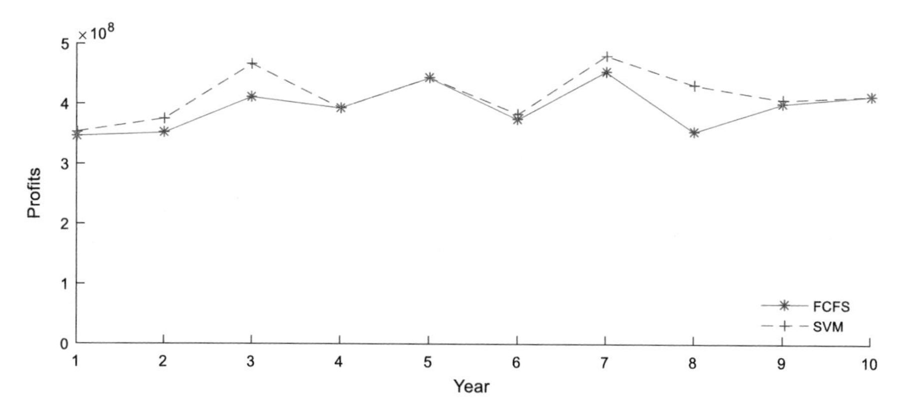

Fig. 9 Experimental results by comparison of FCFS and SVMs

10 years, although ARPO decreases in these years. The SVMs calculation results can obviously help reject the orders with lower profits.

At first, in order to comparison's purpose, the low-profit orders are screened by using the exhaustion method at the end of the year. The 93.33% of low-profit orders are rejected by using SVMs results against all the low-profit orders by using FCFS method. In addition, to compare with other machine learning methods, we applied the Levenberg–Marquardt training method to Artificial Neural Network (ANN) provided by MATLAB. The classification accuracy is 89.78% by using ANN where the weights and biases are set using the training data. SVMs results in our model show slightly higher prediction accuracy than the ANN results. If the training data is limited, SVMs results show relatively higher prediction accuracy. Figure 9 indicates the profit of an SC by using FCFS method and SVMs.

6 Conclusions

In this paper, an MTO SC acceptance order simulation model with stochastic and regular demand based on SVMs has been developed to solve a multiple criteria decision-making problem for order acceptance policy. The decision-making criteria taken into consideration in order acceptance policy include order's size, due date, and occurring probability, and residual production capacity. The effectiveness of the model based on SVMs has been validated by using a numerical simulation example.

The proposed decision-making support model for order acceptance decision problem has several features. First of all, the SVMs model has a high rate to identify lower-profit orders which helps the managers in an SC to quickly make the decision for accepting orders from different SCs. Secondly, the proposed SVMs model is easy to find the optimal result rather than local optimal result compared with other machine learning methods, such as Artificial Neural Network. Thirdly, the computing time of the proposed SVMs model is reasonably short, which supports quick decision-making. Last, the proposed SVMs model can arrive at the same performance as other methods but using much less training data.

The main contributions of this paper are summarized as follows: (1) An order acceptance decision support model based on SVMs in competitive SCs has been proposed in this paper to differentiate the dynamic orders from different SCs; (2) The primary features of an order out of the SC are analyzed, which include order's size, due date, and occurring probability, and the residual production capacity. To the best of our knowledge, this is the first paper that meaningfully applies SVMs to support dynamic order acceptance decision-making in a competitive make-to-order SC.

The order acceptance policy in this study is widely applicable in dynamic decentralized make-to-order SC. First, this model that embedded a machine learning algorithm (SVMs) can be used to filter negative-order from a mass of orders every day for firm managers in SCs effectively and efficiently. The combination of SVM with order characteristics in competitive make-to-order SC might provide an efficient tool for extracting relevant order information. Our study that focuses on dynamic order arrival and due date can be applied to adjust order acceptance policy with orders feature change by using machine learning algorithm (SVMs).

Acknowledgments This research was financially supported by a project grant from the Discovery Grant from the Natural Science and Engineering Research Council of Canada (NSERC) and the Humanities and Social Sciences of Ministry of Education Planning Fund (No: 16YJC630085) in China.

Appendix

Table 4 A partial list of test data

#	Order's size	Order's due date	Residual production capacity	Probability of demand distribution	Reject?
1	3,258,895	18	5,100,000	0.0002	N
2	3,049,658	17	4,800,000	0.0013	N
3	**616,638**	22	6,300,000	0.0228	Y
4	1,570,738	10	2,700,000	0.0001	N
5	941,467	21	6,000,000	0.0001	N
6	679,068	22	6,300,000	0.0228	N
7	2,363,966	17	4,800,000	0.0062	N
8	2,171,252	9	2,400,000	0.0001	N
9	**29,395**	22	4,090,063	0.0001	Y
10	99,421	12	2,928,150	0.0001	N
11	1,792,079	24	4,422,463	0.0001	N
12	590,623	20	3,776,938	0.0001	N
13	2,160,423	9	2,373,975	0.0001	N
14	**507,947**	23	5,504,950	0.6915	Y
15	3,742,646	22	5,270,750	0.0001	N
16	2,277,433	23	2,962,263	0.0001	N
17	3,156,116	23	5,745,788	0.0001	N
18	775,064	15	1,819,300	0.0001	N
19	66,699	7	1,485,700	0.0668	N
20	1,244,439	23	5,493,488	0.0001	N
21	2,823,803	18	5,070,600	0.8413	N
22	**3,203,684**	20	5,089,775	0.0001	Y
23	284,938	5	800,000	0.0013	N
24	2,580,515	16	3,676,163	0.0001	N
25	2,913,047	19	3,716,650	0.0001	N
26	**3,885,999**	16	4,277,638	0.5	Y
27	1,808,830	16	3,910,725	0.0668	N
28	2,208,700	21	4,788,600	0.0001	N
29	2,996,639	24	5,722,050	0.0013	N
30	727,922	10	1,033,000	0.0001	N
31	390,162	12	2,925,238	0.0668	N
32	703,247	11	900,000	0.5	N
33	2,569,261	15	3,599,988	0.5	N
34	131,760	20	3,692,413	0.5	N
35	156,738	5	800,000	0.5	N
36	371,956	16	3,368,350	0.0668	N
37	1,113,993	19	4,400,000	0.5	N

(continued)

Table 4 (continued)

#	Order's size	Order's due date	Residual production capacity	Probability of demand distribution	Reject?
38	872,435	22	4,518,313	0.0001	N
39	1,441,484	12	1,886,238	0.0001	N
40	885,063	8	707,113	0.0013	N
41	439,447	21	4,600,000	0.0013	N
42	215,452	9	1,374,025	0.0001	N
43	1,027,341	9	1,491,063	0.0002	N
44	2,187,526	20	3,478,188	0.0002	N
45	3,089,465	12	1,213,988	0.0001	N
46	**755,160**	7	798,275	0.0013	Y

Note: 'Bold' values and Y: the simulation result of SC will be improved, if the order will be rejected, though these orders satisfy the residual production capacity constraint

Table 5 A partial list of training data

#	Order's size	Order's due date	Residual production capacity	Probability of demand distribution	Reject?
1	121,541	18	5,100,000	0.0002	N
2	1,311,766	17	4,800,000	0.0013	N
3	3,220,450	22	6,300,000	0.0228	N
4	2,994,036	21	6,000,000	0.0001	N
5	188,311	11	3,000,000	0.0013	N
6	3,202,091	22	6,300,000	0.0228	N
7	3,193,943	17	4,800,000	0.0062	N
8	432,184	9	2,400,000	0.0001	N
9	833,881	10	1,800,000	0.0668	N
10	3,211,861	22	4,482,588	0.0001	N
11	268,891	16	802,650	0.0001	N
12	2,771,274	12	2,928,150	0.0001	N
13	2,173,198	24	4,053,963	0.0001	N
14	854,642	10	1,452,575	0.0228	N
15	420,275	20	2,353,913	0.0001	N
16	1,839,503	9	2,373,975	0.0001	N
17	1,819,865	23	5,166,113	0.6915	N
18	3,803,161	22	4,470,750	0.0001	N
19	1,352,529	23	2,581,150	0.0001	N
20	1,591,356	23	5,745,788	0.0001	N
21	**636,190**	15	1,819,300	0.0001	Y
22	121,081	7	1,485,700	0.0668	N
23	1,803,531	23	5,493,488	0.0001	N
24	947,519	10	1,474,488	0.0228	N
25	2,785,258	20	5,089,775	0.0001	N
26	**34,591**	13	2,431,163	0.0001	Y
27	508,148	16	3,448,388	0.0001	N

(continued)

Table 5 (continued)

#	Order's size	Order's due date	Residual production capacity	Probability of demand distribution	Reject?
28	3,020,584	19	3,716,650	0.0001	N
29	1,173,472	16	4,277,638	0.5	N
30	918,410	16	3,910,725	0.0668	N
31	1,418,025	21	4,788,600	0.0001	N
32	**2,808,947**	24	5,722,050	0.0013	Y
33	928,961	13	3,091,850	0.0228	N
34	3,830,172	15	4,200,000	0.5	N
35	1,720,278	20	3,692,413	0.5	N
36	236,122	9	1,600,000	0.0001	N
37	2,803,400	16	3,168,750	0.0668	N
38	1,416,466	19	4,400,000	0.5	N
39	94,530	22	4,481,200	0.0001	N
40	**2,732,755**	21	4,600,000	0.0013	Y
41	3,121,784	20	3,175,713	0.0002	N
42	626,007	7	798,275	0.0013	N
43	1,301,196	6	1,500,000	0.0001	N
44	**3,889,222**	23	5,295,425	0.0002	Y
45	208,769	17	3,449,025	0.0062	N
46	443,237	8	874,550	0.0001	N
47	**1,829,235**	20	4,240,875	0.0062	Y
48	2,185,608	11	2,292,975	0.0002	N

Note: 'Bold' values and Y: the simulation result of SC will be improved, if the order will be rejected, though these orders satisfy the residual production capacity constraint

References

1. Guerrero, H. H., & Kern, G. M. (1988). How to more effectively accept and refuse orders. *Production and Inventory Management Journal, 29*(4), 59.
2. Lee, C., Piramuthu, S., et al. (1997). Job shop scheduling with a genetic algorithm and machine learning. *International Journal of Production Research, 35*(4), 1171–1191.
3. Zhao, W., & Stankovic, J. A. (1989). Performance analysis of FCFS and improved FCFS scheduling algorithms for dynamic real-time computer systems. In *Proceedings. Real-time systems symposium* (pp. 156–165). IEEE.
4. Wang, J., Yang, J., et al. (1994). Multicriteria order acceptance decision support in over-demanded job shops: A neural network approach. *Mathematical and Computer Modelling, 19*(5), 1–19.
5. Miller, B. L. (1969). A queueing reward system with several customer classes. *Management Science, 16*(3), 234–245.
6. Holweg, M., & Bicheno, J. (2002). Supply chain simulation - a tool for education, enhancement and endeavour. *International Journal of Production Economics, 78*(2), 163–175.
7. Lee, Y. H., Cho, M. K., et al. (2002). Supply chain simulation with discrete–continuous combined modeling. *Computers & Industrial Engineering, 43*(1), 375–392.
8. Petrovic, D. (2001). Simulation of supply chain behaviour and performance in an uncertain environment. *International Journal of Production Economics, 71*(1), 429–438.

9. Hans, A. (1994). Towards a better understanding of order acceptance. *International Journal of Production Economics, 37*(1), 139–152.
10. Ono, K., & Jones, C. (1973). A heuristic approach to acceptance rules in integrated scheduling systems. *Journal of Operations Research Society of Japan, 16*(1), 36–58.
11. Ten Kate, H. A. E. (1995). *Order acceptance and production control*. Princeton, NJ: Labyrint Publication.
12. Stern, H. I., & Avivi, Z. (1990). The selection and scheduling of textile orders with due dates. *European Journal of Operational Research, 44*(1), 11–16.
13. Slotnick, S. A., & Morton, T. E. (2007). Order acceptance with weighted tardiness. *Computers & Operations Research, 34*(10), 3029–3042.
14. Barut, M., & Sridharan, V. (2005). Revenue management in order-driven production systems. *Decision Sciences, 36*(2), 287–316.
15. Ivanescu, C. V., Fransoo, J. C., et al. (2002). Makespan estimation and order acceptance in batch process industries when processing times are uncertain. *OR Spectrum, 24*(4), 467–495.
16. Raaymakers, W. H., Bertrand, J. W. M., et al. (2000). Using aggregate estimation models for order acceptance in a decentralized production control structure for batch chemical manufacturing. *IIE Transactions, 32*(10), 989–998.
17. Lei, D., & Guo, X. (2015). A parallel neighborhood search for order acceptance and scheduling in flow shop environment. *International Journal of Production Economics, 165*, 12–18.
18. Nobibon, F. T., & Leus, R. (2011). Exact algorithms for a generalization of the order acceptance and scheduling problem in a single-machine environment. *Computers & Operations Research, 38*(1), 367–378.
19. Charnsirisakskul, K., Griffin, P. M., et al. (2004). Order selection and scheduling with leadtime flexibility. *IIE Transactions, 36*(7), 697–707.
20. Charnsirisakskul, K., Griffin, P. M., et al. (2006). Pricing and scheduling decisions with leadtime flexibility. *European Journal of Operational Research, 171*(1), 153–169.
21. Og, C., Salman, F. S., et al. (2010). Order acceptance and scheduling decisions in make-to-order systems. *International Journal of Production Economics, 125*(1), 200–211.
22. Rom, W. O., & Slotnick, S. A. (2009). Order acceptance using genetic algorithms. *Computers & Operations Research, 36*(6), 1758–1767.
23. Rahman, H. F., Sarker, R., et al. (2015). A real-time order acceptance and scheduling approach for permutation flow shop problems. *European Journal of Operational Research, 247*(2), 488–503.
24. Chen, C., Yang, Z., et al. (2014). Diversity controlling genetic algorithm for order acceptance and scheduling problem. *Mathematical Problems in Engineering, 2014*, 367152.
25. Park, J., Nguyen, S., et al. (2014). Enhancing heuristics for order acceptance and scheduling using genetic programming. In G. Dick et al. (Eds.), *Simulated evolution and learning. SEAL 2014* (Lecture notes in computer science) (Vol. 8886, pp. 723–734). Cham: Springer.
26. Wester, F., Wijngaard, J., et al. (1992). Order acceptance strategies in a production-to-order environment with setup times and due-dates. *The International Journal of Production Research, 30*(6), 1313–1326.
27. Gordon, V. S., & Strusevich, V. A. (2009). Single machine scheduling and due date assignment with positionally dependent processing times. *European Journal of Operational Research, 198*(1), 57–62.
28. Moreira, M. R. A. R., & Alves, R. A. F. (2009). A methodology for planning and controlling workload in a job-shop: A four-way decision-making problem. *International Journal of Production Research, 47*(10), 2805–2821.
29. Rogers, P., & Nandi, A. (2007). Judicious order acceptance and order release in make-to-order manufacturing systems. *Production Planning & Control, 18*(7), 610–625.
30. Yang, W., & Fung, R. Y. (2014). Stochastic optimization model for order acceptance with multiple demand classes and uncertain demand/supply. *Engineering Optimization, 46*(6), 824–841.

31. Aouam, T., & Brahimi, N. (2013). Integrated production planning and order acceptance under uncertainty: A robust optimization approach. *European Journal of Operational Research, 228*(3), 504–515.
32. Kilic, O. A., van Donk, D. P., et al. (2010). Order acceptance in food processing systems with random raw material requirements. *OR Spectrum, 32*(4), 905–925.
33. Boser, B. E., Guyon, I. M., et al. (1992). *A training algorithm for optimal margin classifiers* (pp. 144–152). New York: ACM.
34. Vapnik, V. (1995). *The nature of statistical learning theory* (pp. 15–24). New York: Springer.
35. Vapnik, V. (2013). *The nature of statistical learning theory* (pp. 78–89). New York: Springer.
36. Amari, S., & Wu, S. (1999). Improving support vector machine classifiers by modifying kernel functions. *Neural Networks, 12*(6), 783–789.
37. Carbonneau, R., Laframboise, K., et al. (2008). Application of machine learning techniques for supply chain demand forecasting. *European Journal of Operational Research, 184*(3), 1140–1154.
38. Caruana, R., & Niculescu-Mizil, A. (2006). *An empirical comparison of supervised learning algorithms* (pp. 161–168). New York: ACM.
39. Meyer, D., Leisch, F., et al. (2003). The support vector machine under test. *Neurocomputing, 55*(1), 169–186.
40. Nagurney, A., & Dong, J. (2002). *Supernetworks: Decision-making for the information age* (pp. 33–48). Cheltenham: Edward Elgar Publishing.
41. Robinson, B., & Lakhani, C. (1975). Dynamic price models for new-product planning. *Management Science, 21*(10), 1113–1122.
42. Zhang, D. (2006). A network economic model for supply chain versus supply chain competition. *Omega, 34*(3), 283–295.

Importance of Data Analytics for Improving Teaching and Learning Methods

Mahmood Moussavi, Yasaman Amannejad, Mohammad Moshirpour, Emily Marasco, and Laleh Behjat

Abstract Institutions of higher education have increasingly embraced flipped classroom and online teaching approaches to manage large-scale classes with several hundreds of students. In parallel with growing demand of this type of educational and pedagogical approach, substantial improvements have occurred in related technologies and tools. Current online platforms and tools are generating a considerable volume of data. Educators can use the collected data sets to further improve teaching and learning methods. However, there are some limitations: First, the existing data are hidden between the deep layers of the current platforms and educators may barely be aware of their existence. Second, some of the existing raw data needs a substantial data mining and data analytic effort to convert them to useful information for decision-making purposes. Third, there is a lack of communication between educators and architects of the online teaching and learning management systems and tools.

The focus of this paper is twofold: (1) provide a set of informative recommendations that help educators to use many years of available recorded data on large-scale courses to improve their teaching methods; (2) reveal opportunities for data analytics research that can lead to improvement of current teaching and learning tools and platforms.

Keywords Online courses · Flipped classroom · Large-scale courses · Big data analytics · Scholarship of teaching and learning

M. Moussavi · M. Moshirpour (✉) · E. Marasco · L. Behjat
Department of Electrical and Computer Engineering, University of Calgary, Calgary, AB, Canada
e-mail: moussam@ucalgary.ca; mmoshirp@ucalgary.ca; eamarasc@ucalgary.ca; laleh@ucalgary.ca

Y. Amannejad
Department of Electrical and Computer Engineering, University of Calgary, Calgary, AB, Canada

Department of Mathematics and Computing, Mount Royal University, Calgary, AB, Canada
e-mail: yamannej@ucalgary.ca

R. Alhajj et al. (eds.), *Data Management and Analysis*, Studies in Big Data 65,
https://doi.org/10.1007/978-3-030-32587-9_6

1 Introduction

The flipped classroom format has become increasingly popular among engineering courses [1]. In flipped classrooms, technical instructions and content materials are provided online or via other methods external to scheduled course time. This allows the instructor to use their face-to-face time with the students to facilitate exploratory learning and hands-on application for more in-depth understanding [2, 3]. Various forms of flipped classrooms have been tried in electrical, computer, and software engineering education, from early low-tech activities (Bland 2006) to videos with programming exercises [4] (Talbert 2012). However, there are few reports on flipped classrooms for large cohorts [1], which present their own challenges for scalability, feasibility, and verification of students learning outcomes.

The emergence of online education has led to the development of platforms and tools to support content delivery, usage tracking, and assessment. A learning management system (LMS), such as Blackboard or Brightspace Desire to Learn, can be used to assist instructors with online teaching and learning. The intended goal of these systems is to provide educators with a single system for posting teaching documents and to record course evaluation results, as well as allow them to interact with and respond to learning materials within courses, and across terms. One of the advantages of online teaching is the huge size of invaluable data that is collected as students access the provided online learning resources. LMS tools provide substantial amounts of data regarding student interaction and their study behavior. Mining this data allows educators to analyze student study habits. However, we believe that this aspect of LMS tools is not used to its full extent. This paper aims to raise awareness about the amount of data and research opportunities that exist in this area.

The rest of this paper is organized as follows: Section 2 reviews related work. In Sect. 3, we discuss our research methodology and the case study we have used for this paper. Section 4 provides our findings and discussion. Section 5 concludes the paper and provides possible future directions.

2 Related Work

The collection and analysis of teaching and learning data allows higher education institutions to remain competitive and effective in the development of high quality, rapidly changing education [5]. The analysis of educational data is an emerging field with several benefits and challenges, building on the area of knowledge discovery. Interdisciplinary in nature, knowledge discovery is an area that uses patterns, models, algorithms, and data analysis to extract useful information from a set of data [5]. Analysis and interpretation of educational data provides evidence-based support for educational activities [6]. This allows educators to better understand where students are at when beginning their program, and to better understand student needs [7]. Furthermore, the consequences of evidence-based improvements have practical benefits for learners, educators, and administrators when developing more effective teaching and learning experiences [5, 7].

However, there are some challenges to consider as well. There are currently a lack of standardized measures and indicators for collecting and comparing educational data [5]. In addition, the analysis of aggregate data requires careful interpretation to avoid the loss of individualization [7]. Understanding and using the resulting predictions requires educators to consider the nuances of student behaviors to avoid making collective assumptions for all learners based on the aggregate population [7]. A more individualized approach, however, risks potential ethical issues by identifying specific students, their behaviors, and grades. Educators can mitigate potential risks by using their own judgment and experience when analyzing the data [7].

Initiatives such as the Data Quality Campaign are being developed to provide recommendations for educational data use. Such initiatives recognize the benefit of using data to provide more effective, timely, and evidence-based experiences used to improve education for all students (Data Quality Campaign, 2018).

3 Methodology

In this section, we explain the details of our study. First, we describe the goals of this paper and the research questions that we aim to answer in Sect. 3.1. Next, in Sect. 3.2, we describe the steps involved in our study.

3.1 Goals and Research Questions

The process of teaching and learning is a dynamic process and benefits from receiving continuous feedback about student performance and learning behaviors. Our main objective is to help educators take a student-centric approach to teaching and learning by conducting evidence-based modifications in their courses. To this end, the goals of this study are: (1) to provide a set of informative examples that can help educators to use available recorded data from large-scale courses for improving their teaching methods, and (2) to reveal opportunities for data-oriented research that can lead to the improvement of current teaching and learning tools and platforms. To achieve our goals, we define the following research questions (RQs) for this study:

- *RQ 1*: What is the state of available data in online learning management systems?
  - *RQ 1.1*: What types of data are available in online learning management systems for educators?

  - *RQ 1.2*: How accessible are the data to be used by the educators?
- *RQ 2*: What are the open issues to be addressed by researchers and learning management systems architects?

3.2 Steps Involved in this Study

We have followed four steps in this study. The following figure briefly describes these steps and the rest of this section describes these steps in further details (Fig. 1).

Step 1 To answer our research questions, we first listed important questions that can help educators to improve their online courses. In this step, we have relied on many years of experience of the authors, with a total of over 60 years teaching experience, to list the important questions that educators may need to answer. We have categorized these questions in two main groups.

These two groups and the questions in each category are shown in Fig. 2.

Fig. 1 Flow of this study

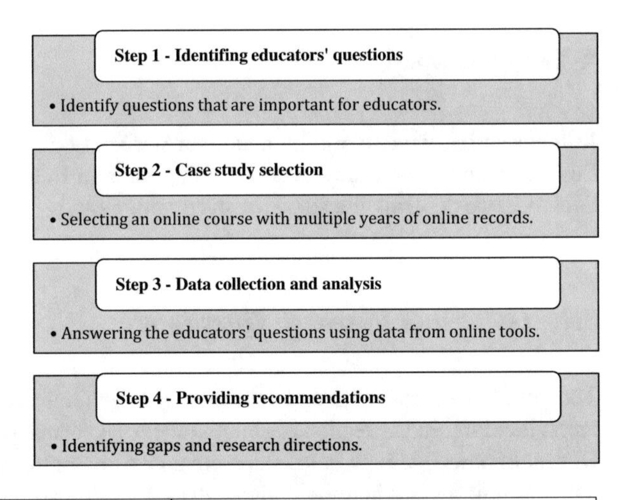

Performance Analysis	Behaviour Analysis
• What is the overall performance of students? • What is the correlation between students' grades and the amount of time they have spent on each component of the course? • What is the correlation between students' performance in each component and the number of evaluation methods such as quizzes or exams?	• What percentage of the students has tried to access the available onlin e documents? • What is the effect of video component length on the time spent by each student? • How many times have students made attempts to visit or revisit a component of the course? • What is the trend of the students' access to the course components during the term? • Which components of the course are more complex for students and require additional resources?

Fig. 2 Important questions for educators

The first category contains questions that analyze student performance in a course.

These questions are usually straight-forward to answer and are used by many educators in traditional and new teaching environments. The second category contains behavioral questions. The questions in this category are usually broader, more diverse, and more interesting for the educators to answer using the new educational platforms. There is less research available in this regard and these questions are normally more complex to answer.

Step 2 To conduct our analysis, we selected a case study course from the many courses that the authors have taught in past. To make the context clear, here we describe the course that we have used in this paper.

For this study, we have selected a first-year introductory programming course at the Schulich School of Engineering titled "Computing for Engineers." This course is a required course for all students enrolled in engineering programs. The aim of the course is to help students explore principles and fundamentals of programming and problem solving. For many years, this course focused on the C++ programming language, and the Blackboard learning management system was used as a content platform to support the traditional lecture-style delivery. In 2015, the course was redesigned to a flipped classroom with a blended learning objective, including a significant regular laboratory component where students are given the opportunity to collaborate with peers and receive coaching from instructors and teaching assistants. The current version of the course uses the processing programming language, which is similar to Java and provides functionalities for easy implementation of graphics and animations. In the past few years, the average total enrolment for this course was over 860 students per year. The course typically runs during a 13-week Fall semester. A second offering is made available in Spring semesters, usually with a much smaller class size. Instructional content in this course is posted weekly using the D2L learning management system. Each content release includes several videos with embedded quiz questions, all developed by the instructors. The video content varies depending on the topic, and includes a combination of PowerPoint slides, real-time handwritten notes, and real-time screen-captured coding. Additional online tutorials are occasionally posted to provide in-depth exploration of particularly difficult topics, as well as links to external media and material. Since Fall 2016, this model is supplemented with scheduled lecture sessions, as studies have shown that students prefer to have the opportunity to ask questions and interact with an instructor while practicing online material (Marasco, 2017). The course concludes with a large design project that combines technical course content with creative thinking. Students are asked to design and program their own interactive games while fulfilling a set of technical requirements. Students are free to work individually or with a partner and no restriction is set on the theme or the type of games. This course has been offered for many years and as a result a tremendous amount of data exist for this course. The data are either entered manually by the course staff or automatically recorded by D2L as students use the course components for their assignments or learning purposes.

Step 3 In this step, we used our learning management system, D2L, and the collected data from this system for the first-year programming course during the academic years of 2016 and 2017. Using the collected data, we tried to provide answers to the questions identified in Step 1, allowing us to investigate which type of questions can be answered by the existing data and what are the gaps that the educational learning management systems need to improve. In Sect. 4 we show our analysis and to the extent that we were able to answer these questions using data available in D2L for our selected course.

Step 4 Using our analysis in Step 3, the authors have provided the areas that require more research and the areas that need the attention of the online learning management architects and developers. These directions and recommendations are provided in Sect. 4.2.

4 Results

In this section, we first show some of our analysis to answer the educators' questions defined in Step 1 of our study. Our results are provided in Sect. 4.1. Based on our analysis, we answer the research questions of this study in Sect. 4.2 and provide some recommendations.

4.1 Analysis of D2L Data to Answer Educators' Questions

In this section, we provide examples of data that we extracted from D2L to answer educators' questions.

Using D2L, we were able to extract information about student performance and learning behavior. Figure 3 shows an example of information that D2L provides for students' study patterns. In this example, educators can see the student access pattern for semester course material and also their performance on the assessed components. This information can help educators to identify students who are struggling with course content despite the amount of time that they are investing in the course.

Another available source of D2L information is the amount of time that students are spending on each course module. As shown in Fig. 4, D2L can provide information per student. For privacy purposes, students' names have been removed from the left column.

D2L also provides aggregated time data spent by all students for each course module. Moreover, the number of visits for each module is provided and allows us to calculate the average amount of time that students spend on each module in every visit. This aggregated time data can provide invaluable insights for educators. For example, average time spent by students for each video content along with the length of each video can be used to identify the complex components of the course, i.e.,

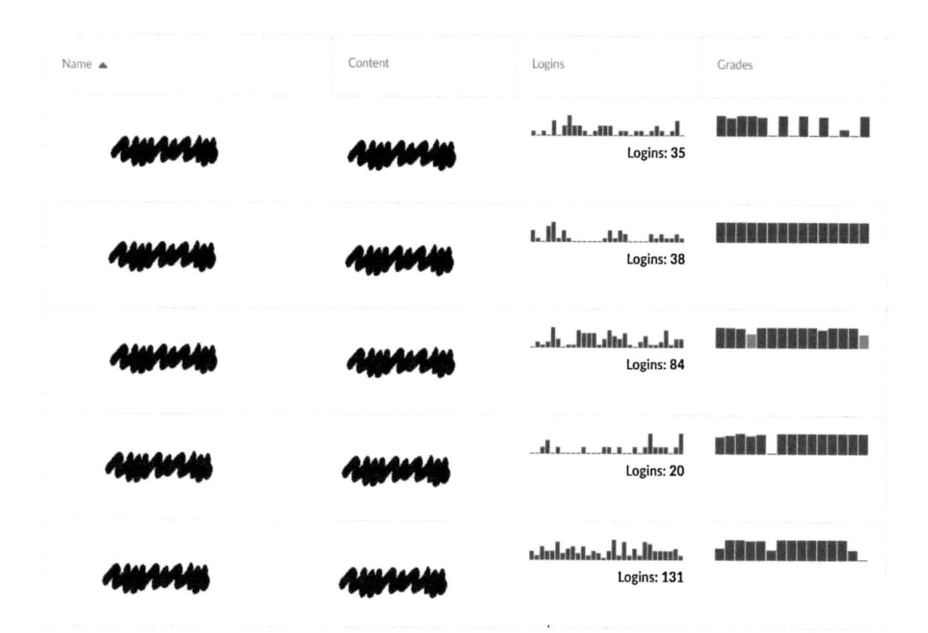

Fig. 3 Student study pattern examples

	Last Name, First Name	Last Visited	Number of Visits	Total Time Spent ▾	Average Time Spent
	[illegible]	Oct 29, 2016	2	4:17:13	2:08:36
	[illegible]	Nov 8, 2016	2	3:37:36	1:48:48
	[illegible]	Oct 30, 2016	2	3:06:54	3:06:54
	[illegible]	Oct 30, 2016	2	2:36:45	2:36:45
	[illegible]	Oct 29, 2016	1	2:27:05	2:27:05
	[illegible]	Oct 28, 2016	1	1:55:48	1:55:48
	[illegible]	Oct 28, 2016	1	1:53:43	1:53:43
	[illegible]	Oct 30, 2016	1	1:41:57	1:41:57

Fig. 4 Time spent by each student on a course module

the components that require students to spend more time. The course schedule and materials for these components can be improved to assist students in their learning process (Fig. 5).

Content	Users Visited	Average Time Spent
I. Arrays Part 1	784	0:14:48
II. Arrays Part 2	787	0:13:17
III. Quiz - Array 2	773	0:02:41
IV. Arrays Part 3	793	0:26:07
V. Quiz - Array 3	774	0:03:22
VI. Arrays Part 4	788	0:33:00
VII. Quiz - Array 4	769	0:04:50
VIII. Arrays Part 5	775	0:27:05
IX. Quiz - Array 5	763	0:03:59
X. Arrays Part 6	757	0:27:17

Fig. 5 Example of aggregated access patterns to the course modules

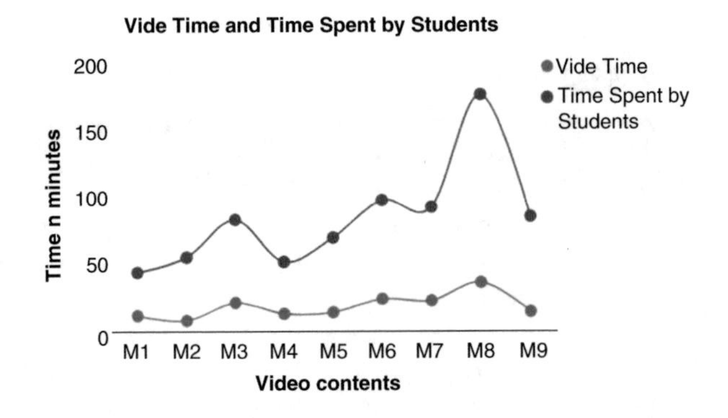

Fig. 6 Relation between time of video contents and the time spent by student

In addition, the time spent by students along with the length of each video can be used by educators to identify the appropriate time for the video contents. Our analysis in this regard is shown in Fig. 6. In this figure, we show the average time spent by students and the length of the video for nine video lectures. A correlation between the length of the videos and time spent by students is demonstrated. As this figure shows, when videos are longer than a certain level, e.g., 8–10 min in this example, the students' completion times rapidly increase. This analysis confirms that pre-class videos should not be too long, with an approximate recommended length of 8–10 min. This range may vary from course to course and requires further analysis by educators for different subject areas.

4.2 Findings of This Study with Regard to the RQS

In this section, we summarize our findings to answer RQ1 and RQ2 based on the data collection and analysis from the case study. We categorize the data available in learning management systems into three main levels:

- *Readily available data*: There are considerable amount of data that can be directly used by educators to answer questions such as:
  - What is the percentage of the students that have tried to access the available online documents?
  - How many times have they made attempts to visit or revisit a component of the course?
  - What is the trend of the students' access to the course components during the term?

  Data in this category are usually recognized by learning management systems. Interfaces are provided by the learning management systems for the educators to access and use the data. An example of this category is the time spent by user data provided by D2L.
- *Data that needs further data mining and supportive efforts*: There are plenty of raw data available hidden in between deeper layers of the learning management systems that require further data mining and analytical planning. These are normally the type of the data that can provide answers to more complex student study pattern questions and their correlation with student performance.
  - What is the correlation between students' study patterns on course modules such as videos and their final performance outcome?
  - What is the correlation between student study time on each subject and their exam marks for midterm, final, lab assignments, or term projects?
  - What is the correlation between students' access time and/or number of access attempts to the course components and their performance?
  - What is the correlation between students' performance and the degrees of complexity of the course material?

  In spite of its remarkable potential value for educators, data in this category is not usually ready to be used by educators. While the learning management systems are collecting the data, they do not provide an easy-to-use interface for educators to access and interpret the data. This category of data may benefit from AI or heuristic-based research and requires attention from these research communities.
- *Data that needs structural revision or customization*: Another group of important data are those that need fundamental restructuring and should be communicated to developers and architects of the online learning and teaching management systems. Access to this data requires a collaborative effort from the major stakeholders of learning systems, which are developers and architects of the system and educators. Moreover, developers of the learning management systems should make their platforms customizable, to some extent, by the educators.

Some examples of the educators' need for fundamental changes in learning management systems are:

- Collected data regarding students' study behavior, such as time spent on the course components, should be customizable by the educators to collect information such as start and end time.
- To remove possibilities of outlier data, the learning management systems should use some techniques to provide more reliable data. For example, if the system has been on idle status for a long time, the recorded time should be flagged and allow the educators to consider them as outliers.

5 Conclusion

The rapid progress in online teaching and learning pedagogical approaches and the advances in current development of big data analytics provides a unique opportunity for educators to use data analytics to improve their online courses. This study aims to address the research opportunities and the importance of data analytic studies in education, and the importance of assisting educators to learn more from available data to improve their teaching practices.

In this paper, we introduced three levels of data that can help educators: (1) Readily available data that can be used with minimal effort by the educators to analyze and improve their teaching practice. (2) Data that exists in deep layers of the learning management system and requires collaboration between system administrators and researchers to be used for extracting useful information. (3) Data that is important to educators but requires further support from learning system developers. The importance of data in this category highlights the necessity of improvements in learning management tools for increased effectiveness in educational applications.

References

1. Velegol, S. B., Zappe, S. E., & Mahoney, E. (2015). The evolution of a flipped classroom: Evidence-based recommendations. *Advances in Engineering Education, 4*(3), n3.
2. Kolb, A., & Kolb, D. (2005). Learning styles and learning space: Enhancing experiential learning in higher education. *Academy of Management Learning & Education, 4*(2), 193–212.
3. Robinson, K., & Azzam, A. M. (2009). Why creativity now? (interview). *Educational Leadership, 67*(1), 22–26.
4. Gannod, G. C. (2007). Work in Progress – Using podcasting in an inverted classroom. In *IEEE Frontiers in Education Conference. Milwaukee, Wisconsin.* IEEE.
5. Daniel, B. (2015). Big data and analytics in higher education: Opportunities and challenges. *British Journal of Educational Technology, 46*(5), 904–920. https://doi.org/10.1111/bjet.12230.

6. Proitz, T. S., Mausethagen, S., & Skedsmo, G. (2017). Investigative modes in research on data use in education. *Nordic Journal of Studies in Educational Policy, 3*(1), 42–55. https://doi.org/10.1080/20020317.2017.1326280.
7. Schouten, G. (2017). On meeting students where they are: Teacher judgment and the use of data in higher education. *Theory and Research in Education, 15*(3), 321–338. https://doi.org/10.1177/1477878517734452.
8. Pears, A., Seidman, S., Malmi, L., Mannila, L., & Adams, E. (2007). A survey of literature on the teaching of introductory programming. In *Working group report on ITiCSE on innovation and technology in computer science education*. New York: ACM. https://doi.org/10.1145/1345443.1345441.
9. UC San Diego. (2018). *Data structures and algorithms specialization*. Mountain View, CA: Coursera. https://www.coursera.org/specializations/data-structures-algorithms#courses.

Prediction Model for Prevalence of Type-2 Diabetes Mellitus Complications Using Machine Learning Approach

Muhammad Younus, Md Tahsir Ahmed Munna, Mirza Mohtashim Alam, Shaikh Muhammad Allayear, and Sheikh Joly Ferdous Ara

Abstract Nowadays, most of the people are suffering from the attack of chronic diseases because of their lifestyle, food habits, and reduction in physical activities. Diabetes is one of the most common chronic diseases being suffered by the people of all ages. As a result, the healthcare sector is generating extensive data containing huge volume, enormous velocity, and a vast variety of heterogeneous sources. In such scenario, scientific solutions offer to harness these massive, heterogeneous and complex datasets to obtain more meaningful information. Moreover, machine learning algorithms can play a tremendous part in creating a statistical prediction-based model. The aim of this paper is to identify the prevalence of diabetes related to long-term complications among patients with type-2 diabetes mellitus. The processing and statistical analysis require machine learning environment known as Scikit-Learn, Pandas for Python, and R-Studio for R. In this work, machine learning approaches such as decision tree, random forest for developing classification system-based prediction model to assess type-2 diabetes mellitus chronic diseases have been studied. Additionally, we have proposed an algorithm which is solely based on random forest and tried to detect the complicated areas of type-2 diabetes patients.

Keywords Healthcare · Machine learning · Diabetes type-2 · Prediction · Decision tree · Random Forest · Classification model

M. Younus (✉)
Department of Electrical and Computer Engineering, University of Calgary, Calgary, AB, Canada
e-mail: muhammad.younus1@ucalgary.ca

M. T. A. Munna · M. M. Alam · S. M. Allayear
Department of Multimedia and Creative Technology, Daffodil International University, Dhaka, Bangladesh

S. J. F. Ara
Department of Microbiology and Immunology, Bangabandhu Sheikh Mujib Medical University, Dhaka, Bangladesh

R. Alhajj et al. (eds.), *Data Management and Analysis*, Studies in Big Data 65,
https://doi.org/10.1007/978-3-030-32587-9_7

1 Introduction

Diabetes mellitus [5] is a group of metabolic diseases characterized by elevated blood glucose levels resulting from the defects in insulin secretion. Diabetes mellitus is classified into two types: type-1 diabetes mellitus and type-2 diabetes mellitus. Type-1 requires daily insulin injection because of the null production of insulin by pancreas. Type-1 diabetes is usually diagnosed during childhood or early adolescence. On the other hand, considering worldwide scenario, type-2 diabetes is considered one of the most prevalent endocrine disorders [7]. This is the most common form of diabetes which is characterized by either inadequate insulin production by beta cells of pancreas or the fact of defective insulin production. As a result, cells in the body are not able to react with it. This form of diabetes is prevalent worldwide and comprises 90% of all diabetic cases. The global prevalence of diabetes [19] for all age groups was estimated to be 2.8% in 2000 and 4.4% in 2030 worldwide. It is projected that the total number of people with diabetes would rise from 171 million in 2000 to 366 million in 2030. Bangladesh has been experiencing an epidemiological transition from communicable diseases to non-communicable diseases [1]. Non-communicable diseases (NCD) are a heterogeneous group that includes major causes of death, such as heart diseases, diabetes, cancer, disability, and mental disorders. NCDs are important cause of disease burden, morbidity, and mortality. At least 25% of the deaths in primary and secondary government health facilities are caused by these diseases. Diabetes mellitus, a chronic disease once thought to be uncommon in Bangladesh but now it has emerged as public health problem. At present it is estimated that about 3.6 million people are affected throughout the country [10]. The prevalence of diabetes in adult varied from 2.2% to 8% and the higher prevalence was found in urban areas predominantly among women. People with type-2 diabetes, women may be at higher risk for coronary heart disease than men. The presence of microvascular disease is also a predictor of coronary heart events [16]. Unfortunately, there is still inadequate awareness about the real dimension of the problem among the general population. There is also lack of awareness about the existing interventions for preventing diabetes and management of complications. Several recent intervention studies have undisputedly proved that type-2 diabetes can be efficiently prevented by lifestyle modification in high risk individuals [6, 8]. Now the major task for public health administrations as well as Government are to identify the causes of individuals who would benefit from intensive counseling.

The healthcare industry has generated large amounts of data driven by record keeping, compliance, regulatory requirements and patients care. While most of the data is stored in hard copy form, the current trend is moving towards rapid digitization of these large amounts of data to support a wide range of medical and healthcare functions, including other clinical decision support, disease surveillance, and population health management. Study says data from US healthcare system alone reached 150 exabyte in 2011. At this growth rate, data for US healthcare will soon reach the zettabyte (1021 gigabytes) scale and not long after it will be yottabyte

(1024 gigabytes) [3] in terms of size. These all are classified both as structured and unstructured data. The massive amount of data is difficult to store, analyze, process, share, visualize, and manage in normal database system. Additionally, the software tools–techniques become obsolete because there is not much capacity to store large data. Nowadays, many tools are available for processing large amount of data like Hadoop, MongoDb, Talend, pentaho, SAP, etc.

In most of the countries, health care costs account for a good percentage of its economy. Health care industry is very critical and vast, unfortunately it is highly inefficient. Till now, common people could not ripe the yield of cutting edge technology in the health care domain. According to Bangladesh demography profile at 2016, 18.24 million people live in Dhaka city. The prevalence of type-2 diabetes in Dhaka is alarmingly high [12] but there are very few studies on Dhaka city about its consequences.

In this paper, we have prepared an analysis of the dataset of urban area's diabetes patients to assess the prevalence of type-2 diabetes mellitus containing long-term complications. Additionally, we have used several machine learning frameworks on Python programming environment such as Pandas, Scikit-Learn, mpl_toolkits, and Matplotlib. We have also used "R" and "Python" programming language for statistical computation of our analysis.

2 Related Studies

The software tools and techniques for big data analytics in health care [17] discuss about how techniques are applied on the data which is growing both in terms of in the volume of data, rate of generation's velocity and variety. Sharmila et al. [13] use the data of diabetes mellitus from different parts of the world for analysis using Hadoop. In their study they have shown death rate caused in particular age group by their diabetes data analysis. Rajesh et al. [11] discuss about the reliable prediction methodology to diagnose diabetes and interpret the data patterns so as to get meaningful and useful information for the healthcare providers. Sharmila et al. [14]surveyed various progress made in the area of big data technology, its latest adoption in Hadoop platform, algorithms used in such platform and listed out the open challenges in using such algorithms in healthcare datasets. They used Pima dataset of Indian Diabetes Database of National Institute of Diabetes and Digestive and Kidney Diseases which has 8 attributes and 768 instances. Authors in [20] have successfully predicted the risk of being affected by type-2 diabetes using random forest model and have achieved decent accuracy level. Another study [2] developed a decision tree model for the diagnosis of type-2 diabetes. They have used public dataset called Pima Indian Dataset for their research. To improve their accuracy level, they have used pre-processing. Most of the research related to this have illustrated whether a person is affected or not affected by diabetes. But, we have gone through a different approach where all the patients were affected with diabetes and we wanted to find out the possible complications for a person after being affected by diabetes.

3 Data Collection and Conceptual Framework

Non-government hospitals in Dhaka City which are under National Health Network (NHN) were selected purposively for the convenience of the survey data collection process. Our survey data collection phase lasted from January 2016 to January 2017. The inclusion criteria for the patients having type-2 diabetes mellitus was chosen at the age greater than or equal to 35 years. All the patients are severely ill. Additionally, they all had diabetes guidebook provided by National Health Network (NHN). We took the two types of glucose level test value from diabetes patients for our analysis. One is fasting blood sugar test, and another is oral glucose tolerance test. Initially, the whole variables have been divided into two parts: dependent variable and independent variable. Independent variable had certain components which supposedly regulated the factors of the dependent variables and they are age, sex, educational status, occupational status, age of onset, duration of disease, types of medications, blood glucose monitoring, regular exercise, cessation of smoking, and use of smokeless tobacco.

The dependent variables are the labels that we have used for our system model and they are cardiovascular complication, neurological complication, ophthalmological complication, and diabetic foot ulcer. Our total population consisted of 26,000 (in the size of this dataset in megabyte 2.1) populations, having 12,824 males and 13,176 female correspondents.

From Figs. 1 and 2, we can observe that all type-2 diabetic complications happened when BMI and HbA1c both rise from 20 and 7 accordingly. Because, if we sum Figs. 1 and 2, we get the resulting sum equivalent to the summation values of frequencies of Fig. 3 for each of the complications, where Fig. 3 includes the prevalence of chronic disease for type-2 diabetic patients of the total population. That is why we may consider for building prediction model's hypothesis that HbA1c and BMI attributes are associated with type-2 diabetes complications.

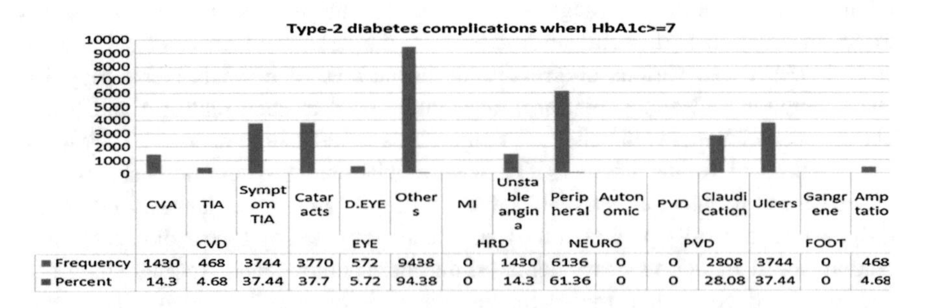

Fig. 1 Frequency and percentage result of various complications among type-2 diabetes patients when HbA1c ≥ 7

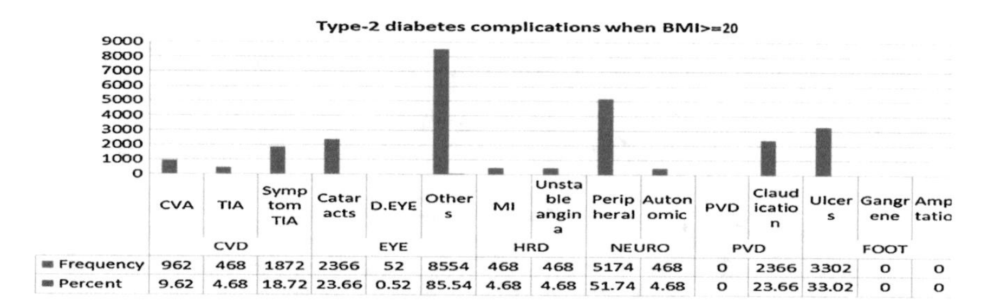

Fig. 2 Frequency and percentage result of various complications among type-2 diabetes patients when BMI $\geq$20

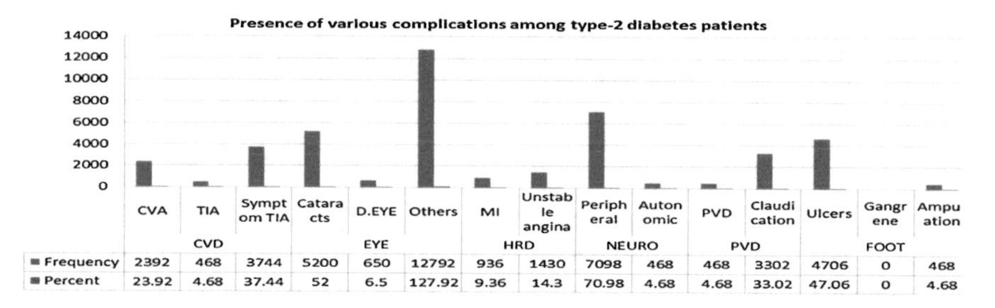

Fig. 3 Frequency and percentage result of various complications among type-2 diabetic patients

4 System Model

Our model is consisted of several components which include data pre-processing, training, analysis, and prediction. We have initiated a survey among diabetes patients having complications. We have gathered a raw dataset contained the information of age, gender, BMI, HbA1c, education, urban living time, smoking, marital status, etc. for both male and female as features. Six key diseases as occurring complications (i.e. cerebrovascular disease (CVD), ophthalmological disease (EYE), cardiovascular disease (HRD), neuropathy disease (NEURO), peripheral vascular disease (PVD), and foot ulcer (FOOT)) because of diabetes have also been stated in the dataset. The block diagram of our system model is provided in Fig. 4.

4.1 Data Pre-processing

We have analyzed the data and came to a conclusion which included only two important factors as featured. These factors are none other than BMI and HbA1c. Furthermore, male and female both varied in terms of weight according to their BMI levels. That is why, our dataset was split in two different categories: male and female. These two categories, which are classified as normal, overweight, and

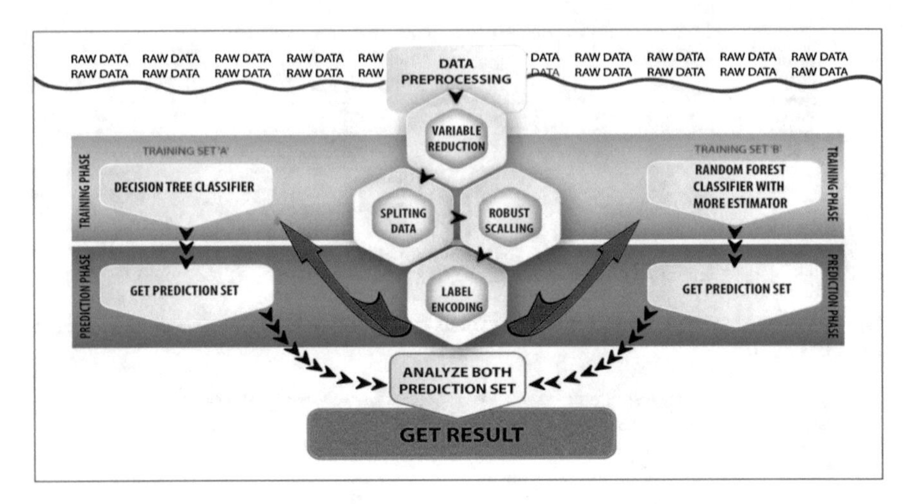

Fig. 4 Prediction model for prevalence of type-2 diabetes mellitus complications

obese, in fact treated differently because of variable body mass index (BMI) [18]. For example, male is considered overweight if the BMI is in between 25 and 30. On the other hand, the BMI of overweight female is ranged in between 18 and 25. We had to apply robust scaling [9] as our dataset contained too much outlier. Robust scalar is responsible for removing the median values. Additionally, it scales the data according to the quintile range [9]. We had applied various label encoding techniques such as factor (R) and one hot encoding (Python: Scikit-Learn) since our dataset was built on six predicted complication namely diseases as labels. A person might get into multiple diseases at the same time. For this reason, in our dataset, we have split and encoded all the labels. Moreover, the main target was to predict the appearance factor of each of the disease after becoming a diabetes patient.

4.2 Training Phase

A. Decision Tree Classification Our training sector is separated into several parts. Firstly, we have applied the decision tree algorithm for initial intuition and grab an overview about what is going on. In fact, decision tree has been illustrated in a way that we could get a tree which shows us various amounts of BMI and HbA1c which led to the diseases. The variants of these two factors led to the different combinations of the diseases stated in the previous section. Ours is a classification problem where the full data is separated into training set and test set. Since the labels are unordered, they are considered as categorical [15]. Our model was trained on the training set which in fact consisted of about 70% of the full dataset. We have tested the result based on the values of test set. Since decision tree obtains a reasonable amount of accuracy along with the inexpensiveness in computation [15], our model was initiated upon decision tree classification algorithm. In a decision tree, a class is considered as a domain consisting of the subset of elements whereas input feature labels the non-leaf nodes.

Additionally, an ark determines either the possible values of the target data or the output labels or a supporting decision based on the input features [4]. In a big data environment, data comes in the form of dependent and independent variables, namely X and Y.

$$X, y(X1, X2, X3, \ldots., Xn; y1, y2, y3, \ldots, yn) \tag{1}$$

We had a wide array of features initially but after analyzing the dataset and the consequences, we have reduced these into only two independent factors BMI and HbA1c. Six diseases are greatly correlated with these two independent variables. That is why we considered these six diseases as the dependent factor individually. These diseases are also called labels for each of the combinational features, namely BMI and HbA1c.

Decision tree is very much likely to be easily visualized and understood [9]. Firstly, this is one of the reasons to use this algorithm as start up. Secondly, there were no missing values in our dataset and it is another reason for using decision tree. Thirdly, decision tree is able to sort our multi-output problem by predicting each of the outputs independently. Here in our case, we had to solve multi-output problem as each of the diseases are non-mutually exclusive. The problem was stated as multi-label mutually non-exclusive problem since each of the disease can occur in an independent basis. For a particular set of BMI and HbA1c it is likely that a disease breaks out alongside with the other diseases and there is no dependency among the diseases. Finally, from this section we have observed our result and predicted diseases by the test set. This data has been kept for later part of comparison. However, we had to make a paradigm shift towards another algorithm which is an improvement over decision trees because of poor generalization and over-fitting [9].

B. Random Forest Classification with High Estimator To get more precise result, we did a paradigm shift to more improved random forest-based system model. Like the decision tree classifier, robust scaling has been used on the features of both training and test set. Since, the complications contained numerical values from 1 to 6 indicating each of the diseases, we have done categorical transformation. Afterwards, encoded the resultant values with OneHotEncoder [9]. Categorical discrete values which have been taken as the matrix of integer transform the output as a sparse matrix and random forest classifier needs the encoding of categorical data [9]. Additionally, we needed each of the complications to be in correspondence individually with the features, namely BMI and HbA1c to get a better intuition and accuracy. That is why, after mapping to OneHotEncoder, we have separated individual column matrix of the complications from Y1 to Y6, which is clearly indicated in algorithm 1. Since random forest calculates the average to control over-fitting and gain a better predictive accuracy level [9], we have used a high estimator number. Here, in our case, estimator is equivalent to decimal 1000. This number represents the total number of trees in the whole forest and we have used bootstrap for drawing the samples with replacement [9]. The detailed work procedure of our random forest classifier-based model has been indicated in Algorithm 1.

Algorithm 1 Prediction Model Algorithm for Prevalence of Type-2 Diabetes Complications

```
1: procedure TRAINTESTSPLIT (X,Y,TestSize)
2:     Xtrain = X(totalSet−testSet)
3:     Xtest = X(testSet)
4:     Ytrain = MapColumnWise(Xtrain)
5:     Ytest = MapColumnWise(Xtest)
6:     Return Xtrain, Ytrain,Xtest,Ytest
7: end procedure
8: procedure ROBUSTSCALING(X)
9:     X = RobustScale.Transform(X)
10:    Return X
11: end procedure
12: procedure CATEGORICALENCODING(Y)
13:    for each CategoricalFeature in Y do
14:        Y= OneHotEncode(Y)
15:    end for
16:    Return Y
17: end procedure
18: Dataset = Input(Directory/FileName)
19: X[EachRow][ZerathColumn] = Dataset[BMI].value
20: X[EachRow][FirstColumn] = Dataset[HbA1c].value
21: X= RobustScaling(X[EachRow][EachColumn])
22: Y= CategoricalEncoding(Y)
23: Y1 = Y[EachRow][ZerothColumn]
24: Y2= Y[EachRow][FirstColumn]
25: Y3= Y[EachRow][SecondColumn]
26: Y4= Y[EachRow][ThirdColumn]
27: Y5= Y[EachRow][FourthColumn]
28: Y6= Y[EachRow][FifthColumn]
29: for each Y in Range (Y1, Y6) do
30:    Xtrain,Ytrain,Xtest,Ytest = TrainTestSplit(X,Y,0.20f)
31:    Classifier= RandomForestClassifier(NEstimators = 1000, bootstrap = True)
32:    Classifier.Train(Xtrain,Ytrain)
33:    Classifier.test(Xtest,Ytest)
34: end for
```

C. Model Training and Evaluating After encoding, for every label of complications which we have separated as a sparse matrix, our model has been trained with a train test ratio of 80:20. We have used sklearns default train_test_split [9] function in order to splitting the training and evaluation set. We have tested the accuracy of our model by evaluating it by the test set. Individual accuracy and graph for each of the complications have been acquired, which is demonstrated in the result section. Finally, we went further to analyze our both prediction-based results to build our intuition. While evaluating results from both Decision Tree and Random Forest, we went further for analyzing our both prediction-based results to build our intuition.

4.3 Build a Conclusion Using Both Results

After getting the result and graphs from random forest classifier, we have made an analysis of both results. The result of the random forest-based complication prediction model is highly backed by the decision tree. In fact, we did come to some sort of conclusion regarding the complications considering BMI and HbA1c. The novelty of our study is, we tried to find out the probable diseases after a person is affected with type-2 diabetes. We tried to point out the strong, average, and weak complication areas for each of the diseases after getting the proper visualization of each of the diabetes complication for both male and female. There are a dense area, average dense area, low dense area, and null dense area in each of the graphs. However, we have tried to visualize and point out each of the areas of interest for the indication of danger and non-danger zones. The algorithm of our visualization procedure has been provided in Algorithm 2.

Algorithm 2 Area visualization

```
1:  DenseArea =NULL
2:  AverageDenseArea = NULL
3:  LowDenseArea = NULL
4:  NullDenseArea = NULL
5:  interator = 0
6:  for each i in Range List(PredictedComplications) do
7:      DenseArea[iterator].Add(Scan(Threshold.InRange(i.Radius())))
8:      AverageDenseArea[iterator].Add(Scan(Threshold.InRange(i.Radius())))
9:      LowDenseArea[iterator].Add(Scan(Threshold.InRange(i.Radius())))
10:     NullDenseArea[iterator].Add(Scan(Threshold.InRange(i.Radius())))
11:     iterator = iterator + 1
12: end for
```

5 Result and Analysis

Our result and analysis part include several graphs and tables of both decision tree and random forest classification algorithm. Firstly, we have visualized a tree after applying the decision tree algorithm to our dataset. The resultant decision tree for the male has been illustrated in Fig. 5.

Alternatively, the decision tree for the predicted complication of the female population has been illustrated in Fig. 6. The resultant visualization of the decision tree for both male and female varied greatly for each of the complications according to their levels of BMI and HbA1c. However, after moving towards the random forest classification-based complication prediction model, we have also visualized by the scatter plot for the predicting results for each of the complication factors for male and females which have been illustrated in Figs. 7 and 8.

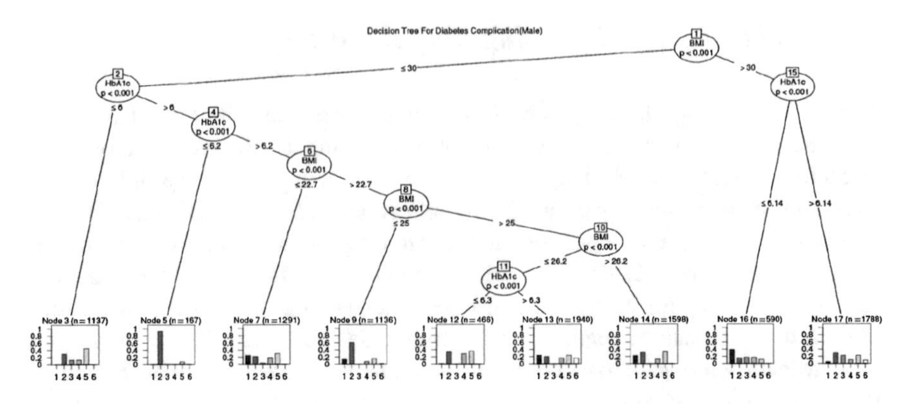

Fig. 5 Classified prediction model for prevalence of type-2 diabetes mellitus complications (male respondents)

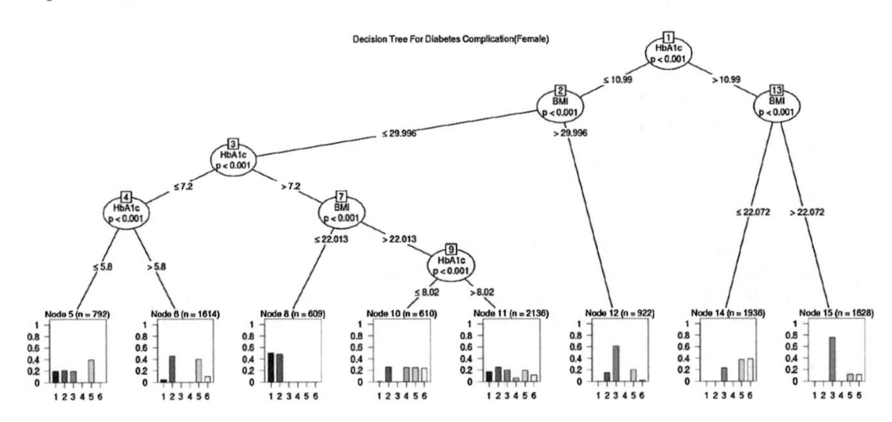

Fig. 6 Classified prediction model for prevalence of type-2 diabetes mellitus complications (female respondents)

The female respondent showed significant different results from the male population because of their class: normal, overweight, and obese varied in terms of BMI.

After doing graphical analysis, we have segmented our prediction results into several areas of graphical co-ordinate. These areas are considered as dense areas, average dense area, lowest dense area, and null dense areas. The main target was to make identification of each of the zones of interest, especially the dense areas, which is consisted of the dense population with the most predictive of a chronic disease for type-2 diabetes patients. Each of the zones was built on the certain BMI and HbA1c range. For example, we can see the dense areas from the graph which is contained in the most populated areas with an overlapping scenario.

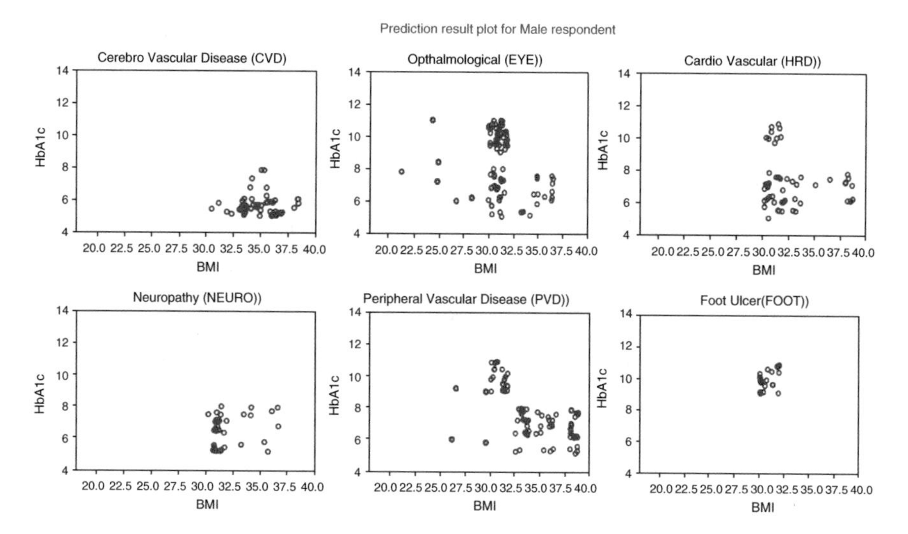

Fig. 7 Prediction results for male respondents

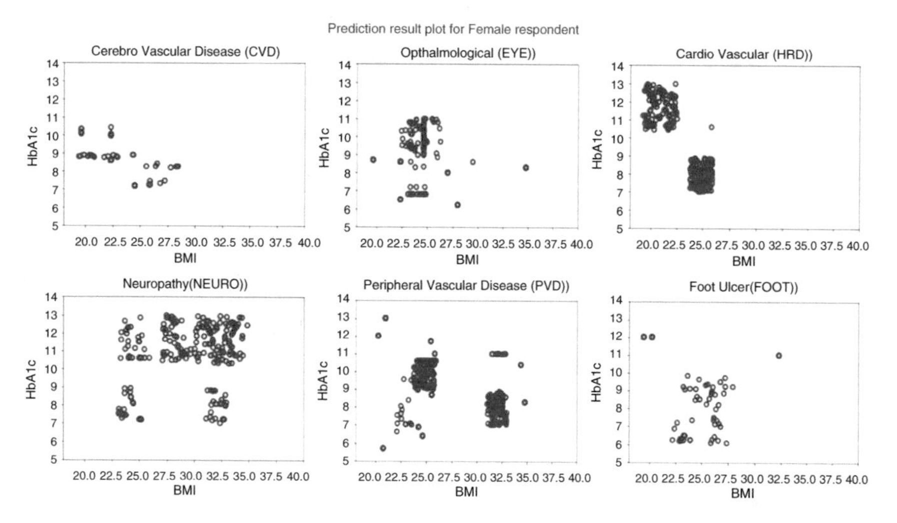

Fig. 8 Prediction results for female respondents

On the other hand, the least populated areas with the less overlapping scenario are considered as the lowest dense areas. Figure 9 represents the zonal ranges of BMI and HbA1c for each disease for male respondent. Alternatively, Fig. 10 represents the zonal ranges for each of the complications for the female population. The accuracy of prediction for each of the complications has been measured and represented in Fig. 11.

Respondent	Cerebro Vascular Disease (CVD)		Ophthalmological (EYE)		Cardio Vascular (HRD)		Neuropathy (NEURO)		Peripheral Vascular Disease(PVD)		Foot Ulcer(FOOT)	
MALE	DENSE AREA		DENSE AREA		DENSE AREA		DENSE AREA		DENSE AREA		DENSE AREA	
	BMI	HbA1c	BMI	HbA1c	BMI	HbA1c	BMI	HbA1c	BMI	HbA1c	BMI	HbA1c
	32.5-33.5 36.0-37.5	5.0-6.0 4.8-5.8	30.0-32.2	9.00-11.0	30.0-32.0	9.8-11.0	31.0-32.0	5.0-6.0	30.0-32.0 33.0-34.8 38.0-39.0	9.0-11.0 6.4-8.0 6.5-7.1	30.0-31.0 32.0-32.5	9.0-10.8 11.0-11.2
	AVEREGE DENSE AREA		AVEREGE DENSE AREA		AVEREGE DENSE AREA		AVEREGE DENSITY AREA		AVEREGE DENSE AREA		AVEREGE DENSE AREA	
	BMI	HbA1c	BMI	HbA1c	BMI	HbA1c	BMI	HbA1c	BMI	HbA1c	BMI	HbA1c
	33.0-36.0	6.0-8.0	30.0-31.3 33.1-36.8	5.0-8.0 5.2-7.8	37.5-39	6.2-8.0	34.0-37.0	5.0-8.0	35.0-37.0	5.2-7.6	31.0-32.5	9.0-11.0
	LOW DENSE AREA		LOW DENSE AREA		LOW DENSE AREA		LOW DENSE AREA		LOW DENSE AREA		LOW DENSE AREA	
	BMI	HbA1c	BMI	HbA1c	BMI	HbA1c	BMI	HbA1c	BMI	HbA1c	BMI	HbA1c
	30.0-32.5 37.7-38.2	5.0-6.2 5.7-6.2	21.0-28.0	6.0-9.0	35.0-36.0	7.0-7.8	33.0-33.5	5.0-5.5	25.0-30.0	6.0-9.0	31.9-32.1	9.0-9.2
	NULL DENSE AREA		NULL DENSE AREA		NULL DENSE AREA		NULL DENSE AREA		NULL DENSE AREA		NULL DENSE AREA	
	BMI	HbA1c	BMI	HbA1c	BMI	HbA1c	BMI	HbA1c	BMI	HbA1c	BMI	HbA1c
	20.0-30.0 39.0-40.0	4.0-14.0 9.7-14.0	32.5-40 20.0-40.0	9.0-14.0 12.0-14.0	20.0-40 20.0-30.0 34.0-40.0	8.2-9.8 4.0-14.0 8.0-14.0	20.0-30.0 37.5-40.0 20.0-40.0	4.0-14.0 4.0-14.0 8.5-14.0	20.0-25.0 20.0-40.0 39.0-40.0	4.0-14.0 12.0-14.0 4.0-40.0	20.0-40.0 20.0-40.0 32.5-40.0	4.0-9.0 11.0-14.0 4.0-14.0

Fig. 9 Area visualization results for prevalence of type-2 diabetes mellitus complications (male respondents)

Respondent	Cerebro Vascular Disease (CVD)		Ophthalmological (EYE)		Cardio Vascular (HRD)		Neuropathy (NEURO)		Peripheral Vascular Disease(PVD)		Foot Ulcer(FOOT)	
FEMALE	DENSE AREA		DENSE AREA		DENSE AREA		DENSE AREA		DENSE AREA		DENSE AREA	
	BMI	HbA1c	BMI	HbA1c	BMI	HbA1c	BMI	HbA1c	BMI	HbA1c	BMI	HbA1c
	19.0-20.5 21.9-23.0	8.8-9.1 8.7-9.0	22.5-25.0 23.0-25.0	6.8-7 9.0-11.0	19.0-22.5 23.0-26.0	10.5-13.0 7.0-9.0	27.0-34.5	10.5-13.0	24.0-26.0 31.0-33.0 31.0-33.2	8.5-10.5 7.0-8.7 11.0-11.2	22.5-27.5	8.0-10.0
	AVEREGE DENSE AREA		AVEREGE DENSE AREA		AVEREGE DENSE AREA		AVEREGE DENSE AREA		AVEREGE DENSE AREA		AVEREGE DENSE AREA	
	BMI	HbA1c	BMI	HbA1c	BMI	HbA1c	BMI	HbA1c	BMI	HbA1c	BMI	HbA1c
	24.8-28.0	7.2-8.4	23.0-25.0	7.0-8.0	–	–	23.0-25.0 23.0-24.8 31.0-33.0	10.5-13.0 7.0-9.0 7.0-9.0	22.0-25.0	6.5-9.5	23.0-24.5 26.0-27.5 21.8-22.5	6.0-6.4 6.0-8.0 6.0-7.0
	LOW DENSE AREA		LOW DENSE AREA		LOW DENSE AREA		LOW DENSE AREA		LOW DENSE AREA		LOW DENSE AREA	
	BMI	HbA1c	BMI	HbA1c	BMI	HbA1c	BMI	HbA1c	BMI	HbA1c	BMI	HbA1c
	19.0-22.0	9.9-10.5	25.0-30.0	6.0-9.0	22.0-22.5 26.0-26.3	13.0-13.2 10.4-10.7	–	–	20.0-26.0	11.0-13.0	20.0-21.0	12.0-12.2
	NULL DENSE AREA		NULL DENSE AREA		NULL DENSE AREA		NULL DENSE AREA		NULL DENSE AREA		NULL DENSE AREA	
	BMI	HbA1c	BMI	HbA1c	BMI	HbA1c	BMI	HbA1c	BMI	HbA1c	BMI	HbA1c
	29.0-40.0 20.0-40.0	5.0-14.0 11.0-14.0	20.0-40.0 30.0-40.0 27.5-40.0 19.0-22.0	11.0-14.0 5.0-8.0 9.0-11.0 5.0-8.0	19.0-24.0 26.0-40.0 20.0-40.0	5.0-10.0 5.0-14.0 13.2-14.0	20.0-40.0 20.0-40.0 19.0-22.5 35.0-40.0 20.0-40.0	5.0-6.5 9.0-10.4 5.0-14.0 35.0-40.0 13.0-14.0	26.0-31.0 35.5-40.0 20.0-40.0	5.0-14.0 5.0-14.0 12.0-14.0	19.0-22.0 12.3-14.0 20.0-40.0 27.5-40.0	5.0-11.9 12.3-14.0 5.0-5.9 5.0-14.0

Fig. 10 Area visualization results for prevalence of type-2 diabetes mellitus complications (female respondents)

Accuracy Measurement Table												
Disease Name	Cerebro Vascular Disease (CVD)		Ophthalmological (EYE)		Cardio Vascular (HRD)		Neuropathy (NEURO)		Peripheral Vascular Disease(PVD)		Foot Ulcer(FOOT)	
	Training Accuracy	Test Accuracy	Training Accuracy	Test Accuracy	Training Accuracy	Test Accuracy	Training Accuracy	Test Accuracy	Training Accuracy	Test Accuracy	Training Accuracy	Test Accuracy
Male	87	83	81	74	98	91	88	86	81	77	97	94
Female	92	89	90	86	98	95	98	93	82	78	90	84

Fig. 11 Accuracy measurement table for prevalence of type-2 diabetes mellitus complications (both respondents)

6 Conclusion

With the growing of digitization of health-care industry, an enormous amount of health-care data has been generated and size is increasing at a bizarre rate. To deliver the best evidence-based, generalized and patient-centric care, the medical data from industry must be analyzed to discover deep knowledge and values. Type-2 diabetes is one of the most prevalent endocrine disorders worldwide nowadays, by using machine learning prediction model among all the complications discussed in this work, here we able to identify higher percentage where the HbA1c level is $\geq$7 and BMI value is $\geq$20 which indicates the actuality of this model. So, this model can be recommended for researching medical data to controlling HbA1c and BMI which in further could be helpful for improving knowledge and consciousness of participants. More research is needed to evaluate the benefits of low-cost screening tools with efficacy, cost-effectiveness, and sustainability of culturally appropriate interventions in institutions. It would be more helpful to improve the current situation and beneficial for public health in future.

References

1. Ahmed, K. R. (2009). Incidence of diabetic retinopathy: A 15 year follow up in a hospital population (Bangladesh). Master's thesis.
2. Al Jarullah, A. A. (2011). Decision tree discovery for the diagnosis of type II diabetes. In *2011 International Conference on Innovations in Information Technology* (pp. 303–307). Piscataway: IEEE.
3. Cottle, M., Hoover, W., Kanwal, S., Kohn, M., Strome, T., & Treister, N. (2013). Transforming health care through big data strategies for leveraging big data in the health care industry. Institute for Health Technology Transformation. http://ihealthtran.com/big-data-in-healthcare.
4. Friedman, J., Hastie, T., & Tibshirani, R. (2001). *The Elements of Statistical Learning*. Springer Series in Statistics (Vol. 1). New York: Springer.
5. Hersen, M., & Thomas, J. C. (2007) *Handbook of Clinical Interviewing with Adults*. Los Angeles: Sage Publications.
6. Knowler, W. C., Barrett-Connor, E., Fowler, S. E., Hamman, R. F., Lachin, J. M., Walker, E. A., et al. (2002). Reduction in the incidence of type 2 diabetes with lifestyle intervention or metformin. *The New England Journal of Medicine, 346*(6), 393–403.
7. Mahmoodi, M., Hosseini-zijoud, S. M., Nabati, S., Modarresi, M., Mehrabian, M., Sayyadi, A., et al. (2013). The effect of white vinegar on some blood biochemical factors in type 2 diabetic patients. *Journal of Diabetes and Endocrinology, 4*(1), 1–5.
8. Pan, X. R., Li, G. W., Hu, Y. H., Wang, J. X., Yang, W. Y., An, Z. X., et al. (1997). Effects of diet and exercise in preventing NIDDM in people with impaired glucose tolerance: The Da Qing IGT and diabetes study. *Diabetes care, 20*(4), 537–544.
9. Pedregosa, F., Varoquaux, G., Gramfort, A., Michel, V., Thirion, B., Grisel, O., et al. (2011). Scikit-learn: Machine learning in Python. *Journal of Machine Learning Research, 12*, 2825–2830.
10. Rahim, M. A. (2002). Diabetes in Bangladesh: Prevalence and determinants. Master's thesis.

11. Rajesh, K., & Sangeetha, V. (2012). Application of data mining methods and techniques for diabetes diagnosis. *International Journal of Engineering and Innovative Technology (IJEIT), 2*(3), 224–229.
12. Saquib, N., Khanam, M. A., Saquib, J., Anand, S., Chertow, G. M., Barry, M., et al. (2013). High prevalence of type 2 diabetes among the urban middle class in Bangladesh. *BMC Public Health, 13*(1), 1032.
13. Sharmila, K., & Manickam, S. (2016). Diagnosing diabetic dataset using Hadoop and k-means clustering techniques. *Indian Journal of Science and Technology, 9*(40), 1–5.
14. Sharmila, K., & Vethamanickam, S. (2015). Survey on data mining algorithm and its application in healthcare sector using Hadoop platform. *International Journal of Emerging Technology and Advanced Engineering, 5*(1), 2250–2459. ISSN 2250-2459.
15. Srivastava, A., Han, E. H., Kumar, V., & Singh, V. (1999). Parallel formulations of decision-tree classification algorithms. In *High Performance Data Mining* (pp. 237–261). Berlin: Springer.
16. Vaz, N. C., Ferreira, A., Kulkarni, M., Vaz, F. S., & Pinto, N. (2011). Prevalence of diabetic complications in rural Goa, India. *Indian Journal of Community Medicine: Official Publication of Indian Association of Preventive & Social Medicine, 36*(4), 283.
17. Wang, L., Ranjan, R., Kołodziej, J., Zomaya, A., & Alem, L. (2015). Software tools and techniques for big data computing in healthcare clouds. *Future Generation Computer Systems, 43*(C), 38–39.
18. Wikipedia Contributors. (2018). Body mass index — Wikipedia, the free encyclopedia. https://en.wikipedia.org/w/index.php?title=Body_mass_index&oldid=893812047. Accessed 24 April 2018.
19. Wild, S., Roglic, G., Green, A., Sicree, R., & King, H. (2004). Global prevalence of diabetes: Estimates for the year 2000 and projections for 2030. *Diabetes Care, 27*(5), 1047–1053.
20. Xu, W., Zhang, J., Zhang, Q., & Wei, X. (2017). Risk prediction of type II diabetes based on random forest model. In *2017 Third International Conference on Advances in Electrical, Electronics, Information, Communication and Bio-Informatics (AEEICB)* (pp. 382–386). Piscataway: IEEE.

Face Reconstruction from Profile to Frontal Evaluation of Face Recognition

Salim Afra and Reda Alhajj

Abstract One of the main challenges in face recognition is handling extreme variation of poses which may be faced for images collected in labs and in the wild. Recognizing faces in profile view has been shown to perform poorly compared to using frontal view of faces. Indeed, previous approaches failed to capture distinct features of a profile face compared to a frontal one. Approaches to enhance face recognition on profile faces have been recently proposed following two different trends. One trend depends on training a neural network model with big multi-view face datasets to learn features of faces by handling all poses. The second trend generates a frontal face image (face reconstruction) from any given face pose and applies feature extraction and face recognition on the generated face instead of profile faces. Recent methods for face reconstruction use generative adversarial networks (GAN) learning model to train two competing neural networks to generate authentic frontal view of any pose preserving person's identity. For the work described in this paper, we trained a feature extraction neural network model to learn representation of any face pose which is then compared with each other using Euclidean distance. We also used two recent face reconstruction techniques to generate frontal faces. We evaluated the performance of using the generated frontal faces against the posed counterparts. In the conducted experiments, we used three face datasets that contain several challenges for face recognition having faces in a variety of poses and in the wild.

Keywords Face recognition · Pose-invariant recognition · Face reconstruction · Face frontalization

S. Afra (✉)
Department of Computer Science, University of Calgary, Calgary, AB, Canada
e-mail: salim.afra@ucalgary.ca

R. Alhajj
Department of Computer Science, University of Calgary, Calgary, AB, Canada

Department of Computer Engineering, Istanbul Medipol University, Istanbul, Turkey
e-mail: alhajj@ucalgary.ca

R. Alhajj et al. (eds.), *Data Management and Analysis*, Studies in Big Data 65,
https://doi.org/10.1007/978-3-030-32587-9_8

1 Introduction

Face recognition has received significant interest in the past few decades due to its various important real-world applications, including identity verification, video surveillance, monitoring, etc. Advances in face recognition resulted in continuously redefining the problem as new technologies and data become more available. Early face recognition work focused on recognizing people faces in controlled conditions where images are collected in a lab setting with defined parameters such as illumination, face rotation, pose variation, background, and occlusion. The approaches described in [1, 2] handled face recognition by designing methods for extracting local descriptors from face images. They achieved good results for testing on face images taken in controlled environment.

Research on face recognition then evolved to identify faces in unconstrained environments. For this purpose, several benchmark datasets, such as labeled faces in the wild (LFW) [3], have been proposed for this problem where previous face recognition algorithms performance dropped significantly. Current methods, e.g., [4–8] used recent development in deep learning, especially convolutional neural networks (CNN), to learn a network model which extracts faces. Deep learning has proved to provide very accurate results in differentiating and identifying people faces in unconstrained environment. They reported around 99% accuracy, which is better than what humans can achieve (97%) [9].

The current challenge facing face recognition is the ability to recognize faces not only in an unconstrained environment, but also with varied and extreme poses of faces. This problem is referred to as pose-invariant face recognition (PIFR). Though LFW dataset was collected in an unconstrained environment, most faces are near frontal and do not reflect much pose variation. Applying state-of-the-art algorithms resulted in 10% performance loss when applied on frontal to profile faces as shown in [10]; human performance drops slightly. This is due to the nature of profile faces. Having more than half of a face not shown may lead to a dramatic increase in intra-person variances where different people can look the same for the recognizing algorithms.

Recently, several methods, e.g., [11–14], have been proposed to tackle pose variation in face recognition by applying face frontalization, which refers to the process of synthesizing frontal face images given a face image of any pose in any environment. For the work described in this paper, we evaluate the performance of using different face frontalization techniques and their effect on face recognition compared to training a CNN model to learn features from any pose. We first train a face recognition model based on [5]. A deep neural model is learned from faces collected from CASIA-WebFace [15] to extract features of faces. Then, we experiment whether any of the newly designed methods for face frontalization could improve the performance of face recognition compared to using profile faces in face verification. We used several challenging datasets for the conducted experiments, namely FEI [16], FERET [17], and IJB-A [18] face datasets which provide pose variance and faces collected in unconstrained environment.

The rest of this paper is structured as follows. Section 2 presents related work on face recognition and face frontalization methods for face identification techniques. The methodology for face recognition using different face frontalization methods is described in Sect. 3. Section 4 covers the experiments conducted to test the performance of face recognition in uncontrolled and multi-view environments using three datasets on frontalized and original faces. Section 5 is conclusions.

2 Related Work

Recent methods proposed for pose-invariant face recognition can be classified into two main categories. One category aims at developing a model that learns pose-invariant features given a face image of any pose. The other category applies face frontalization or face rotation to get a frontal view of any pose face image which will then be used for face recognition.

Several methods attempted to apply pose aware face recognition either by training one model, e.g., [5, 7] or multiple pose specific models, e.g., [19]. Methods which use one joint model for training pose aware face recognition handle pose variations and the effect of profile faces by learning a deep neural network where face images in order of tens of millions are used for training. These are private images that the community does not have access to. Other methods such as Masi et al. [19] tackle pose variation by training multiple pose-aware specific models (PAMs). They use deep convolutional neural networks to learn representations of faces for different pose values. First, they apply landmark detection on an input face to classify it into profile or frontal face. Then they extract corresponding features at different PAMs to fuse the features.

Other approaches used face frontalization techniques either by applying face rotation using 2D [20, 21] and 3D [11, 22] alignment techniques or by learning deep neural network [12, 23]. The work described in [11] used 3D modelling by first extracting location of features on the face and then applying hard frontalization by having a 3D model of a general face and map the extracted features into a face. The method described in [22] meshes a face image into a 3D object and eliminates the pose and expression variations using an identity preserving 3D transformation. Then they apply an inpainting method based on Poisson editing to fill the invisible region caused by self-occlusion. The work described in [12] applies face rotation by training a deep neural network which takes a face image and a binary code encoding a target pose and generates a face image with the same identity viewed at the target pose. Experiments are within ± 45 poses of faces; they did not consider extreme poses. Frontalized faces generated from these neural network models, however, are with no significant details in faces, making the generated faces very general. This leads to losing texture information and hence poor performance for using these faces in experiments.

The latest face frontalization methods, e.g., [13, 14] use variations of the learning model created by Goodfellow et al. [24], called generative adversarial network (GAN), which is used to generate new images by estimating a target data distribution [25]. GAN is implemented by training two neural networks (generator, discriminator) continuously in a min-max two player game fashion. The generator model learns to generate new images by mapping from a latent space to a particular data distribution. The discriminator learns to classify whether an image belongs to the original set of images or it is generated by the generator.

Generator network objective is to increase the error rate of the discriminator such that the generated images are very close to the original ones. The discriminator network objective is to successfully classify images into either artificial (from generator) or real (original). This is why it is called adversarial learning as both are being trained to compete against each other. Several architectures of GAN have been recently proposed and successfully applied in computer vision tasks, such as image super resolution [26, 27], image synthesis [25, 28], and image to image translation [29].

Motivated by the success of GANs in generating realistic images, couple of works [13, 14] have been proposed to apply face frontalization using GAN network architecture. The work described in [14] proposed synthesizing frontal faces by using a two pathway GAN (TF-GAN) to process global and local features. Local features correspond to detecting four landmarks on a face (left eye, right eye, nose tip, mouth) and then aggregating the positions of these landmarks into a general face model. The global path uses an encoder–decoder structure to extract features of all the face. After that, feature map fusion is used to merge the features into one single frontal face, which is then fed to light CNN [30] for face identification and verification. The work described in [13] proposed a disentangled representation learning GAN (DR-GAN) to perform both face frontalization, and to learn a generative representation of a non-frontal face. They proposed an encoder–decoder GAN structure to learn face representation using the encoder. This representation is used with noise and pose degree to generate a frontalized face. They trained DR-GAN using Multi-PIE [31] and CASISA-Web Face [15]. They evaluated the results on Multi-PIE (faces angled between ±60 °), CFP [10], and IJB-A [18] datasets.

3 Methodology

The overall methodology followed for face frontalization and recognition is depicted in Fig. 1. The methodology consists of three major components.

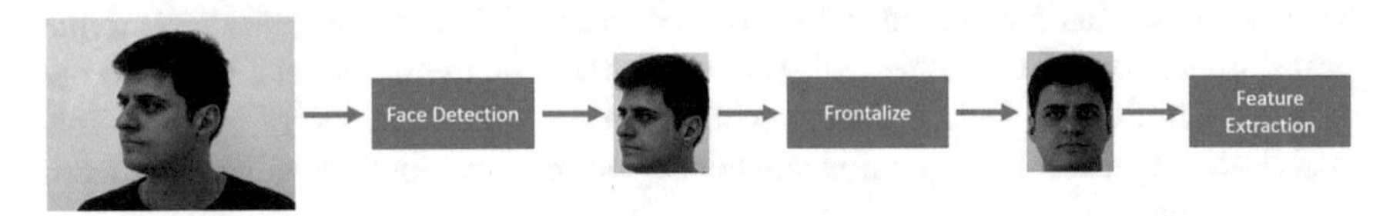

Fig. 1 The overall methodology for face frontalization from any pose into a frontal one. First face detection is applied to get face boundaries, after that the face is frontalized to get frontal view features of the image which are then used for recognition

3.1 Face Detection

Face detection refers to the problem of identifying boundaries of faces in complex images which may contain several people or objects in the background. Early face detection work developed by Viola and Jones [32] provided fast and accurate face detection. Their method used boosted cascade detectors and Haar features extraction to locate face regions. Other methods such as histogram of oriented gradient (HOG) [33] was also proposed by dividing an image into grid cells, and then computing the feature vector of the image using the gradient descriptor. While these early methods provided fast and accurate detection rates for frontal images, they failed to detect faces in a multi-view scene or in an uncontrolled environment. The works described in [34–36] focused on enhancing these detectors to be able to detect profile faces by creating multiple face detectors for different face poses.

Recent techniques for face detection use deep convolutional neural networks (DCNN) as the architecture to detect and extract features of faces. Indeed, the success of using deep neural networks in speech recognition and image classification encouraged researchers to apply it for face detection. Zhang et al. [37] work was one of the first to use DCNN for face detection. They collected around 120,000 face images from different datasets containing different poses of faces. They used the collected faces to train a DCNN with 4 layers. Other convolutional neural network (CNN) methods, such as [38] trained a model based on fine-tuning AlexNet [39] network with face images datasets. Their method recorded a receiver operating characteristic (ROC) value of around 80% on FDDB dataset [40]. In another work, Li et al. [41] created a cascade of six CNNs for face detection. The first CNN (called 12-net) used a sliding window of size 12 to extract regions from a test image. Then, a CNN is used for alignment. They repeat these two procedures for 34-net and 48-net CNNs. Their method recorded a ROC value of around 85%.

Girshick et al. [42] proposed a region-based CNN called R-CNN. Their work is based on region proposal and object identification using CNN. Given an input image, the first step uses a region proposal method, such as Selective Search [43] or EdgeBox [44], to extract regions, where each region might contain an object desired to be detected. Each extracted region is warped and fed into the trained CNN model which decides whether the region contains the desired object or not. Later, the authors introduced Fast R-CNN in [45] to make the detection process faster than the original R-CNN by forwarding the entire test image to CNN only once, instead of forwarding every extracted region. First, the region proposal method is applied on the test image, then the whole image is fed to CNN where the extracted regions are mapped from the original image to the convolutional feature maps inside CNN. Faster R-CNN has then been proposed in [46] to make the whole process even faster by incorporating the region proposal method into a convolutional layer. They avoided using any external method that will make the process slower. Faster R-CNN is applied on the face detection problem in [47].

As our approach is intended to perform face recognition in multi-view face images, a multi-view face detector is required as the first step. We trained a CNN

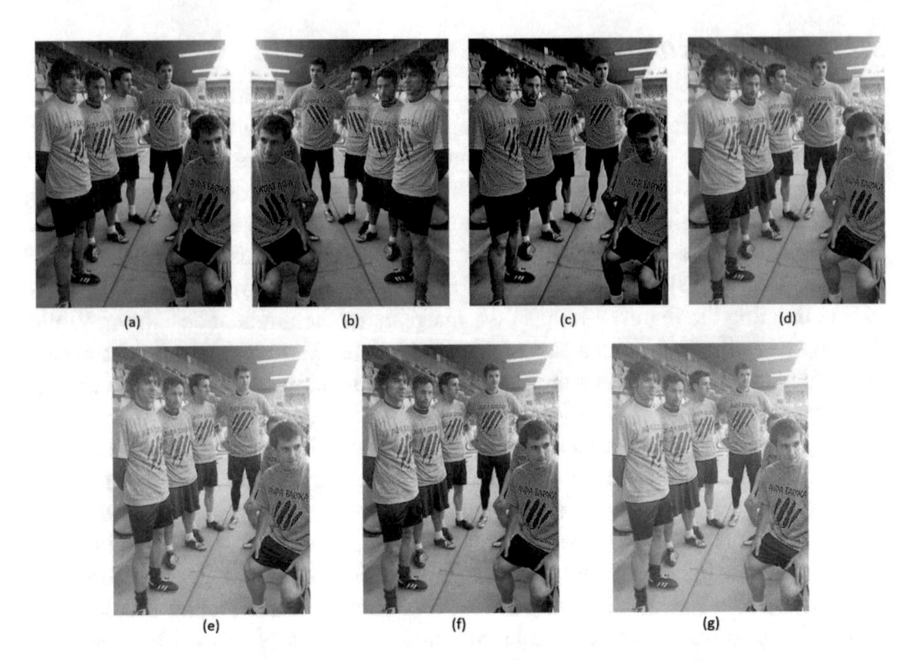

Fig. 2 Image manipulation for training: (**a**) an original image from WIDER dataset; (**b**) a rotated version of the image shown in (**a**); (**c**)–(**g**) versions of the image in (**a**) using different gamma levels, namely 0.5, 1.5, 2, 2.5, and 3, respectively

model to perform face detection on WIDER face dataset [48]. WIDER dataset contains thousands of face images collected under extreme cases with varying scale, pose, occlusion, and illumination of faces. We used the recently proposed MobileNet-v1 [49] CNN network architecture to train a neural network on WIDER dataset. MobileNet-v1 has been designed using depth-wise separable convolutions to provide drastic decrease in model size and training/evaluation time without affecting detection performance. To get better detection accuracy, we pre-processed every image in the training data of WIDER dataset before training our detector model. We generated four different views for every image in the dataset, and then fed the images to the learning model. The various image types we generated from every image are listed below. They are illustrated in Fig. 2.

- Adjust Gamma Degree: The gamma degree controls the lightning effect in an image. For our training, we adjusted the gamma level to these five values: 0.5, 1.5, 2, 2.5, and 3 to have variety of effects ranging from dark to light illumination. This leads to images covering different periods of a day.
- Rotate Image: We also rotated images to get different angles of faces in the training set.

By using these pre-processing steps for training, we improved the performance of the detector on WIDER dataset from 75% to 80%.

3.2 Face Frontalization

After detecting the face region, we applied face frontalization to get a frontal and aligned face image from any given face pose. Extracting features of the frontalized face and evaluating its performance will test how realistic the generated frontalized faces are. Different face frontalization techniques were discussed in Sect. 2. For our study described in this paper, we have chosen DRGAN [13] and effective frontalization (EF) [11] techniques which are publicly available.

- DRGAN [13]: This method uses GAN learning architecture to generate frontal face images along with a feature vector extraction method. They modified the original GAN architecture by introducing a generator encoder–decoder structure, not only to learn realistic frontal face generation, but also to learn feature vector representation for faces. The target is to have closer cosine similarity between vectors of various views of the face of the same person. In our study, we use DRGAN for feature extraction and also to generate a frontal face. This generated face is then used as input to our feature extraction technique.
- Effective Frontalization [11]: This method as illustrated in Fig. 3 rotates any given face into frontal one by first applying landmark detection to locate local features of the face (eyes, mouth, nose, chin). It then estimates a 3D shape of the face, get what parts of the face are invisible, completes the face by using symmetry of visible parts.

3.3 Feature Extraction

Before applying person verification which corresponds to check whether two face images belong to the same person or not, feature extraction is needed such that faces of the same person have more similar representation than those of different people. Various feature extraction techniques exist, they can be divided into two categories: hand-crafted and learned features.

Algorithms for hand-crafted features take an input image of a face and follow some predefined steps to locate key-points in the image. They extract features based on the location of the key-points. Hand-crafted feature extraction techniques such as SIFT [50], SURF [51], and LBPH [1] have been used by several studies, e.g., [52–55].

For techniques which incorporate leaned features, a model is trained based on an image dataset to automatically extract features of a certain object. Recent learned face image representations use neural network model due to its great performance in other object recognition domains [56]. Taigman et al. introduced DeepFace [6] which uses a neural network model to learn face representation from large training datasets (order of millions). The innovation of their method is that they implement 3D modelling for all faces as a pre-processing step to align faces before feeding them to the neural network to learn better face representation. Schroff et al.

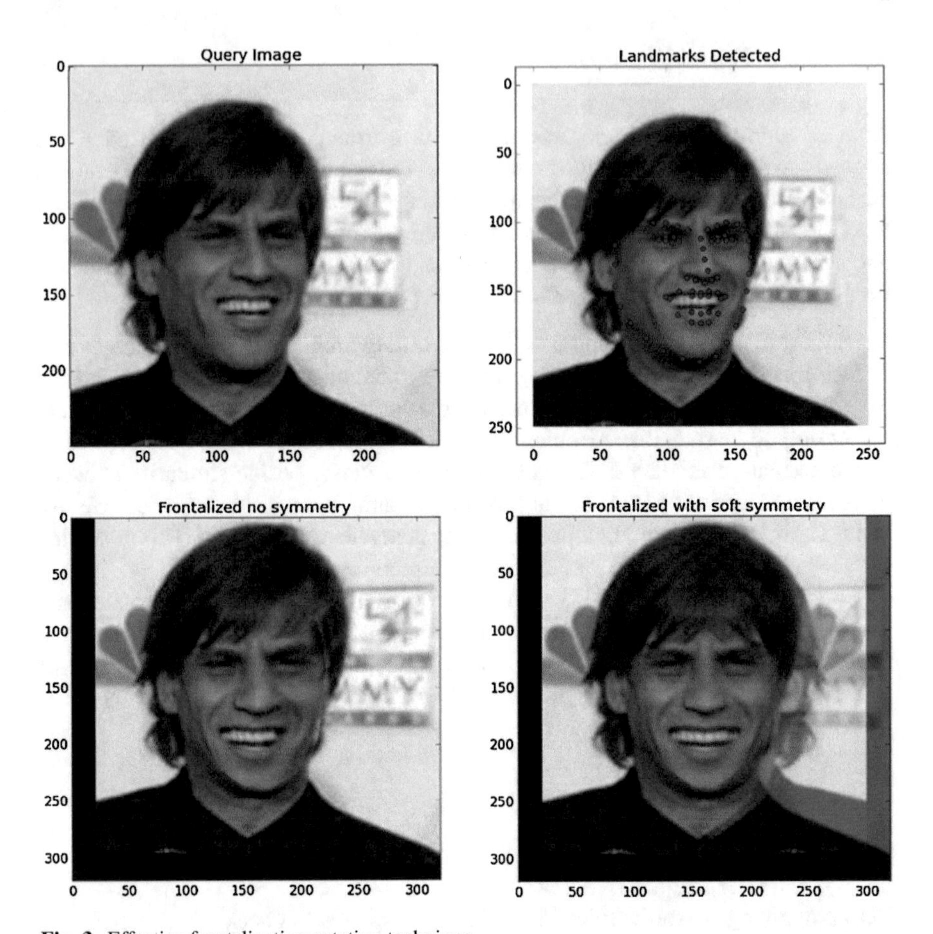

Fig. 3 Effective frontalization rotation technique

created a face feature extraction technique based on a neural network model called FaceNet [5]. Like DeepFace, their model is trained on million of private images where faces are taken in an uncontrolled environment. However, the difference is that FaceNet does not use any kind of 2D or 3D alignment. Instead, they use simple scaling and translation techniques on the images. Further, the method uses a triplet loss learning technique on each learning step of the neural network so that the representation is a vector. Then, the Euclidean distance between the vectors is the distance between the images. Both DeepFace and FaceNet achieve a state-of-the-art accuracy of $\tilde{9}7\%$ on face identification on LFW dataset.

For this work, we trained our own CNN. In particular, we trained the Inception-Resnet-v1 [57] network architecture on MS-Celeb-1M [58] face dataset. The training implementation follows the method described in FaceNet [5], and using the triple loss learning technique for our training.

4 Experiments and Results

In this section, we explain the conducted experiments and show evaluation results of different face frontalization techniques. We report on their effect on face recognition compared to not using any frontalization. In the rest of this section, we will list the datasets used in the evaluation, types of the conducted experiments, and the obtained results.

4.1 Datasets

We have used three datasets for the evaluation described below. Samples of these datasets are shown in Fig. 4.

- FEI [16]: The FEI face dataset contains a set of face images taken between June 2005 and March 2006 in a lab environment. There are 14 images for each of 200 individuals, a total of 2800 images. Images were collected with a homogeneous background taken in 180 degrees covering all views of the face, The age of people in the collected images is between 19 and 40 years old with distinct appearance and hairstyle.

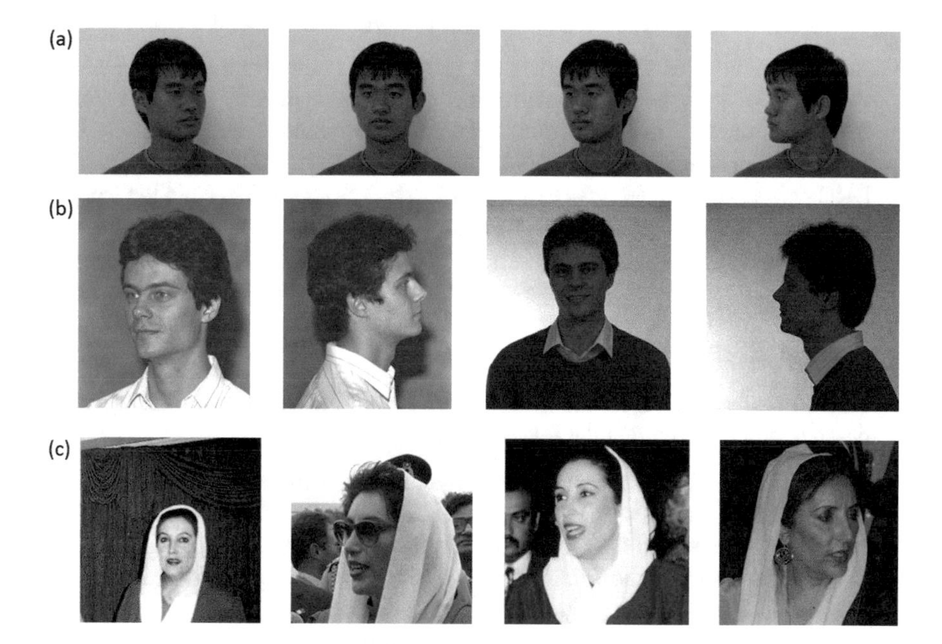

Fig. 4 Sample of the image datasets used; variations in each dataset are illustrated. (**a**) A sample of FEI dataset where images are taken in a controlled environment. (**b**) Corresponds to FERET dataset where images are taken in controlled environment and at different time sessions. (**c**) Sample from the IJB-A dataset where faces are collected in the wild with different poses and facial appearance

- FERET [17]: The FERET database was originally collected to provide large face database to the research community. It was collected between August 1993 and July 1996. The database contains 1564 sets of images for a total of 14126 images that includes 1199 individuals and 365 duplicate sets of images. Every set is collected for a person with several images ranging from pose degree $-90°$ to $90°$. A duplicate set is a second set of images of a person already in the database where images in the latter set were taken on a different day. Images of some people are taken over the span of 2 years. This ensures different facial features of the same person to be included in the experiments.
- IJB-A [18]: The IARPA Janus Benchmark-A (IJB-A) contains 25,813 images of 500 subjects collected in an uncontrolled environment. Faces in IJB-A dataset contain several poses with semi-profile faces unlike LFW [3] dataset which contains mostly frontal poses. This dataset is considered one of the most challenging face datasets since images are collected in an uncontrolled environment (illumination, background, pose variation, etc.) with varying pose of individuals and facial appearance.

4.2 Experiments

To evaluate the performance of the face frontalization techniques mentioned in Sect. 3.2, for every test face image we apply the following alignment steps:

- No Alignment: This step considers the face image output from the face detector without applying any face frontalization technique. It directly extracts features from the image. This step is important to check whether not using any face frontalization technique is actually better.
- DRGAN: We use the features extracted (DR-FV) from DRGAN and the frontalized image (DR-Image) to extract its features using our trained feature extraction technique.
- Effective Frontalization: We use two rotated images output for a given face as shown in Fig. 3, namely symmetric (EF-Sym) and nonsymmetric face (EF-NonSym).

For FEI and FERET datasets, we evaluated the performance of the face frontalization technique by running the following tests.

- Frontal Faces: We generate a subset of the datasets using only frontal faces. We evaluated the accuracy of this subset of faces by getting one random frontal face from every person and then testing all these subset images whether they belong to the same person or not. Using this evaluation subset, the performance of the methods is expected to be high since the faces are frontal.
- Profile Faces: We followed the same procedure as for frontal faces described above, but this time using profile faces subset from these datasets. The performance in this subset is where most face feature extraction techniques fail and we are trying to improve.

- Angled Faces: In this experiment, we split faces into subsets depending on the angle of every face, such that every face with the same angle is in the same subset. We then compare all these subsets of angled faces to a set of one frontal face of every person and calculate the accuracy of every angle set. In this experiment, extreme poses are expected to perform lower than other poses.

As for the IJB-A face dataset, it provides 10 splits of face verification instances. Each split contains tens of thousands of face images pairs. Face verification is done when two images are fed to a system which should decide if these two images belong to the same person or not. From the result, we can derive the confusion matrix of the verification system to calculate the accuracy of the different frontalization techniques on each split.

A sample of original faces with their corresponding generated faces are shown in Fig. 5. We show samples for two different people taken from the FEI dataset ranging from −90 to +90 degrees of face pose. The effective frontalization method as shown in Fig. 5 (Sym and NonSym faces) performs poorly for angles greater than 45 degrees as the 3D modelling fails to complete the missing half of the face. However, it performs reasonably good when most of the face is visible. DRGAN has not reported good results even for frontal faces; the output of the method is mostly a new generated face which sometimes may be very off.

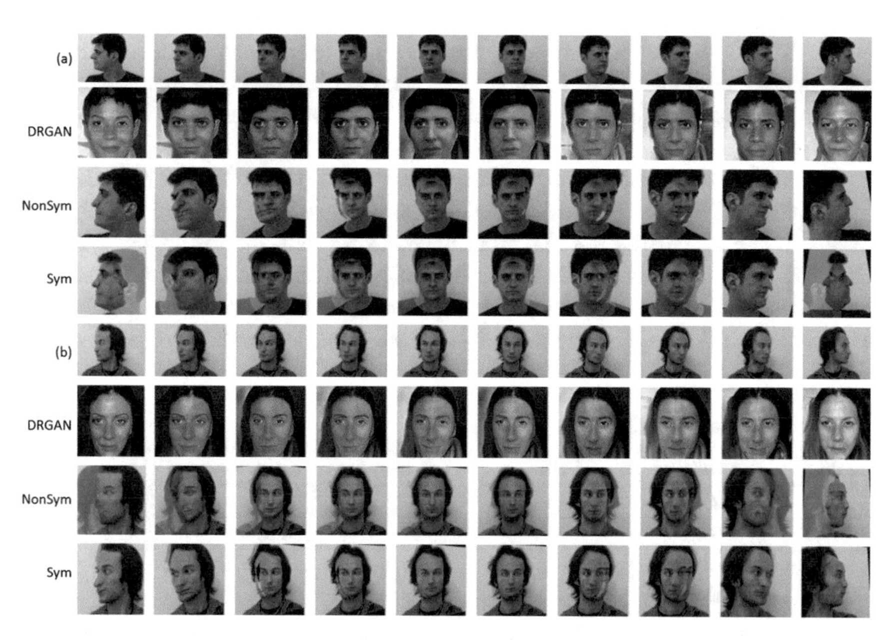

Fig. 5 Sample of the different face frontalization techniques output using two people's set of images

4.3 Results

Table 1 reports accuracy results for frontal face subsets of FEI and FERET datasets. These accuracy results (100% and $\tilde{9}7\%$, respectively) are the best for both datasets when faces are directly used (with no alignment). This is something expected for frontal faces. Using DRGAN, the feature extraction technique (DR-FV) performed second best with accuracy of 92.55% on FERET dataset. On the other hand, using the faces generated from this method reported slightly lower accuracy, 90.14%. However, by using the effective frontalization technique, accuracy levels dropped into the range of 70% for FERET dataset. Accuracy is higher on FEI dataset compared to FERET because the latter dataset contains face images taken at different time instances. This resulted in different facial features, and made it a harder dataset for face recognition.

Table 2 shows accuracy results for profile faces from FEI and FERET datasets. As expected, the performance is lower on profile faces than it is on frontal ones. The results reported in Table 2 demonstrate how using unaligned faces has produced high accuracy on both datasets comparable to using frontal ones ($\tilde{9}9\%$). However, for frontalized faces, the performance dropped significantly to around 80% when DRGAN was used and to around 40% by using effective frontalization method on FERET dataset. From experimenting with FEI and FERET datasets, it can be easily realized that using a neural network feature extraction method on any pose image performs well and better than using frontalization techniques when trained on a large dataset. Although frontalization techniques performed lower than the original images, DRGAN performed well enough on both datasets, around 98 and 82%, respectively.

Tables 3 and 4 show in detail at what angles of faces does different frontalization techniques perform for FEI and FERET datasets, respectively. From the reported results, it can be easily seen that from angle 45 to −45, the results are good for DRGAN and no rotation, while FR performed poorly in general. Going to extreme poses at 90 and −90, the accuracy of no rotation is the best followed by the features extracted from DRGAN, while using frontalized faces performed very poorly.

Table 1 Frontal set accuracy

Frontal	No alignment	DR-FV	DR-image	EF-NonSym	EF-Sym
FEI	100	99	99	98	94.5
FERET	96.88	92.55	90.14	78.67	71.23

Table 2 Profile accuracy

Frontal	No alignment	DR-FV	DR-Image	EF-NonSym	EF-Sym
FEI	99.5	99.5	98	74.5	69
FERET	98.05	93.84	82.38	45.62	36.43

Table 3 FEI angular results

Angle	No alignment	DR-FV	DR-image	EF-NonSym	EF-Sym
−90	82	71	43	14	8.5
−75	100	94	76.5	28	16
−45	100	98.5	91.96	42.7	45.68
−25	99.5	99	95.5	64.5	49
25	100	99.5	95.5	63.5	63
45	100	99	93.5	44	44.5
75	99	95.98	81.9	18.1	17.59
90	93.5	75.5	58.5	11.5	6.5

Table 4 FERET angular results

Angle	No alignment	DR-FV	DR-image	EF-NonSym	EF-Sym
−90	56.66	40.41	22.46	4.63	2.71
−45	95.39	85.12	62.05	18.22	12.46
−15	98.6	88.82	84.63	54.29	44.11
15	99.2	91.42	84.83	56.29	45.91
45	95.54	83.28	60.76	23.3	14.05
90	55.35	41.05	23.36	7.97	3.6

Table 5 IJBA verification results

Split	No alignment	DR-FV	DR-image	EF-NonSym	EF-Sym
1	86.71	21.16	83.63	42.99	44.26
2	88.39	18.81	85.48	45.22	46.69
3	90.26	16.16	87.92	40.74	43.23
4	87.54	20.07	84.78	42.46	44.79
5	89.71	18.58	86.48	42.57	44.03
6	89.05	17.62	86.53	42.43	44.00
7	88.81	17.43	86.53	41.48	43.69
8	89.45	18.02	86.27	42.87	44.54
9	88.13	18.75	85.35	41.78	44.06
10	88.19	18.79	85.17	43.82	45.52

Table 5 shows recognition results of IJB-A across the ten splits. Some interesting results have been reported for this dataset. Using frontalized images, DRGAN performed comparably very good ($\tilde{8}5\%$) across all splits compared to using no alignment ($\tilde{8}8\%$). On the other hand, feature vector extraction from DRGAN (which performed well for the previous datasets) reported very poor ($\tilde{1}9\%$) in an uncontrolled environment (wild). The effective frontalization technique, however, reported on average around ($\tilde{4}4\%$) for both symmetric and nonsymmetric faces output from the method.

5 Conclusion

Interest in face recognition has evolved in recent years to tackle the problem of identifying faces in the wild. Faces in the wild are captured in an uncontrolled environment (public places) where faces can be captured in an any pose, occluded, cluttered, etc. Early face recognition methods that reported good results for faces captured under certain prespecified conditions are not directly applicable to current datasets which contain faces in uncontrolled environments and in multi-view scenarios. To satisfy this purpose, recent methods are capable of handling the multi-view face recognition problem either by training one neural network model with huge number of faces to extract representative features of every person or by applying face frontalization to get a frontal face of any given input face. A frontal face can be later fed into a feature extraction model. Challenges facing face frontalization techniques include generating a frontal face that has enough details and representation of the human face even in extreme poses where more than half of the face is not visible. Face frontalization methods either use 3D modelling of a face and try to complete a face from existing facial features or use neural networks to generate new frontal face images (GAN).

In this study, we analyzed the performance of recent face frontalization techniques compared to using profile faces as it is the case in different types of challenging datasets. The results reported in Sect. 4.3 demonstrated that using frontalized faces leads to better performance in controlled environments and with several pose variations. However, the same process performs poorly when the angle of the face is more than 75° compared to the good accuracy result given while using no alignment for the face. Also, using frontalized faces from uncontrolled environment has produced poor performance. This shows that still for face recognition, training one model to extract features of faces is expected to perform better than current methods for frontalized faces. While frontalized faces can be considered as a visualization technique for analysts to better view of the identity and not for face recognition purposes.

References

1. Ahonen, T., Hadid, A., & Pietikainen, M. (2006). Face description with local binary patterns: Application to face recognition. *IEEE Transactions on Pattern Analysis and Machine Intelligence, 28*(12), 2037–2041.
2. Turk, M. A., & Pentland, A. P. (1991). Face recognition using eigenfaces. In *IEEE Computer Society Conference on Computer Vision and Pattern Recognition, 1991. Proceedings CVPR'91* (pp. 586–591). Piscataway: IEEE.
3. Huang, G. B., Ramesh, M., Berg, T., & Learned-Miller, E. (2007). Labeled faces in the wild: A database for studying face recognition in unconstrained environments. Technical report, Technical Report 07-49, University of Massachusetts, Amherst.
4. Cao, Z., Yin, Q., Tang, X., & Sun, J. (2010). Face recognition with learning-based descriptor. In *2010 IEEE Conference on Computer Vision and Pattern Recognition (CVPR)* (pp. 2707–2714). Piscataway: IEEE.

5. Schroff, F., Kalenichenko, D., & Philbin, J. (2015). Facenet: A unified embedding for face recognition and clustering. In *Proceedings of the IEEE Conference on Computer Vision and Pattern Recognition* (pp. 815–823).
6. Taigman, Y., Yang, M., Ranzato, M., & Wolf, L. (2014). Deepface: Closing the gap to human-level performance in face verification. In *Proceedings of the IEEE Conference on Computer Vision and Pattern Recognition* (pp. 1701–1708).
7. Sun, Y., Wang, X., & Tang, X. (2014). Deep learning face representation from predicting 10,000 classes. In *Proceedings of the IEEE Conference on Computer Vision and Pattern Recognition* (pp. 1891–1898).
8. Sun, Y., Liang, D., Wang, X., & Tang, X. (2015). Deepid3: Face recognition with very deep neural networks. Preprint arXiv:1502.00873.
9. Kumar, N., Berg, A. C., Belhumeur, P. N., & Nayar, S. K. (2009). Attribute and simile classifiers for face verification. In *2009 IEEE 12th International Conference on Computer Vision* (pp. 365–372). Piscataway: IEEE.
10. Sengupta, S., Chen, J.-C., Castillo, C., Patel, V. M., Chellappa, R., & Jacobs, D. W. (2016). Frontal to profile face verification in the wild. In *2016 IEEE Winter Conference on Applications of Computer Vision (WACV)* (pp. 1–9). Piscataway: IEEE.
11. Hassner, T., Harel, S., Paz, E., & Enbar, R. (2015). Effective face frontalization in unconstrained images. In *Proceedings of the IEEE Conference on Computer Vision and Pattern Recognition* (pp. 4295–4304).
12. Yim, J., Jung, H., Yoo, B., Choi, C., Park, D., & Kim, J. (2015). Rotating your face using multi-task deep neural network. In *Proceedings of the IEEE Conference on Computer Vision and Pattern Recognition* (pp. 676–684).
13. Tran, L., Yin, X., & Liu, X. (2017). Disentangled representation learning GAN for pose-invariant face recognition. In *CVPR* (Vol. 3, p. 7).
14. Huang, R., Zhang, S., Li, T., He, R., et al. (2017). Beyond face rotation: Global and local perception GAN for photorealistic and identity preserving frontal view synthesis. Preprint arXiv:1704.04086.
15. Yi, D., Lei, Z., Liao, S., & Li, S. Z. (2014). Learning face representation from scratch. Preprint arXiv:1411.7923.
16. Thomaz, C. E. (2012). Fei face database. http://fei.edu.br/~cet/facedatabase.html. Accessed 2 October 2012.
17. Phillips, P. J., Moon, H., Rizvi, S. A., & Rauss, P. J. (2000). The feret evaluation methodology for face-recognition algorithms. *IEEE Transactions on Pattern Analysis and Machine Intelligence, 22*(10), 1090–1104.
18. Klare, B. F., Klein, B., Taborsky, E., Blanton, A., Cheney, J., Allen, K., et al. (2015). Pushing the frontiers of unconstrained face detection and recognition: IARPA Janus Benchmark A. In *Proceedings of the IEEE Conference on Computer Vision and Pattern Recognition* (pp. 1931–1939).
19. Masi, I., Rawls, S., Medioni, G., & Natarajan, P. (2016). Pose-aware face recognition in the wild. In *Proceedings of the IEEE Conference on Computer Vision and Pattern Recognition* (pp. 4838–4846).
20. Huang, G., Mattar, M., Lee, H., & Learned-Miller, E. G. (2012). Learning to align from scratch. In *Advances in Neural Information Processing Systems* (pp. 764–772).
21. Wolf, L., Hassner, T., & Taigman, Y. (2009). Similarity scores based on background samples. In *Asian Conference on Computer Vision* (pp. 88–97). Berlin: Springer.
22. Zhu, X., Lei, Z., Yan, J., Yi, D., & Li, S. Z. (2015). High-fidelity pose and expression normalization for face recognition in the wild. In *Proceedings of the IEEE Conference on Computer Vision and Pattern Recognition* (pp. 787–796).
23. Zhu, Z., Luo, P., Wang, X., & Tang, X. (2014). Multi-view perceptron: A deep model for learning face identity and view representations. In *Advances in Neural Information Processing Systems* (pp. 217–225).

24. Goodfellow, I., Pouget-Abadie, J., Mirza, M., Xu, B., Warde-Farley, D., Ozair, S., et al. Generative adversarial nets. In *Advances in Neural Information Processing Systems* (pp. 2672–2680).
25. Denton, E. L., Chintala, S., Fergus, R., et al. (2015). Deep generative image models using a Laplacian pyramid of adversarial networks. In *Advances in Neural Information Processing Systems* (pp. 1486–1494).
26. Ledig, C., Theis, L., Huszár, F., Caballero, J., Cunningham, A., Acosta, A., et al. (2016). Photo-realistic single image super-resolution using a generative adversarial network. arXiv preprint.
27. Yu, X., & Porikli, F. (2016). Ultra-resolving face images by discriminative generative networks. In *European Conference on Computer Vision* (pp. 318–333). Berlin: Springer.
28. Reed, S., Akata, Z., Yan, X., Logeswaran, L., Schiele, B., & Lee, H. (2016). Generative adversarial text to image synthesis. Preprint arXiv:1605.05396.
29. Isola, P., Zhu, J.-Y., Zhou, T., & Efros, A. A. (2017). Image-to-image translation with conditional adversarial networks. arXiv preprint.
30. Wu, X., He, R., Sun, Z., & Tan, T. (2015). A light CNN for deep face representation with noisy labels. Preprint arXiv:1511.02683.
31. Gross, R., Matthews, I., Cohn, J., Kanade, T., & Baker, S. (2010). Multi-pie. *Image and Vision Computing, 28*(5), 807–813.
32. Viola, P., & Jones, M. (2001). Rapid object detection using a boosted cascade of simple features. In *Proceedings of the 2001 IEEE Computer Society Conference on Computer Vision and Pattern Recognition, 2001. CVPR 2001* (Vol. 1, pp. I–I). Piscataway: IEEE.
33. Dalal, N., & Triggs, B. (2005). Histograms of oriented gradients for human detection. In *IEEE Computer Society Conference on Computer Vision and Pattern Recognition, 2005. CVPR 2005* (Vol. 1, pp. 886–893). Piscataway: IEEE.
34. Wu, B., Ai, H., Huang, C., & Lao, S. (2004). Fast rotation invariant multi-view face detection based on real Adaboost. In *Sixth IEEE International Conference on Automatic Face and Gesture Recognition, 2004. Proceedings* (pp. 79–84). Piscataway: IEEE.
35. Huang, C., Ai, H., Li, Y., & Lao, S. (2005). Vector boosting for rotation invariant multi-view face detection. In *Tenth IEEE International Conference on Computer Vision, 2005. ICCV 2005* (Vol. 1, pp. 446–453). Piscataway: IEEE.
36. Jones, M., & Viola, P. (2003). Fast multi-view face detection. *Mitsubishi Electric Research Lab TR-20003-96, 3*, 14.
37. Zhang, C., & Zhang, Z. (2014). Improving multiview face detection with multi-task deep convolutional neural networks. In *2014 IEEE Winter Conference on Applications of Computer Vision (WACV)* (pp. 1036–1041). Piscataway: IEEE.
38. Farfade, S. S., Saberian, M. J., & Li, L.-J. (2015). Multi-view face detection using deep convolutional neural networks. In *Proceedings of the 5th ACM on International Conference on Multimedia Retrieval* (pp. 643–650). New York: ACM.
39. Krizhevsky, A., Sutskever, I., & Hinton, G. E. (2012). Imagenet classification with deep convolutional neural networks. In *Advances in Neural Information Processing Systems* (pp. 1097–1105).
40. Jain, V., & Learned-Miller, E. G. (2010). Fddb: A benchmark for face detection in unconstrained settings. *UMass Amherst Technical Report.*
41. Li, H., Lin, Z., Shen, X., Brandt, J., & Hua, G. (2015). A convolutional neural network cascade for face detection. In *Proceedings of the IEEE Conference on Computer Vision and Pattern Recognition* (pp. 5325–5334).
42. Girshick, R., Donahue, J., Darrell, T., & Malik, J. (2014). Rich feature hierarchies for accurate object detection and semantic segmentation. In *Proceedings of the IEEE Conference on Computer Vision and Pattern Recognition*, (pp. 580–587).
43. Uijlings, J. R. R., Van De Sande, K. E. A., Gevers, T., & Smeulders, A. W. M. (2013). Selective search for object recognition. *International Journal of Computer Vision, 104*(2), 154–171.
44. Zitnick, C. L., & Dollár, P. (2014). Edge boxes: Locating object proposals from edges. In *European Conference on Computer Vision* (pp. 391–405). Berlin: Springer.

45. Girshick, R. (2015). Fast R-CNN. In *Proceedings of the IEEE International Conference on Computer Vision* (pp. 1440–1448).
46. Ren, S., He, K., Girshick, R., & Sun, J. (2015). Faster R-CNN: Towards real-time object detection with region proposal networks. In *Advances in Neural Information Processing Systems* (pp. 91–99).
47. Jiang, H., & Learned-Miller, E. (2016). Face detection with the faster R-CNN. Preprint arXiv:1606.03473.
48. Yang, S., Luo, P., Loy, C.-C., & Tang, X. (2016). Wider face: A face detection benchmark. In *Proceedings of the IEEE Conference on Computer Vision and Pattern Recognition* (pp. 5525–5533).
49. Howard, A. G., Zhu, M., Chen, B., Kalenichenko, D., Wang, W., Weyand, T., et al. (2017). Mobilenets: Efficient convolutional neural networks for mobile vision applications. Preprint arXiv:1704.04861.
50. Lowe, D. G. (2004). Distinctive image features from scale-invariant keypoints. *International Journal of Computer Vision, 60*(2), 91–110.
51. Bay, H., Tuytelaars, T., & Van Gool, L. (2006). Surf: Speeded up robust features. *Computer Vision-ECCV 2006* (pp. 404–417).
52. Geng, C., & Jiang, X. (2009). Face recognition using sift features. In *2009 16th IEEE International Conference on Image Processing (ICIP)* (pp. 3313–3316). Piscataway: IEEE.
53. Bicego, M., Lagorio, A., Grosso, E., & Tistarelli, M. (2006). On the use of sift features for face authentication. In *Conference on Computer Vision and Pattern Recognition Workshop, 2006. CVPRW'06* (pp. 35–35). Piscataway: IEEE.
54. Du, G., Su, F., & Cai, A. (2009). Face recognition using surf features. In *Sixth International Symposium on Multispectral Image Processing and Pattern Recognition* (pp. 749628–749628). International Society for Optics and Photonics.
55. Chan, C.-H., Kittler, J., & Messer, K. (2007). Multi-scale local binary pattern histograms for face recognition. In *Advances in Biometrics* (pp. 809–818).
56. Sharif Razavian, A., Azizpour, H., Sullivan, J., & Carlsson, S. (2014). Cnn features off-the-shelf: An astounding baseline for recognition. In *Proceedings of the IEEE Conference on Computer Vision and Pattern Recognition Workshops* (pp. 806–813).
57. Szegedy, C., Ioffe, S., Vanhoucke, V., & Alemi, A. A. (2017). Inception-v4, inception-resnet and the impact of residual connections on learning. In *AAAI* (Vol. 4, p. 12).
58. Guo, Y., Zhang, L., Hu, Y., He, X., & Gao, J. (2016). MS-Celeb-1M: A dataset and benchmark for large scale face recognition. In *European Conference on Computer Vision*. Berlin: Springer.

A Data Management Scheme for Micro-Level Modular Computation-Intensive Programs in Big Data Platforms

Debasish Chakroborti, Banani Roy, Amit Mondal, Golam Mostaeen, Chanchal K. Roy, Kevin A. Schneider, and Ralph Deters

Abstract Big Data analytics or systems developed with parallel distributed processing frameworks (e.g., Hadoop and Spark) are becoming popular for finding important insights from a huge amount of heterogeneous data (e.g., image, text, and sensor data). These systems offer a wide range of tools and connect them to form workflows for processing Big Data. Independent schemes from different studies for managing programs and data of workflows have been already proposed by many researchers and most of the systems have been presented with data or metadata management. However, to the best of our knowledge, no study particularly discusses the performance implications of utilizing intermediate states of data and programs generated at various execution steps of a workflow in distributed platforms. In order to address the shortcomings, we propose a scheme of Big Data management for micro-level modular computation-intensive programs in a Spark and Hadoop-based platform. In this paper, we investigate whether management of the intermediate states can speed up the execution of an image processing pipeline consisting of various image processing tools/APIs in Hadoop Distributed File System (HDFS) while ensuring appropriate reusability and error monitoring. From our experiments, we obtained prominent results, e.g., we have reported that with the intermediate data management, we can gain up to 87% computation time for an image processing job.

Keywords Data management · Modular programming · Computation-intensive program · Big Data · Distributed environment · Intermediate state

---

D. Chakroborti (✉) · B. Roy · A. Mondal · G. Mostaeen · C. K. Roy · K. A. Schneider · R. Deters
Department of Computer Science, University of Saskatchewan, Saskatoon, SK, Canada
e-mail: debasish.chakroborti@usask.ca; banani.roy@usask.ca; amit.mondal@usask.ca; golam.mostaeen@usask.ca; chanchal.roy@usask.ca; kevin.schneider@usask.ca; ralph.deters@usask.ca

R. Alhajj et al. (eds.), *Data Management and Analysis*, Studies in Big Data 65,
https://doi.org/10.1007/978-3-030-32587-9_9

1 Introduction

With the rapid advancement of Big Data platforms, software systems [11, 13, 14, 23, 28] are being developed to provide an interactive environment for large-scale data analysis to the end users in the area of scientific research, business, government, and journalism. Big Data platforms such as Hadoop, Spark, and Google Dataflow provide us a high-level abstract interface for implementing distributed-cluster processing of data. Recently, many researchers [5, 13, 24, 29] have focused on developing architectures and frameworks for large-scale data analysis tools utilizing these platforms. Most of these architectural frameworks are adopting workflows or pipelines [18, 21, 23] for data analysis to provide flexible job creation environment. Workflows, in general, connect a sequence of interoperating tools to accomplish a task. For example, in order to find features from images of a large crop field, different image processing tools such as *image registration, stitching, segmentation, clustering, and feature finding tools* are needed to be connected in order to form a workflow. In such workflow management systems, modularization is important to support scalability and heterogeneity. Thus, a wide range of tools is incorporated where each tool is treated as an independent process or module or service and can be implemented using different programming languages. Traditionally, researchers and data analysts require to run same workflows frequently with different algorithms and models that causes overwhelming efforts even with the moderate size of data by running all of the modules in the workflows. Utilization dimensions of those modules can be increased by storing their outcomes as intermediate states in such systems. In other words the possibility to use the transformed data in later stages to reduce computation time, to enhance reusability, and to ensure error recovery can be increased by a proper data management.

Modular programming is a software design approach that draws attention to uncoupling the functionalities of a script towards independent, interchangeable, reusable units [17]. On the other hand, data modularity is always anticipated for quick and flexible access to a dataset. In this paper, the intermediate states of data are being recognized as modular data which are outcomes of modular programs. The dynamic management of datasets is another ground to have intermediate states for a huge amount of data [1]. Some other common benefits of intermediate data are sustainability, scalability, quick construction, and cost savings [1, 8, 16, 26]. In many circumstances of a data-intensive distributed application, image processing is an inevitable part where contemporary technologies of image analysis are pertinent for processing a large set of image data. However, special care is needed for both image data and program to process a huge amount of data with such emerging technologies. To make users' tasks more realistic in real time for Big Data analytics in image processing, intermediate modular data states can be an appreciable settlement to design and observe pipelines or workflows. In image-based tasks, the common execution operations (such as pre-processing, transformation, model fitting, and analysis) can be wrapped up as modules, and their outputs can be used for both observation and post-processing. Another important aspect of Big Data analytics is to store lots of data in a way that can be accessed in a low-cost [10], thus data management with the reusable intermediate data and program states might be a great deal to restore program state by reflecting the lower cost.

A distributed image processing system requires huge storage and data processing time for high-resolution large files. For such a system, stored intermediate states can be fruitful rather than transmitting raw files for a paralleled task. Spark itself generates some intermediate states of data in its processing engine to reduce IO cost [31]. Hence, in our modular programming paradigm, if we introduce a mechanism of storing intermediate states and manage them, we can reuse our data from various modules without computation which eventually minimizes total cost of processing. Many researchers and organizations are now pointing up on long time data processing with distributed parallel environments for low cost and convenient system to handle a large amount of data [20]. Following the trends, a machine/deep learning-based algorithm with heterogeneous data is another emerging practice to analyze a large amount of data for agricultural and other data-intensive tasks [22]. Considering the current technologies and trends, our scheme would be a contemporary package to analyze a large amount of image data.

Although a few studies [1, 8, 9, 16, 26] focused on propagated results in the intermediate states in Big Data management, to the best of our knowledge none reflected the performance implications of reusability of intermediate data and model in distributed platforms. Moreover, these studies do not show how the intermediate states across various image processing workflows can be reused. To fill the gap, in this paper we investigated whether the intermediate states generated from modular programs can speed up the overall execution time of workflows in Hadoop/Spark-based distributed processing units by assuring enhanced reusability and error recovery. Here our idea was that loading intermediate states from Hadoop Distributed File System (HDFS) might take longer than generating them in memory during the execution of a workflow. In order to figure out the actual situations, we developed a web-based interactive environment where users can easily access intermediate states and associated them across various workflows, e.g., some outcomes of the image segmentation pipeline are reusable to the image clustering and registration pipelines. We found that even though it takes some time to load intermediate states from an HDFS-based storage, a workflow can be executed faster in a system of handled intermediate states in persistent memory than a system of no intermediate states in persistent memory. Our finding is described in Fig. 5 for various workflows. In the figure, we illustrate if we can skip some modules with the help of stored intermediate states, we can get better performance than the case of without storing intermediate states. Details of the performance and reusability have been discussed in Sect. 5. The rest of the paper is organized as follows. Section 2 discusses the related work, Sect. 3 presents our proposed scheme of intermediate data management, Sect. 4 describes our experiment setup, Sect. 5 compares our proposed scheme with the usual technique of intermediate data handling by using various image progressing pipelines, Sect. 6 describes some valuable findings towards data management for modular programming and, finally, Sect. 7 concludes the paper.

2 Related Work

A number of studies [3, 7, 13, 29] have investigated recent techniques of file system to process Big Data and some studies [4, 12, 18, 19, 24] were presented with application of data or image processing in such file systems with metadata management. Similarly, various databases, algorithms, tools, technologies, and storage systems are acknowledged in a number of studies while solving the problem of Big Data processing for image analysis and plant-based research in distributed environments. Studies related to phenotyping, image processing, and intermediate states in distributed environments are considered to compare with our work, and some of them are presented below in three subsections.

2.1 Study on File Systems of Big Data Processing

Blomer [3] investigates various file systems of computer systems and compared them with parallel distributed file systems. Benefits of both distributed and core file systems of computer systems are discussed. As well as, a distributed file system as a layer of the main file system has been addressed with common facilities and problems. In their work, data and metadata management's key points are also discussed for map-reduce-based problems and fault tolerance concept. Luyen et al. [13] experiment on different data storage systems with a large amount of data for phenotyping investigation. Their work on a number of heterogeneous database systems and technologies such as MongoDB, RDF, and SPARQL explores possibilities of interoperability and performance. Similar to the above studies, Donvito et al. [7] discuss and compare various popular distributed storage technologies such as HDFS, Ceph, and GlusterFS. Wang et al. [29] propose a technique of metadata replication in Hadoop-based parallel distributed framework for failure recovery. By emphasizing metadata replications in slave nodes for reliable data access in Big Data ecosystem, the proposed metadata replication technique works in three stages such as initialization, replication, and failover recovery. Similarly, Li et al. [12] propose a log-based metadata replication and recovery model for metadata management in a distributed environment for high performance, balanced load, reliability, and scalability. In their work, caching and prefetching technologies are used for the metadata to enhance performance. While above studies focus on metadata management in various file systems, our study is fundamentally different with an investigation of a scheme of intermediate data management for distributed file systems considering reusability, error recovery, and execution at a lower cost.

2.2 Big Data in Terms of Image Processing

Minervini et al. [14] discuss different challenges in phenotyping by addressing the current limitations in image processing technologies, where collaboration is emphasized from diverse research group to overcome the challenges. Collaboration is an essential part of a scientific workflow management system (SWfMS) to overcome the limitations of managing data from diverse domains. In this study, we overcome the limitations of managing heterogeneous data by proposing a data management scheme for a SWfMS. The main focus of this study is the association of intermediate states with micro-level modular computational-intensive programs while composing workflows in a distributed environment. Some other studies on phenotyping concentrate on the costs of processing and appropriate usage of current technologies to reduce the costs such as Minervini et al. [15] propose a context-aware-based capturing technique for JPEG images that will be processed by distributed receivers in a phenotyping environment. Singh et al. [22] provide a comprehensive study on ML tools in phenotyping area for appropriate and correct application of them in plant research. Coppens et al. [4] emphasize data management for automated phenotyping and explore the image metadata potentiality for synergism (usage of metadata with main features). Sensor's metadata of imaging technique could be used by appropriate filtering for the synergism is also addressed in their work. Smith et al. [24] address the importance of metadata in Big Data ecosystems to migrate and share data or code from one environment to another. Data consolidation, analysis, discovery, error, and integration also have been scrutinized from metadata usage perspective in the Big Data environment. Pineda-Morales et al. [19] emphasize on both file metadata and task metadata to propose a model for filtering hot metadata. After categorizing and analyzing both hot and cold metadata, they recommend for distributing hot metadata (frequently accessed) and centralizing cold metadata in a system of data management. Although the above works show the behavior and direction of metadata, none of them analyze the processed data or intermediate data as metadata for efficient management. In our work, modular outcomes of computational intensive programs are analyzed, and a scheme is proposed to store those intermediate outcomes for efficiency in a SWfMS.

2.3 Study on Intermediate-Data

Becker et al. [1] survey on current Big Data usage and emphasize on intermediate data behavior for iterative analysis at every stage of processing to minimize the overall response time with an algorithmic perspective. Besides, intermediate data can be saved in persistent storage at checkpoints was considered for error recovery. Similarly, Heit et al. [9] explained the nature of intermediate data while proposing a Big Data processing framework for statistical models. They also stated that intermediate data should be independent in a system to use them in different components. Intermediate data management is considered by Tudoran et al. [26], where they pointed out storing of intermediate-data for rollback purposes from the application level. Intermediate data for checkpoints analysis are also considered by Mistrik and Bahsoon in their work [16]. Likewise, how intermediate data are dispatched in parallel distributed systems such as Spark, Hadoop is discussed by Han and Hong [8] in their book by bringing together and analyzing various areas of Big Data processing.

Although, some of the above works were discussed with the fault-tolerant concept using intermediate states, none of them discussed the possibility and necessity of storing intermediate data for Big Data analytics in a distributed environment. Reviewing the above works, we realized that in a distributed environment efficient data access mechanism is a big concern and time implications for both data storing and loading are needed to be observed in a distributed environment. Focusing these, we investigate the possibility of a data management mechanism by storing intermediate states with the help of modularized programs for enhancing processing time, reusability, and error recovery.

3 Proposed Method

Modular programming for computation-intensive tasks is already a proven technology for reusability of code [2, 6, 25, 27], but for large raw data transaction and loading from distributed systems, we cannot fully use the proficiency of modularity. On the other hand, processed data require less memory, transaction, and loading time. Having both these knowledge, we store processed intermediate data with other program data and want to explore three research questions in a SWfMS, such as

- **RQ1:** Does the system support data reusability that ultimately reduces time and efforts?
- **RQ2:** Does it have any error recovery mechanism that could construct workflows quicker if errors occur?
- **RQ3:** and How the system is supporting fast processing for frequently used workflows?

Answers to these three research questions have been presented in Sect. 5. To use both of these intermediate data and modular programs, and explore the usability of modular outcomes in our full system a modularized data access mechanism is introduced. We have an interactive web interface, which is used for accessing datasets of various modules' input and output. A dedicated distributed data server where images and intermediate data are stored was used in our system for parallel processing. From the web interface, image processing workflows can be built, and modules of the workflows can be submitted to a distributed processing master node as jobs, by this way distributed image data are processed with specified modules from the workflows.

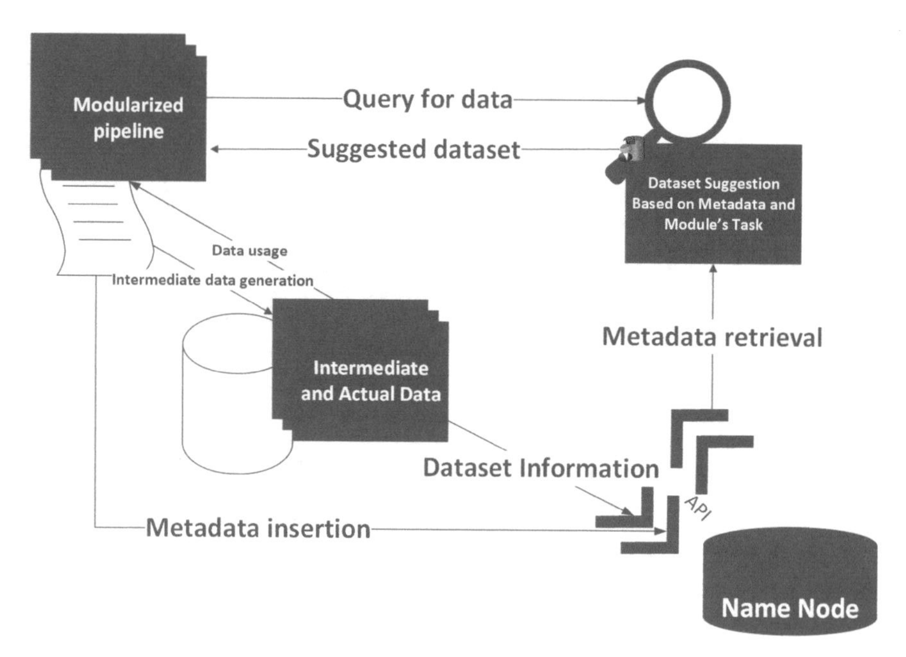

Fig. 1 Proposed data management scheme

Two major types of metadata of image processing environment are file-structure-metadata and result-metadata [19]. In our system, we managed both kinds of metadata using APIs that retrieve and store information on a dedicated Hadoop server. This dedicated server is designed to facilitate various parallel processing from different modules of pipelines or workflows. When a SHIPPI's (Spark High-throughput Image Processing Pipeline) module needed to be executed for a task, available data or intermediate data states are suggested from a web interface with the help of the metadata and HDFS APIs (e.g., Fig. 1). SHIPPI is our designed library that provides cloud-based APIs for the modular functionality of image processing [17]. Details of the SHIPPI has been described in the experimental setup section, i.e., Sect. 4. Our system at first tries to find suitable datasets for a modular task with task information and information from the metadata server, suggested datasets are presented on a web interface to be selected for a particular task from our distributed storage system, i.e., HDFS. Suggested datasets can be an intermediate or raw data, but the intermediate states will always have a higher priority to be selected if available. Another important task of our system is to keep track of metadata and intermediate data. After every execution, there are a few outputs from a single module such as analysis results and intermediate data. Intermediate data are stored in a distributed file system with actual data, and analysis results are stored in a server as metadata for future use.

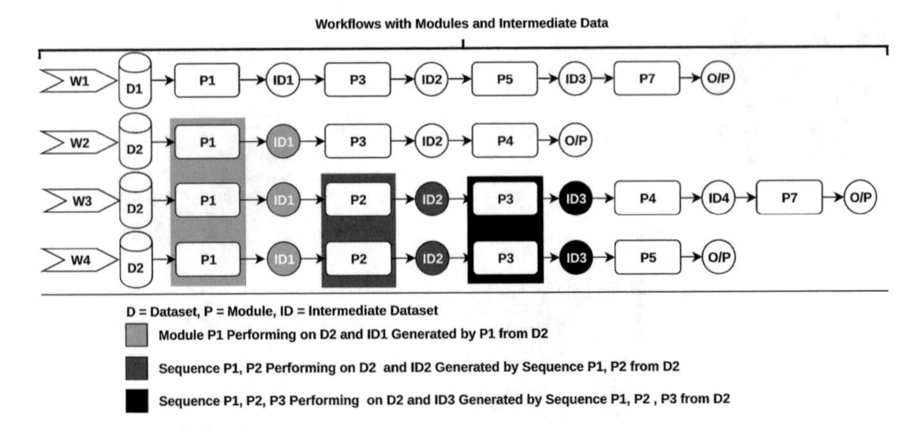

Fig. 2 Reusable intermediate data in workflows

How the proposed scheme of data management by modular programs and intermediate data can introduce reusability, error recovery and faster processing in a Scientific Workflow Management System (SWfMS) is described with simple workflows (Fig. 2). In the figure, four workflows are illustrated with modules and intermediate data. All black and gray marked processes (Ps) and intermediated data (IDs) represent more than the one-time existence of them in the four workflows and possibility to be reused of them. This reusability of them means they are likely to be reused later in either for the same workflow with different tools or the other workflows in a SWfMS. Different intensities of black and gray colors represent the same modules or intermediate states from different workflows in different groups. A particular group is formed for the same operations on the same dataset or for the intermediate states that are being generated for the same operation of module sequences on them with same input dataset. In workflow 1, we have four modules (P1, P3, P5, and P7). These modules perform operations sequentially on dataset D1 and produce three intermediate datasets (ID1, ID2, and ID3), where the last outcome is desired output (O/P). All workflows have some processing modules to perform operations on specific datasets or intermediate datasets for generating desired intermediate outcomes or final results. The intermediate states are usually used by intermediate modules sequentially (N. B. For simplicity we are considering only sequential module processing in workflows.) in workflows. Workflow 2 has three modules (P1, P3, and P4) that generate two intermediate datasets (ID1 and ID2). Workflows 3 and 4 have five and four processing modules with four and three intermediate stages, respectively. Last three workflows in the figure are working on the same dataset D2, and a few modules such as P1, P2, and P3 are frequently used for building those workflows. This scenario opens the possibility of reusability of intermediate states, as it is common in a SWfMS that same modules can be used in different workflows. As well as, the same sequence of operations on the same or different dataset can be occurred in various workflows by supporting the possibility of program reusability. In the workflow 2, an operation by module P1 is performed on dataset D2 and generates intermediate dataset ID1. This operation and the outcome (ID1) are the same in the other three workflows for the same module sequence and same dataset. Same sequence $P1 \rightarrow P2 \rightarrow P3$ in workflow 3 also occurs in workflow 4 with the same input dataset D2. Thus, ID3 (intermediate dataset) from workflow 3 can be directly used in workflow 4 for skipping the first three module operation to analyze with only last module or increase the performance. To introduce this type of efficiency and performance enhancement in a system of workflow management, modules outcome is needed to be stored with appropriate access mechanism. Furthermore, if failures occur in any workflow, stored intermediate states (IDs) can be used to recover the workflow by addressing the issues only in faulty modules. In a distributed environment, data are partitioned and replicated on different nodes, and the transition time of data is not as simple as it is a single file system. Data transfer time from slave nodes to master nodes is needed to be considered for both storing and retrieving. So, for storing and retrieving intermediate data from such distributed systems, experiments are necessary regarding transition and computation time. Our experimental section (Sect. 5) is designed in that way to investigate the actual scenario of I/O operation and computation time for the micro-level modular computation-intensive programs in a distributed environment and explore the possibility of reusability.

4 Experimental Setup

In our experiments, for evaluating a full system performance with the proposed scheme, a web platform is used, a web interface is designed with current web technologies and Flask (A Python micro-framework) web framework. From the web interface, SHIPPI's APIs are called to execute a job in an OpenStack-based Spark-Hadoop cluster (e.g., five-node, 40 cores, and total 210 GB RAM). It provides cloud-based APIs for the modular functionality of image-processing pipeline and automatically parallelizes different modules of a program. Each API call is modularized into four sections such as conversion, estimation, model-fitting, analysis-transform. Figure 4 shows the block diagram of SHIPPI, which represents the relation among different libraries and modules of the framework. In our testing environment, HDFS is used to store our image data for parallel processing. To store intermediate states, we used the Pickle library of Python, and we designed three image processing pipelines—Segmentation, Clustering, and Leaves Recognition following our proposed model discussed in Sect. 3. Every pipeline was tested at least five times and an average of their execution time was recorded. For testing purposes, we mainly used three datasets—*Flavia* [30], *2KCanola*, *4KCanola*. Each of those datasets has more than 2000 images, where *Flavia* is a known dataset used for leaves recognition system, and *2KCanola* and *4KCanola* datasets are from the P2IRC (Plant Phenotyping and Imaging Research Centre) project of University of Saskatchewan used for various purposes of image analysis. The three pipelines are illustrated in Fig. 3, where a single job such as leaves recognition,

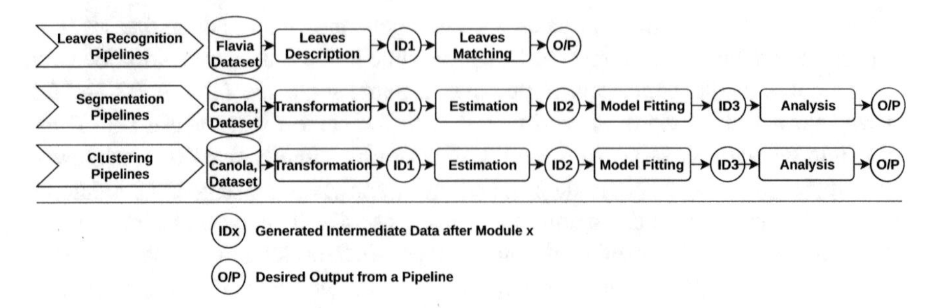

Fig. 3 Pipeline building with image processing tools

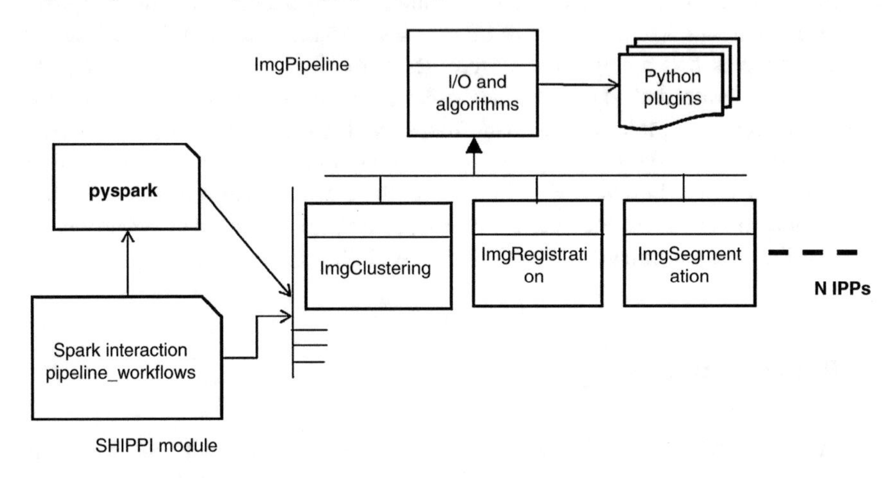

Fig. 4 Block diagram of components of SHIPPI

segmentation, or clustering is built by their respective modularized parts. The first module (Leaves Description) of the leaves recognition pipelines extracts features and prepares data for the next module leaves matching. The next module (Leaves Matching), which is the final module in the leaves recognition pipelines, does the job of comparing those features and reports a classification result of leaves. Similarly, image segmentation and clustering pipelines are modularized by four common modules such as *transformation, estimation, model fitting, and analysis*. Transformation is used for mainly color conversion, estimation is used for feature extraction, model fitting is used for training an algorithm and setting parameters, and the final module analysis is used for testing and result preparation. Pipelines can be built by selecting modules and parameters for submitting a desired task in the distributed environment on the web interface, where each module works as a job in the distributed environment and their outcomes are gathered from a master node and distributed file system for further analysis (Fig. 4).

5 Results and Evaluation

We developed a Spark High-throughput Image Processing Pipeline framework known as SHIPPI, which is an image processing pipeline library to abstract map reduce, data loading, and low-level complexity of image operations. SHIPPI was written in Python 2.7 and Spark 2.0.1, four modules of our modular program paradigm of a pipeline using SHIPPI can be modified based on image processing operations concerning the desired purpose. Furthermore, these modules are parallel with the help of PySpark library, and each output of a module is used in the next module. In a spark-based solution all data are in main memory, so to reuse those processed data, we store them as intermediate states in Hadoop distributed file system from those modules that give reusable data. This system designed not only for reusability but also for error recovery (for the higher failure rate of a long-running program or pipeline with a huge amount of data). Thus, if we store intermediate data, there is a chance for us to recover a system at low cost.

Total eight distinct modules of the three image processing pipelines have been implemented with current technologies, and all of them are designed for both without intermediate and with intermediate data concept. Both transformation and estimation modules in the pipelines use the same technology, and they are similar in the last two pipelines. Figure 5 is the execution-time comparison graph of both of the concepts for the three pipelines in distributed and ubuntu file systems. Although saving intermediate states is a memory overhead task for all of the pipelines in the figure, but there are possibilities to use stored data and skip some processing steps for executing a pipeline at low cost. Skipping procedure eventually increases the flexibility and reusability to analyze fractions of pipelines in low cost. Pipelines

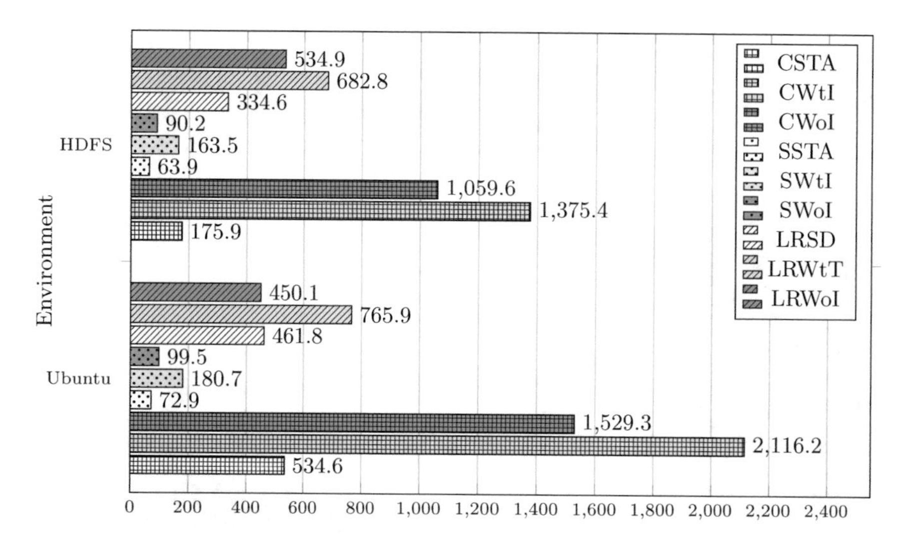

Fig. 5 Performance comparison of workflows with-intermediate and without-intermediate data

with skipped modules by using intermediate data are presented with the improved performance in the figure. Another major concern of our investigation was to explore the trade-off scenario between computation time and data loading/storing time of modules in distributed systems. For investigating this, previously we assumed that a data and metadata transition time among slave and master nodes would be more than a module computation time in a distributed environment. But the experimental results for the pipelines of skipped modules show improved performance and contradict with our assumption regarding time implication of data transfer. Hence, a system of workflow management with distributed processing unit is capable of handling intermediate states, and a scheme is possible to introduce in such systems for reusability, error recovery, and performance enhancement. We organize our experiment into three sections to answer the research questions of our system's usability. All of the three pipelines of image processing are considered in each section for their respective illustrations. Below are the three main subsections of our experiments.

5.1 *Experiment for Reusability*

A collaborative SWfMS is used for design and job submission of the image processing pipelines to a distributed parallel processing system. Figures 6 and 7 show the configuration interface for the image recognition pipelines, which is implemented with SHIPPI's four-phase modular architecture where only two modules are considered for simplicity. Intermediate state from the first module of this pipeline can be reusable to image matching modules. So, an outcome of the

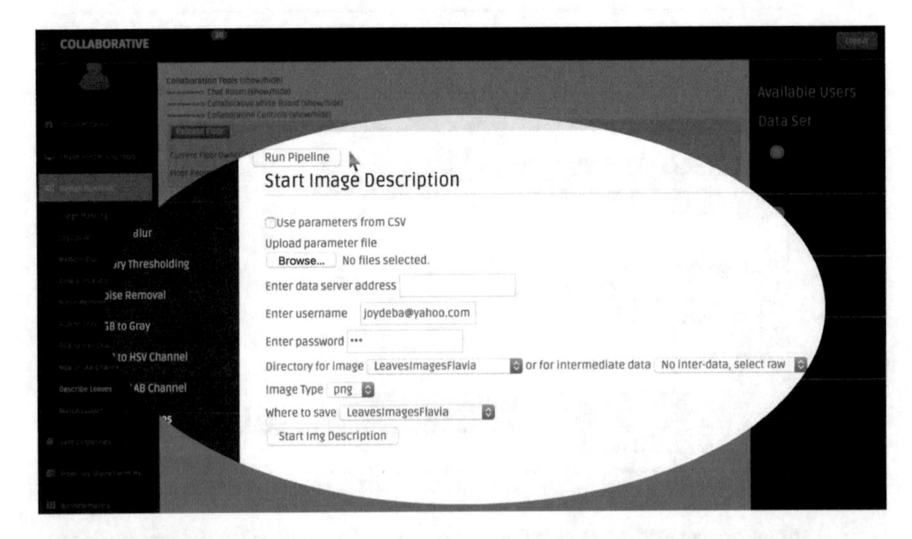

Fig. 6 Image description module in our interactive workflow composition environment

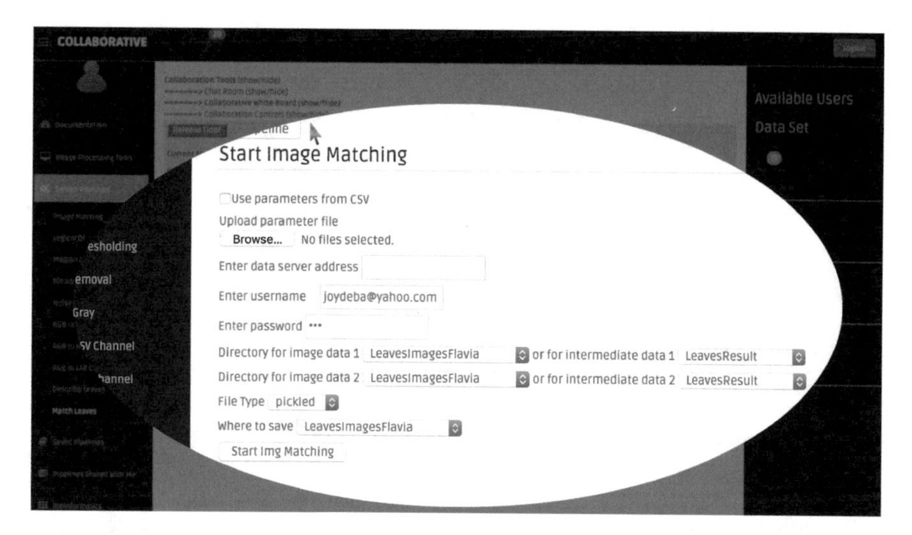

Fig. 7 Image matching module in our interactive workflow composition environment

Table 1 Time gain for the reusable intermediate data

Pipeline tool	Step 1	Step 2	Gain
Leaves description	1163.7 s + 35.7 s	–	–
Leaves matching	Can be skipped	175.9 s	1199.5 s

image description stage is important for an image matching technique and needed to be stored for reuse. In Fig. 7 of the image matching technique, there is an option to use intermediate states for the reuse. Possibility to use intermediate states is the reusability model we are using in our system, an outcome of a module can be used in other modules if available and appropriate for those modules. Consider another situation, when image files are huge in size for high resolution, then pipelines take a large portion of total execution time for only data transferring and loading in a distributed parallel processing system. Thus, stored features or descriptors as intermediate states can help to reduce the transfer time up to a certain level. From Table 1, we can see that module at step 1 (Image Descriptor) required more than 1199.4 s to accomplish the feature extraction part. In a pipeline design, we can skip this step if we can use intermediate states and can gain up to 1199.4 s.

5.2 *Experiment for Error Recovery*

While a pipeline is running in a cluster, it is common that all the steps/modules may not be succeeded and the pipeline may fail to produce the desired output. But in a system of workflow management stored intermediate states can be helpful to recover a workflow execution by applying appropriate module configuration. If we store intermediate data and necessary parameters for modules and if there is an

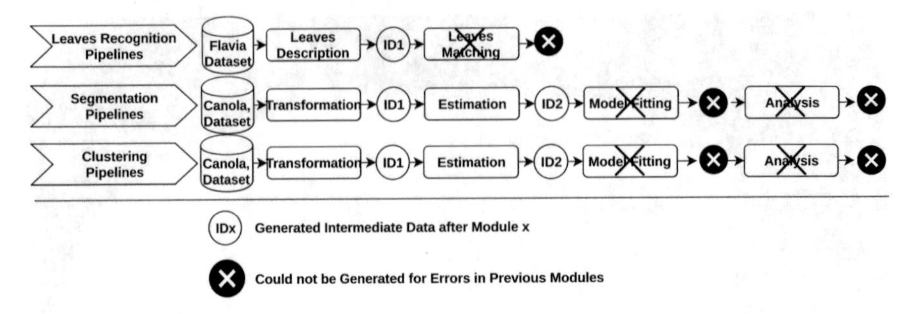

Fig. 8 Common error occurrences in workflow execution

error in a module operation, still data and configuration up to the previous module can be used for stored intermediate data and parameters. So, configuring the failed module with the stored parameters and intermediate data, next run of the pipeline will only take time for the failed modules. For example, in our case (Fig. 8), image recognition pipeline is divided into two modules using SHIPPI library, the second stage sometimes fails for too many comparisons and I/O operations, but using intermediate states we can quickly re-run the second stage by only reconsidering the error issues in that module. Similarly, both segmentation and clustering pipelines are error-prone at the model fitting stage for lots of computation, in that case, up to two stages of computation can be saved if we can reuse stored data with appropriate parameters, and this is possible from our web interface. Besides, in a distributed environment when computation and data are enormous, the failure rate is high for various tasks of a job due to memory overhead and access limitations of different libraries. So, our proposed approach can be a feasible solution in such type of computation-intensive tasks to avoid errors or failures.

5.3 *Experiment for Fast Processing*

Both distributed and ubuntu file systems are considered for the execution time experiments of our scheme, where pipeline design is considered with both with-intermediate and without-intermediate data. Table 1, Figs. 5, and 9 are presented with those execution time experiments. Examining the table, we can say that for the intermediate states, possibilities of skipping execution steps can make pipeline execution time shorter than the normal execution. Figure 5 illustrates the execution time comparisons and performances for the three image processing pipelines in our SWfMS. These image processing pipelines are categorized by three techniques of workflow building for two file systems. The techniques are execution of workflows by storing intermediate data, by not storing intermediate data, and by skipping some module operations. So, there are nine experiments in each file system that makes total eighteen execution scenarios in our system for both file systems. Short forms of the above techniques are given below.

- Leaves recognition workflow without storing intermediate data (LRWoI)
- Leaves recognition workflow with storing intermediate data (LRWtI)
- Leaves recognition workflow by skipping descriptor operation (LRSD)
- Segmentation workflow without storing intermediate data (SWoI)
- Segmentation workflow with storing intermediate data (SWtI)
- Segmentation workflow by skipping transformation and analysis (SSTA)
- Clustering workflow without storing intermediate data (CWoI)
- Clustering workflow with storing intermediate data (CWtI)
- Clustering workflow by skipping transformation and analysis (CSTA)

The gridded dark-gray, gray, and white bars in Fig. 5 represent leaves recognition system performance in two different file systems. If we skip the feature extraction part of this leaves recognition pipeline by using the associated intermediate state (Fig. 6), the execution time of the pipeline is reduced significantly, the gridded white bars in Fig. 5 presents the improved performance of the pipeline. Same goes for the clustering and segmentation pipelines, dotted and lined bars in the figure represent segmentation and clustering algorithms' performances respectively, and white bars of these patterns represent the skipping of modules and improved performance. Furthermore, from Fig. 5, we can have an idea of quantitative values of performance for three different pipelines where gray colors represent all modules computation time of pipelines with or without intermediate states, and white colors represent the computation time of the pipelines that can skip some modules' operation for the availability of intermediate states. So, it can be interpreted from the chart that, if we can skip some module operations for the intermediate states, system or pipeline can be executed at a low cost in both of the file systems. However, there are some delays to store data in a storage system, but for the reusability, a system can really work fast for already processed data. In a SWfMS, amount of data is increased frequently for processing of various workflows. So, without proper data management, volume and velocity of Big Data cannot be addressed efficiently. As well as, different types of data exist in a SWfMS without proper annotation and association variety of Big Data processing cannot be granted. All of the three Vs of Big Data can be appropriately handled in a system of scientific workflow management by using a data-centric component management. Data-centric component development for large-scale data analysis is a current trend to reduce error rates and increase usability, and our system can provide such kind of facilities using stored intermediate data.

6 Discussion and Lesson Learned

From our experimental studies, we figured out that although loading intermediate states from HDFS takes some extra time, the solution and possibility of using intermediate states shows better performance than loading raw large image files

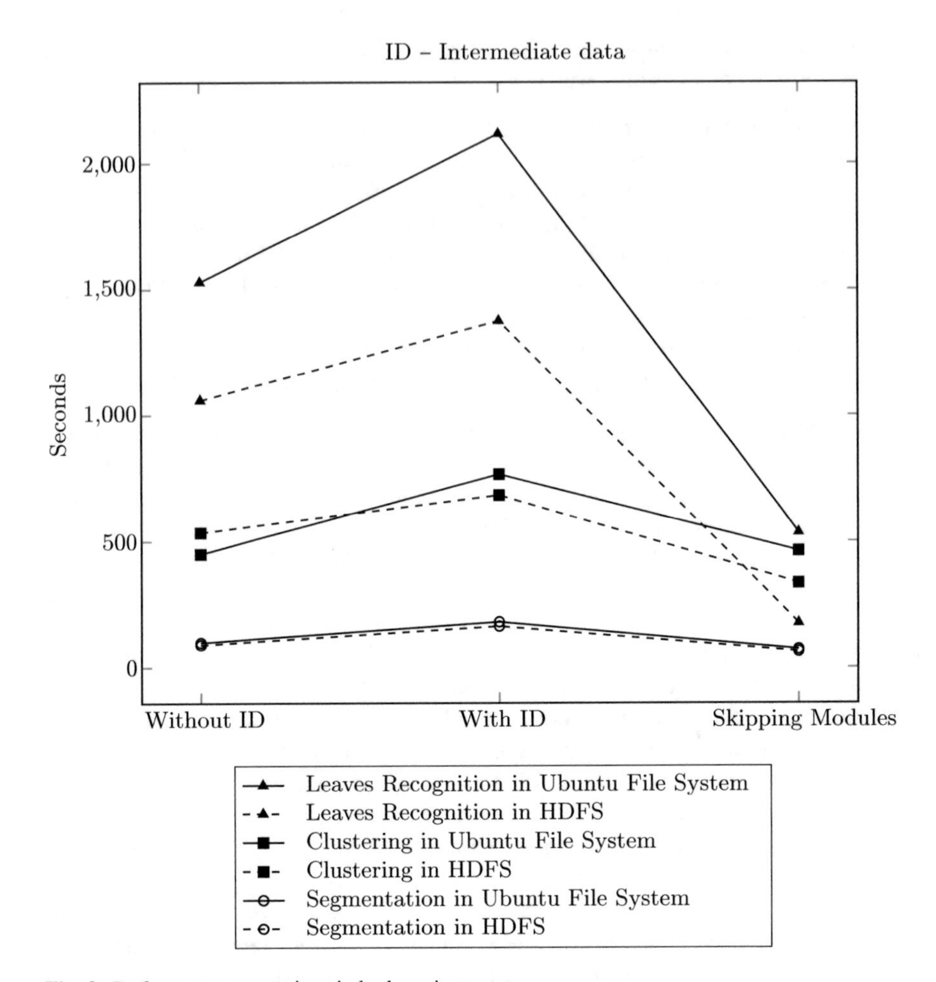

Fig. 9 Performance comparison in both environments

for the execution of image processing workflows. In Fig. 9, normal execution to modules skipping performances have been illustrated for all of the three image processing pipelines. For each pipeline, gain by skipping modules is directly proportional to their normal execution time, as much as the computation time increases, the gain is increased for the time too. This increment directly portraits that the proposed scheme is more effective for computationally intensive tasks than the average workload of pipelines.

We also experienced that discovering data reusability across various image processing tasks are challenging, and significant analysis is required in this regard. In this situation, breaking up an image processing task into micro-level tasks and offering APIs for each task with the micro-level modular programming concept is a viable solution. We learned in a system of modular programming a user has more control over a task configuration such as if a user wishes, certain steps can be used, or some can be skipped with respect to the required functionalities and data availability. Some other common benefits of modular program design that we experienced are easy bug detection, less computation error, easy program handling, and modular testing. Although we noticed this kind of modularity hampers performance, with the appropriate reusability of intermediates states, it is possible to recover the loss. In order to figure out matching intermediate states across various image processing tasks, applying machine learning algorithms might be another solution. In this case, we need to tag intermediate states with metadata to associate them with the tasks they might be used. A system should automatically suggest users for using intermediate states during compositions of workflows.

While we are working in our cluster, we gathered some valuable knowledge of a distributed processing framework such as for parallel processing the cores of different nodes are busy with different tasks of a specific job. So, if anyone wants to store any processed data, it needs to happen on a master node. To store any states, some data transition time from different nodes will be added to the storing procedure, which eventually increases a program's execution time. Another common problem of a distributed system is memory overhead exception. If a master node does not have enough main memory, programs cannot execute operations on a large dataset. For example, in our case, 30GB RAM of the master node could not process 4K images, later which was increased to 90GB and then 4K images were processed with a clustering algorithm. Another problem of a Spark-based distributed system is, for rapid file system access program it throws IO exceptions or SSH library file loading exceptions. Although there are various challenges to process a large dataset in a distributed environment but to facilitate the real-time experience for Big Data, distributed processing environments are inevitable.

7 Conclusion

We devised a data management scheme for our image processing pipeline framework, where we considered to store intermediate data and program state to reuse processed data and recover a pipeline failure with the data. When a dataset has a large number of images and associate programs need long computational time, there is a chance of high error rate. In spite of that, existing models have not concentrated on an organization of intermediate states except raw data and metadata. Considering the above statements, we proposed a model of intermediate state and showed that using intermediate state, it is easy to recover failures quicker and increase reusability in a SWfMS. In addition, intermediate states can be used in other pipelines to reduce the time cost, which eventually increases data reusability. To provide end users an interactive environment for processing Big Data in a parallel distributed framework and at the same time give them reusability with more control is a challenging job. Only a modularization of a program or task might not be a feasible solution in many cases. So, our model with data modularization or intermediate data state at every stage of a modular program will give a user more control of usability. Above all, our study contributes to Volume, Velocity, and Variety creation in Big Data image processing. In the current practice of workflow or pipeline design, high computation capability resources may not facilitate users if users do not have more control over data usability. Hence, using the proposed model of intermediate states of data, resource utilization can be increased up to a certain level. Our experimental results were presented with such utilization, which makes possible the practical use of our system.

Acknowledgement This work is supported in part by the Canada First Research Excellence Fund (CFREF) under the Global Institute for Food Security (GIFS).

References

1. Becker, T., Cavanillas, J., Curry, E., & Wahlster, W. (2016). *Big Data Usage, New Horizons for a Data-Driven Economy*. Cham: Springer.
2. Bezzo, N., Park, J., King, A., Gebhard, P., Ivanov, R., & Lee, I. (2014). Demo abstract: ROSLab A modular programming environment for robotic applications. In *ACM/IEEE International Conference on Cyber-Physical Systems (ICCPS)*, Berlin (pp. 214–214).
3. Blomer, J. (2015). Experiences on file systems: Which is the best file system for you? *Journal of Physics: Conference Series, 664*(4), 042004.
4. Coppens, F., Wuyts, N., Inz, D., & Dhondt, S. (2017). Unlocking the potential of plant phenotyping data through integration and data-driven approaches. *Current Opinion in Systems Biology, 4*, 58–63.
5. Depardon, B., Mahec, G. L., & Seguin, C. (2013). Analysis of Six Distributed File Systems [Research Report]. pp. 44, hal-00789086.
6. Desprez, F., & Dutot, P. F. (2016). Euro-Par 2016: Parallel processing workshops. In *Euro-Par 2016 International Workshops*, Grenoble, August 24–26, Lecture Notes in Computer Science.
7. Donvito, G., Marzulli, G., & Diacono, D. (2014). Testing of several distributed file-systems (HDFS, Ceph and GlusterFS) for supporting the HEP experiments analysis. *Journal of Physics: Conference Series, 513*(4), 04.
8. Han, Z., & Hong, M. (2017, 27 April). *Signal Processing and Networking for Big Data Applications*. Cambridge: Cambridge University Press.
9. Heit, J., Liu, J., & Shah, M. (2016). An architecture for the deployment of statistical models for the big data era. In *IEEE International Conference on Big Data*, Washington, DC (pp. 1377–1384).
10. Kaseb, A. S., Mohan, A., & Lu, Y. H. (2015). Cloud resource management for image and video analysis of big data from network cameras. In *International Conference on Cloud Computing and Big Data (CCBD)*, Shanghai (pp. 287–294).
11. Kim, M., Choi, J., & Yoon, J. (2015). Development of the big data management system on national virtual power plant. In *10th International Conference on P2P, Parallel, Grid, Cloud and Internet Computing (3PGCIC)*, Krakow (pp. 100–107).
12. Li, B., He, Y., & Xu, K. (2011). Distributed metadata management scheme in cloud computing. In *6th International Conference on Pervasive Computing and Applications*, Port Elizabeth (pp. 32–38).
13. Luyen, L. N., Tireau, A., Venkatesan, A., Neveu, P., & Larmande, P. (2016). Development of a knowledge system for Big Data: Case study to plant phenotyping data. In *Proceedings of the 6th International Conference on Web Intelligence*. New York: ACM, Article 27, 9 pages.

14. Minervini, M., Scharr, H., & Tsaftaris, S. (2015). Image analysis: The new bottleneck in plant phenotyping [applications corner]. *IEEE Signal Processing Magazine, 32*(4), 126–131.
15. Minervini, M., & Tsaftaris, S. A. (2013). Application-aware image compression for low cost and distributed plant phenotyping. In *18th International Conference on Digital Signal Processing (DSP)*, Fira (pp. 1–6).
16. Mistrik, I., & Bahsoon, R. (2017). *Software Architecture for Big Data and the Cloud.* ISBN 9780128054673, Jun 12.
17. Mondal, A. K., Roy, B., Roy, C. K., & Schneider, K. A. (2018). *Micro-level Modularity of Computation-intensive Programs in Big Data Platforms: A Case Study with Image Data*, Technical Report, University of Saskatchewan.
18. Pineda-Morales, L., Costan, A., & Antoniu, G. (2015). Towards multi-site metadata management for geographically distributed cloud workflows. In *IEEE International Conference on Cluster Computing*, Chicago, IL (pp. 294–303).
19. Pineda-Morales, L., Liu, J., Costan, A., Pacitti, E., Antoniu, G., Valduriez, P., et al. (2016). Managing hot metadata for scientific workflows on multisite clouds. In *IEEE International Conference on Big Data (Big Data)*, Washington, DC (pp. 390–397).
20. Prasad, S. K., et al. (2017). Parallel processing over spatial-temporal datasets from geo, bio, climate and social science communities: A research roadmap. In *IEEE International Congress on Big Data (BigData Congress)*, Honolulu, HI (pp. 232–250).
21. Roy, B., Mondal, A. K., Roy, C. K., Schneider, K. A., & Wazed, K. (2017). Towards a reference architecture for cloud-based plant genotyping and phenotyping analysis frameworks. In *IEEE International Conference on Software Architecture (ICSA)*, Gothenburg (pp. 41–50).
22. Singh, A., Ganapathysubramanian, B., Singh, A. K., & Sarkar, S. (2016). Machine learning for high-throughput stress phenotyping in plants. *Trends in Plant Science, 21*(2), 110–124. ISSN 1360-1385.
23. Skidmore, E., Kim, S., Kuchimanchi, S., Singaram, S., Merchant, N., & Stanzione, D. (2011). iPlant atmosphere: A gateway to cloud infrastructure for the plant sciences. In *Proceedings of the 2011 ACM Workshop on Gateway Computing Environments* (pp. 59–64). New York, NY: ACM.
24. Smith, K., Seligman, L., Rosenthal, A., Kurcz, C., Greer, M., Macheret, C., et al. (2014). "Big Metadata": The need for principled metadata management in big data ecosystems. In *Proceedings of Workshop on Data analytics in the Cloud.* New York, NY: ACM, Article 13, 4 pages.
25. Sun, W., Wang, X., & Sun, X. (2012). Ac 2012-3155: Using modular programming strategy to practice computer programming: A case study. American Society for Engineering Education.
26. Tudoran, R., Nicolae, B., & Brasche, G. (2017). Data multiverse: The uncertainty challenge of future big data analytics. In *Semantic Keyword-Based Search on Structured Data Sources.* Lecture Notes in Computer Science (Vol. 10151). Cham: Springer.
27. Uti, A. M., Brand, M. V. D., Verhoeff, T. (2017). Exploration of modularity and reusability of domain-specific languages: An expression DSL in MetaMod. *Computer Languages, Systems and Structures, 51*, 48–70. ISSN 1477-8424.
28. Walter, A., Liebisch, F., & Hund, A. (2015). Plant phenotyping: From bean weighing to image analysis. *Plant Methods, 11*(1), 14.
29. Wang, F., Qiu, J., Yang, J., Dong, B., Li, X., & Li, Y. (2009). Hadoop high availability through metadata replication. In *Proceedings of the First International Workshop on Cloud Data Management* (pp. 37–44). New York: ACM.
30. Wu, S. G., Bao, F. S., Xu, E. Y., Wang, Y. X., Chang, Y. F., & Shiang, C. L. (2007, December). A leaf recognition algorithm for plant classification using probabilistic neural network. In *IEEE 7th International Symposium on Signal Processing and Information Technology*, Cairo.
31. Yang, X., Liu, S., Feng, K., Zhou, S., & Sun, X. H. (2016). Visualization and adaptive subsetting of earth science data in HDFS: A novel data analysis strategy with Hadoop and Spark. In *IEEE International Conferences on Big Data and Cloud Computing (BDCloud)*, Atlanta, GA (pp. 89–96).

A Vertical Breadth-First Multilevel Path Algorithm to Find All Paths in a Graph

Maninder Singh, Vaibhav Anu, and Gursimran S. Walia

Abstract This paper presents a novel approach called *vertical breadth-first tree* that utilizes vertical data structures to find all-length paths (including shortest paths) for all pairs of vertices in a graph. Identifying all available paths, including shortest paths is a relevant research problem as this concept can help solve a range of complex problems (e.g., routing problems in computer networks). The advancement of technology, complex computer networks, and extensive exchange of internet communications have resulted in massive increase in data. The conventional path finding algorithms do not scale well with the massive volume of data being communicated over the network and this motivates the need to develop some scalable and efficient path finding algorithms.

Our approach is an advancement of breadth-first algorithm and uses logical operations for path identification. Using vertical data structure, our approach identifies all paths of varying lengths in a graph and stores those paths in the form of a *multilevel bit vector tree* (MBVT). This MBVT results in faster computation of shortest path from source vertex to target vertex with the use of *indexes*. Additionally, our proposed algorithm with vertical data structures is more suitable in distributed processing. Our proposed approach allows addition or removal of any edge in the graph without creating the need to re-generate the multilevel bit vector tree. The results of the implementation of our approach on three sample graphs show that vertical breadth-first approach performed shortest path computations compared with existing approaches (Dijkstra's and all-pair shortest path). The results also show that, when queried about the shortest path between any two vertices, our

M. Singh (✉)
Department of Computer Science, Saint Cloud State University, St Cloud, MN, USA
e-mail: msingh@stcloudstate.edu

V. Anu
Department of Computer Science, Montclair State University, Montclair, NJ, USA
e-mail: anuv@montclair.edu

G. S. Walia
Department of Computer Science, North Dakota State University, Fargo, ND, USA
e-mail: gursimran.walia@ndsu.edu

R. Alhajj et al. (eds.), *Data Management and Analysis*, Studies in Big Data 65,
https://doi.org/10.1007/978-3-030-32587-9_10

algorithm just needs to perform a simple look-up in multilevel bit vector tree via indexes which significantly improves the overall efficiency of shortest-path identification.

Keywords Graph · Path analysis · Shortest path · Vertical data structure · Multilevel bit vectors · All-length paths · Path update

1 Introduction

In recent years, identification of all paths (including the shortest paths) in graphs has received attention because of their application in navigation and location-based services [1]. Path analysis is extensively applied in multi-processor interconnected networks (specifically those networks that can be represented using graphs) to improve fault tolerance. Identifying these alternate paths can help at avoiding congestion and in accelerating transmission rate [2]. Finding all paths is an active research area in bioinformatics to study gene–gene interactions as well [3]. Additionally, shortest-path identification has applications in various other fields like social media (e.g., common friend recommendation), collaboration network (e.g., finding connected scientists), and webpage linkage [4–6].

There has been an extensive increase in data communicated nowadays through computer networks. Existing path finding techniques in a network are efficient, but are not scalable when applied to a very large network. Even though the multilevel tree approach can improve the efficiency of shortest-path identification, there has not been much research done at implementing this technique on larger graphs [1]. Our approach incorporates *vertical bit vectors* into the multilevel tree approach to form a hybrid path-identification approach that can be traversed faster than traditional path identification approaches. The term "*vertical bit vector*" represents the vertical column of adjacency matrix of a graph (details in Sect. 3.7). Our approach also uses logical operations (AND/OR/NOT) on vertical bit vectors to generate new paths in a graph. We hypothesize that our vertical bit vector approach makes the processing of graph data faster when compared to existing algorithms like Dijkstra's approach [7, 8]. Processing of data in bit-form speeds up computation because the bitwise operations on bit vector of *any length* can be done in $O(1)$ time [8]. We report an extension of well-known *breadth-first search* (BFS) to find shortest paths that exist between all pair of vertices (vertices in a graph represent potential location of interest, whereas edge joining two vertices represents existing path between them) through vertical data structure. Implementation details of BFS using vertical vectors appear in Sect. 3.

Problem Formulation The existing algorithms [9, 10] do not scale well (when it comes to efficiency) as data size increases. These existing algorithms are not applicable for distributed processing due to increased pre-processing requirements and complexity. When using the existing algorithms, any addition of new edges to existing graph requires re-identification of paths between all vertices and re-computation of relevant metrics from scratch.

Motivation Vertical data structure have been used successfully in machine learning applications like exploring scalability in semantic web data management [11, 12] and classification using nearest neighbor classifiers [13], and have shown improvement in efficiency and accuracy [14]. Vertical bit vectors are processed independent of each other and this makes them an ideal fit for distributed processing.

Proposed Solution Our proposed approach is shown in Fig. 1 and can be explained using the following steps:

- *Step 1*: Initial vertical bit vectors are obtained from adjacency matrix and are labeled for each vertex. That is, for a graph with four vertices, each column of adjacency matrix represents four initial vertical bit vectors ($E1$, $E2$, $E3$, and $E4$ are the four initial vertical bit vectors in Fig. 1).
- *Step 2*: Next, we apply a combination of breadth-first approach and logical operations to further explore existing paths from initial vertical bit vectors (more details appear in Fig. 5).
- *Step 3*: The algorithm keeps exploring until no new paths are found and then all the explored paths are grouped into levels to form a multilevel path tree (details in Fig. 6).
- *Step 4*: The paths explored are indexed and stored in index list to enable faster look-up.
- *Step 5*: The shortest paths can be found by querying the index list that was created in Step 4.

Our proposed solution does not require re-computation when new edges are added in a graph, thereby avoiding useless extra computations.

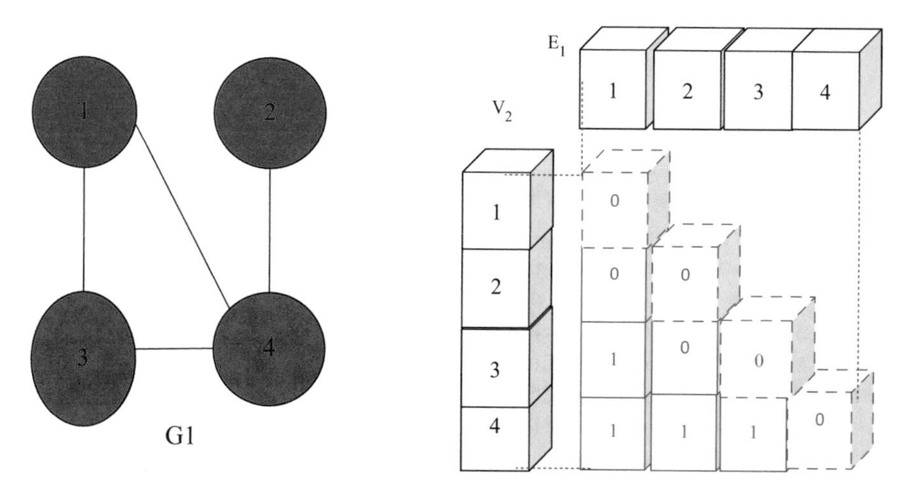

Fig. 1 Graph G1 (four vertices and four edges) and lower triangular matrix representation

Contributions We evaluated our algorithm on undirected and unweighted graphs because, in an undirected graph, the edge runs both ways between two vertices [15]. Implementation of our proposed algorithm on undirected graphs can be helpful in analyzing graphs of social networks, social communities, internet networks, etc., to mine social relations.

Our contribution is demonstrated by the ability of our proposed algorithm to accommodate addition or deletion of an edge within the social media network, without re-computation. The breadth-first approach is versatile and can also be implemented in depth-first manner to suit distributed processing algorithms without excessive pre-processing overhead. The proposed algorithm presents a mathematical formulae that are generalized for any size of graph, i.e., our algorithm is scalable.

Similar Terms The terms *multilevel bit vector tree* (MBVT) and *Allpath* algorithm are used interchangeably in this paper. Throughout this paper, the term graph refers to unweighted bidirectional graph. The major advantage of using this sort of the graph is that when analyzing a social network graph, the presence of undirected link shows the existence of some relation between two persons [4, 5]. So, adding weight to the link does not represent any physical distance of separation among two vertices and is not relevant to our study.

Paper Organization Section 2 provides background on previous research on shortest-path identification, followed by Sects. 3 and 4 that provide a description of important terminology related to the proposed approach. Sections 5 and 6 describe the proposed Allpath algorithm. Section 7 describes the study results wherein the proposed Allpath algorithm was implemented using three sample graphs and the time taken to find shortest path by Allpath algorithm was compared with the time taken by two existing approaches (Dijkstra's and Floyd's). Section 8 discusses validity threats and its impact of the study results. Section 9 provides the anticipated application areas of the proposed Allpath algorithm, and Sect. 10 provides conclusions and future work.

2 Background

This section describes work that is most closely related to our study. Past studies related to shortest path and their complexities have been discussed by [5–9, 16]. The algorithm discussed by Spira in [17], presents a new algorithm for finding shortest path between each pair of nodes in directed positive weighted graph and this algorithm runs in $O(n^2 \log^2 n)$ [18]. Ittai et al. [1], presented their approach on finding shortest paths based on multilevel partition approach in graphs. The authors used multilevel approach to update new edges and vertices in $O(K^3 \log n)$ time, where K is the tree width and n is number of vertices. Their study presented pre-processing of the network to store processed results in a data structure that is faster to look-up and update whenever there is new addition of edge.

Two widely used algorithms that describe an approach to calculate shortest paths are Dijkstra's and Floyd's algorithms [18]. Dijkstra's algorithm takes $O(n^2)$ time to find shortest path from a given source vertex to destination vertex, where n is the total number of vertices. Floyd's algorithm takes $O(n^3)$ time to find a shortest path from one vertex to all other vertexes, where n is number of vertices in a graph [18]. We contrasted our proposed algorithms with Dijkstra and Floyd's algorithm w.r.t. execution time. Shortest paths from all vertices to all other vertices with Dijkstra's and Floyd's are NP-Complete Problem. Along with Dijkstra and Floyd there is another algorithm called A_* that follows greedy approach of minimizing the cost function [9, 18]. The only difference between Dijkstra's algorithm and A_* is that the later selects a labeled vertex v with the smallest value of cost function to scan next node [9].

The existing algorithms (Dijkstra, Floyd, and A_*) are not time-efficient when new nodes are added to the graph or when nodes are removed from the graph, as they have to re-compute all paths and only then can they identify the shortest path. Moreover, these algorithms are also not scalable with larger graph data sets. Our proposed approach (i.e., Allpath algorithm) on the other hand avoids such unnecessary re-computations by creating and storing indexes of all the paths that are computed from each source node to destination node. There exists some other work in literature that discusses path search algorithms but they again face the scalability issue for big graph data.

Therefore, we believe that the Allpath/MBVT algorithm will find applications in areas such as social networks where nodes are added and removed on a frequent basis. Our proposed approach explores the graph vertices with vertical data structure that is most scalable and efficient to use with distributed processing and larger graphs.

3 Graph Terminology

This section provides some necessary details regarding terminology associated with graphs and vertical bit vector approach. The graph G1 is shown in Fig. 1 with four vertices, four edges and its lower triangular matrix representation.

Please note that the graph G1 in Fig. 1 is used as reference to explain various terminologies defined below:

3.1 Vertices and Edges

The "v" in graph G1 represents set of vertices and "e" represents set of edges that joins any two vertices. In graph G1, v contains 1, 2, 3, and 4 labeled vertices and e contains edges 1-3, 1-4, 2-4, and 3-4. Each edge is a pair (x, y) where $x, y \in v$.

3.2 Loop and Subgraph

With respect to graphs, a *loop* is an edge from a vertex to itself. A graph that has a cycle is called *cyclic* graph and *acyclic* otherwise. An undirected graph without any loop is called a *simple graph*. Various terminologies associated with graphs such as for H to be a subgraph of G, it has to satisfy a condition such that $H = (vH, eH)$ if $vH \subseteq v, eH \subseteq e$.

3.3 Undirected Graph

The graph in which direction of edges is not considered, i.e., an edge is considered both ways. For example G1 is undirected graph, where an edge 1➔3 $\approx$ 3➔1.

3.4 Clique

A *subgraph* is called a *clique* if there is an edge between all pairs of nodes. It is an *N*-clique, if *N* vertices within a clique have edges between each possible pair. For example in G1, The edges connecting vertices 1, 3, and 4 makes a *3-clique* because every vertex is reachable directly from any other vertex.

3.5 Degree of a Graph

Degree of a vertex in undirected graph is generally denoted as $v_i \in v$, where v_i is the number of edges incident on that vertex. For example, degree of vertex-4 is 3.

3.6 Adjacency Matrix

This is simply a matrix-style representation to denote existence of an edge between all vertices of a graph. The elements of the matrix indicate whether pairs of vertices are adjacent or not in the graph, e.g., in Fig. 1, presence of an edge between a pair of vertices, is shown with 1 if there is an edge and 0 otherwise. The adjacency matrix has all zeros on its diagonal for a simple graph. This matrix is symmetric if the graph is undirected.

3.7 Vertical Data Structure

Vertical data structure refers to horizontal processing of vertical columns of an adjacency matrix. For the graph G1 (Fig. 3), the vertical data structure is built from each column of adjacency matrix. The vertical columns ($E1$, $E2$, $E3$, $E4$) in Fig. 3 represent the vertical data structures corresponding to each node in graph G1. Each vertical column (e.g., $E1$) represents the vertices that can be reached from vertex-1. One of the advantages of vertical data structure (explained in Sect. 5) is that it can be independently explored to find all the paths from any starting vertex. The computational overhead and update of vertical data structure (with addition) of an edge is described in Sect. 7.4.

Ideally, in a connected graph, the connecting edge between two vertices should be considered only once to avoid repetition and extra work. Our algorithm avoided this extra pre-processing by using lower triangular matrix representation (Fig. 1). Moreover, we marked the edge between vertexes "v" to itself with a 0 because our algorithm does not include any cycle during path generation.

4 Terminology Associated with Proposed Work

This section presents a detailed discussion on underlying mathematics and working of our proposed algorithm. The proposed algorithm operates over vertical bit vectors that generates a new path vectors (also in vertical form) using logical operations to form subsequent levels of a multilevel path tree. Hence, this algorithm is referred to as multilevel bit vector tree (MBVT) in this paper. The overall working of our proposed algorithm is shown in Fig. 2.

The MBVT represents the paths in a graph, so in this paper, it is interchangeably referred to as multilevel path trees or path trees or Allpath trees algorithm. The adjacency matrix (defined in Sect. 3.6) serves as a root in path tree algorithm and newly generated bit-vectors (or paths) become subsequent levels (explained later in this section). The paths are generated and added at appropriate levels of MBVT until the algorithm reaches stopping condition (details in Sect. 5). The final MBVT is the basis to search for the shortest path when the source and destination nodes are given (discussed in Sect. 6). The advantage of MBVT is that it does not require re-computation with the addition and removal of a node from the graph (see Sect. 9).

The proposed algorithm is explained by using graph G1 shown in Fig. 1 (also in Fig. 3). Ideally, in a connected graph, the connecting edge between two vertices should be considered only once to avoid repetition [11]. The graph G1 shown in Fig. 3 has four vertices and four edges. This graph has been chosen from a simplicity point of view, so as to enable the authors in describing the working of the proposed algorithm.

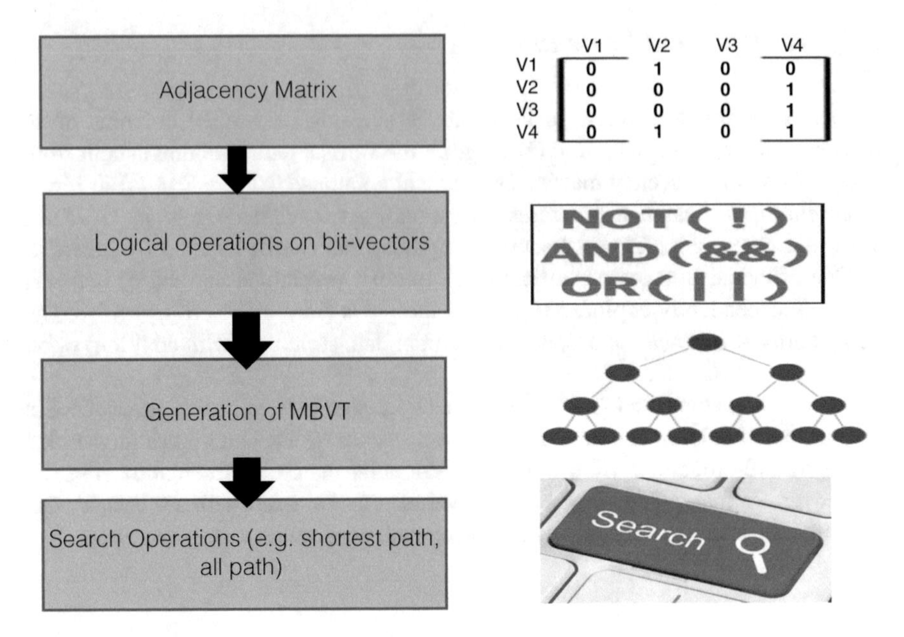

Fig. 2 Overall working of proposed algorithm

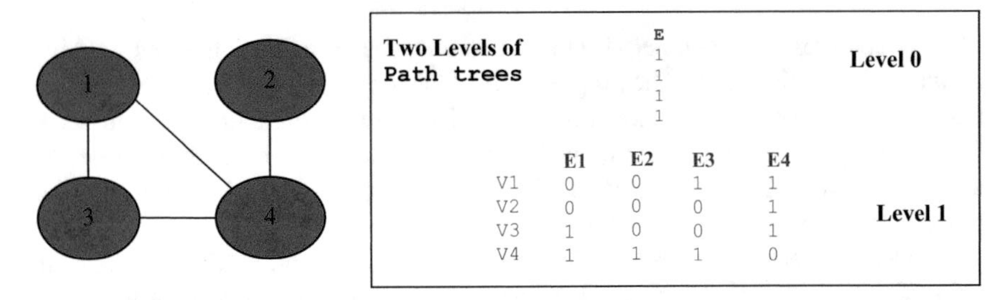

Fig. 3 Two levels of path tree of graph G1

4.1 Definitions and Acronyms

The following definition and acronyms have been used in this paper.

- *Edgepath*: It is denoted as a vertical bit vector and shows the presence of every edge from vertex "v_i" to vertex "v_j" in a graph containing N vertices ($i, j \in N$). *Edgepaths* are defined for each vertex as (E_1, ….., E_n); if N is 2 then there is a single edge (one path) connecting two vertices and if $N \geq 2$, then there are N edgepaths corresponding to each vertex.

  For example, if $N = 3$ then there are three edgepath vectors (E_1, E_2, E_3) and there can be at most two path/two edges starting from vertex 1 to vertex 3. The value of edgepath E_1 (0, 0, 1) means there is only one edge from vertex-1 to vertex-3, i.e., presence of 1 in an edgepath vector shows the existence of a path.

Since the edgepath is corresponding to vertex-1 (i.e., E_1) and 1 is at index 3 (i.e., 001), there is a path from vertex-1 to vertex-3. In a similar way, if edgepath of vertex-2 is E_2 (1, 0, 1) then it means there are two edges from vertex-2; one edge runs from vertex-2 to vertex-1 and another from vertex-2 to vertex-3.

- *Vector Length (VL)* in our approach refers to the number of vertices present in the graph. For example, graph G1 in Fig. 1 has four vertices so the *vector length (VL)* is 4 for this graph.
- *Multilevel path tree*: It is the path tree that contains all the paths reachable from each vertex. This tree is generated in the form of a hierarchy, where the root is an adjacency matrix and subsequent hierarchies are generated through logical operations (more details appear later).
- *Level* defines the hierarchy within multilevel path tree, e.g., graph G1 in Fig. 3, *Level*-1 represents all the paths that are at one edge distance from a specific source vertex. So, edges from V1 (1 is source vertex in this case) in Level-1 are [(V1, V3), (V1, V4)].

  Similarly, Level-2 would show all the paths that are at 2-edge distance from the source vertex. If the source vertex is 1 then from Fig. 3, the edges in level 2 are [(V1, V3, V4), (V1, V4, V3), (V1, V4, V2)].

4.2 Generation of Edgepath Vectors

In our all-path tree algorithm, each edge in the graph is generated with a mathematical formula. Edge path vector $E_k(V_m)$ in Eq. (1) below has been used to generate all the edges present in a graph G1, where k, $V_m \in$ VL (Vector Length).

$$E_k\left(V_m\right) = \begin{cases} 1, \text{ if } \forall_{k,m}, \exists \text{an edge between } V_k \text{ and } V_m \text{ and } V_k \neq V_m,\ k, m \in \text{VL} \\ 0, \qquad\qquad \text{otherwise} \end{cases} \tag{1}$$

The generation of edgepaths vectors (E_1, E_2, E_3, and E_4) at level-1 in Fig. 3 follows conversion formulae in Eq. (1).

4.3 Generation of Vertex Mask Path Vector

The mask vector corresponding to each vertex acts as a filtering condition to exclude source vertex in the MBVT during all-path generation. The $M_k(V_m)$ in Eq. (2), is used to label mask for each vertex in the graph G1 where k, $V_m \in$ VL (see Fig. 4).

$$M_k\left(V_m\right) = \begin{cases} 1, \text{ if } \forall_{k,m}, \text{for bit number} = k \text{ and } k, m \in \text{VL} \\ 0, \qquad\qquad \text{otherwise} \end{cases} \tag{2}$$

Edges	E
1, 1	0
1, 2	0
1, 3	1
1, 4	1
2, 1	0
2, 2	0
2, 3	0
2, 4	1
3, 1	1
3, 2	0
3, 3	0
3, 4	1
4, 1	1
4, 2	1
4, 3	1
4, 4	0

E1	E2	E3	E4	M1	M2	M3	M4	M'1	M'2	M'3	M'4
0	0	1	1	1	0	0	0	0	1	1	1
0	0	0	1	0	1	0	0	1	0	1	1
1	0	0	1	0	0	1	0	1	1	0	1
1	1	1	0	0	0	0	1	1	1	1	0

Fig. 4 Path tree form of graph G1

Additionally, the complement of vertex mask (denoted by M'_h, where $h \in$ VL) is used to exclude already generated vertices in MBVT during all-path generation. The step-by-step details of the operation are explained next.

4.4 Multilevel Path Tree Algorithm

The all-path algorithms use tree like data structure that stores data in vertical bits (i.e., column wise). The multilevel vertical bit-vector tree (MVBT) data structure is known as path tree (see Fig. 3).

In Fig. 3, the edge mask E_k (V_m) at level-1, consists of vertical bit vectors in the form of 0 and 1 (for $\forall$ $V_m \in$ VL). The value of 0 means there is no path from vertex k to vertex m and 1 means that there is a path from vertex k to vertex m $\forall_k$, $V_m \in$ VL. A level-0 in Fig. 3 represents the structure of bit vectors at the top of the tree.

For example: At level-0, the value 1 for all the vertices show that every vertex is reachable within the graph, i.e., there is at least one path from a vertex k to some other vertex m in level-1. Similarly, the presence of 0 at level-0 for any *index* would show isolated vertex in a graph. The notation for edge mask and vertex mask in the following section is going to be E_k and M_k for the sake of simplicity instead of writing $E_k(V_m)$ and $M_k(V_m)$ where k, $V_m \in$ VL.

5 Proposed Algorithm

The proposed algorithm (all-path) starts with generation of adjacency matrix of the graph G1 (see Fig. 4) followed by the creation of the edgepath vectors E_k and vertex mask vectors M_k. Compliments of vertex mask (i.e., M'_k) are created for the graph G1 to restrict the already generated vertices during generation of all the paths.

In Fig. 4, the edge mask E_k is shown as a vertical bit vector. The length of E_k is equal to vertex length (VL), which is 4 in this case. Similarly, M'_k and M_k are written into vertical bit vectors. The all-path algorithm is developed to find all 2-length paths, 3-length paths up to the longest path present in the graph without having the need to re-compute during addition or deletion of a vertex. The underlying mathematical formulae of proposed algorithm is discussed next.

5.1 Generalized Formulae for All-Length Paths

In this section, a generalized mathematical expression for finding all-length paths in a graph has been explained. Our proposed algorithm makes use of breadth-first approach but on vertically structured data. Our algorithm is generalized and it can be implemented in depth-first manner. The advantage of using vertical vector representation is that the algorithm is scalable to graphs of all sizes.

$$
\begin{aligned}
&k = \{\text{Index of } m, \quad \text{where } m = 1 \text{ in ListE}_{i\ldots j} \\
&N\text{-length path } E_{h,k} = E_k \&\& M'_h, \left(\forall \text{other } k, E_{\neg h,k} = 0\right), \text{ and } N = 2 \\
&N\text{-length path } E_{h,i\ldots j,k} = E_k \&\& M'_{i\ldots j}, \left(\forall \text{other } k, E_{\neg h,i\ldots j,k} = 0\right), \text{ and } N \geq 3
\end{aligned} \tag{3}
$$

The mathematical expression works by computing the logical AND between E_k and $M'j$ (see Eq. (3)). These values are obtained from a list, which is denoted as $\text{ListE}_{i,\ldots j}$ (see Eq. (3)). $\text{ListE}_{i,\ldots j}$ has the index values of vertices that has 1 in their edgepaths. The steps to generate all-length paths using generalized formulae is explained with an example as follows:

- *Step 1*: To explain the working, an edgepath vector E_1 $(0, 0, 1, 1)^T$ from level-1 is considered from graph G1 (see Fig. 4). Here the superscript T is transpose that will represent the vector E_1 in vertical form. This example first compute 2-length path and that is why the general formulae $E_{h,\,k}$ is used to compute it (3).
- *Step 2*: To generate level-2 for E_1, the value of 1 is present at index 3 and 4. That shows that there is a path from 1➔3 and 1➔4 (This is also visible in adjacency matrix). The ListE_1, in this case contains the values {3, 4}. These values represents k in generalized formulae.
- *Step 3*: The values of k are read one at a time to generate next level path vectors, i.e., for level-2 starting at source vertex 1. The paths through vertex 3 (1➔3➔?) and vertex 4 (1➔4➔?) are explored and represented as edgepaths E_{13} and E_{14}. The symbol "?" is the vertex at level-2 yet to explore (see Fig. 5).
- *Step 4*: Next, E_k and M'_h values are calculated. The first value of k from the ListE_1 is 3 (see step 3 above), so the E_k becomes E_3 and h is the starting vertex, i.e., vertex 1. So, the value of M'_h becomes M'_1. Once, these values have been generated, the logical AND is performed between bit vector E_k and M'_h as shown in Fig. 5. The resultant edgepath vector from logical AND process is E_{13} $(0001)^T$

For h=1, 1-LengthListE1= {0, 0, 1, 1} K= {3, 4}

E_k && M'_h

E3	&&	M'1=	E13
1		0	0
0		1	0
0		1	0
1		1	1

E_k && M'_h

E4	&&	M'1=	E14
1		0	0
1		1	1
1		1	1
0		1	0

Fig. 5 The 2-Length paths from vertex 1

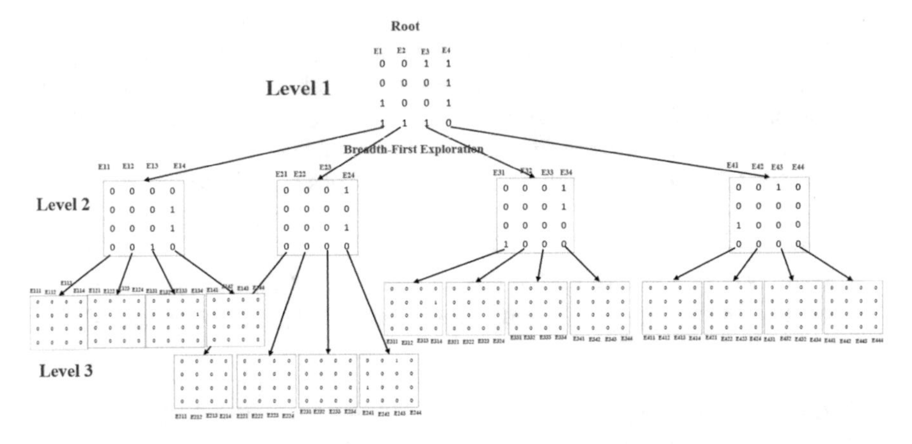

Fig. 6 Generation of multilevel bit vector tree (MBVT)

and E_{14} $(0110)^{\mathrm{T}}$. The edgepath vector E_{13} has 1 at index 4, and the path is read as 1➔3➔4.

- *Step 5*: The 2-length edgepath E_{13} $(0001)^T$ is explored to generate 3-length path for the MBVT approach using the formulae $E_{h,\, i\ldots j,\, k}$ as shown in Eq. (3). E_{13} has a value of 1 at index 4, so, the value of k is 4, $i \ldots j$ is 3 and h is 1. The logical AND between E_4, M'_3, and M'_1 yields the edgepath E_{134} $(0100)^T$ displaying the path as 1➔3➔4➔2. If the edgepath E_{134} is further explored to obtain 4-length path using the same formulae then it results in E_{1342} $(0000)^T$ and this is the stopping condition for further exploration.

Observation The versatility of the algorithm lies in its capability to find all the paths by using logical AND operation over the MBVT, where the 1-length paths can be easily calculated from the level-1 of E_k. Whereas, 2-length and 3-length paths are calculated recursively from their immediate predecessors (as explained in step 1–5 above). The working of formulae in Eq. (3) is shown in Fig. 6 that explains how the algorithm explores path from vertex-1 (i.e., $h = 1$) until stopping condition is met. In a similar way, edgepath vector E_{142} and E_{143} can be recursively explored.

Any loop formed at any level of path tree will not be explored while generating next level edgepaths because logical AND operation for such a case will always generate output bit vector containing all 0s. The complement of M_j makes sure that the immediate vertex j, just traversed from a given source vertex is not added again in path tree while generating subsequent levels from that source vertex. In generalized formulae, the subscript $(i\ldots j)$ represents all the vertices to which the existing path from the starting vertex have been counted. The proof of general formulae for all-path lengths $\forall N$, $N \geq 3$, has explained in Theorem 1 below.

Theorem 1 *The N-length path $E_{h,\, i\ldots j,\, k}$ in a given graph $\forall_N$, $N \geq 3$ can be found by performing logical AND between the vertical bit vectors of E_k AND $M'_{i\ldots j}$ for $\forall_k$, where $k \in (N\text{-}1)$-length List $E_{i\ldots j}$.*

Proof For $N = 1$, 1-length path is obtained from the basic path vectors of E_k, $\forall k$, $k \in$ VL, so 1-length paths are calculated from the adjacency matrix formed for every vertex to every other vertex and that is why there is no logical AND operations involved in calculating 1-length paths. For $N = 2$, there is only one most recent visited vertex (in this case from source vertex), so logical AND is performed between E_k and M'_h, $i\ldots j$ ($i\ldots j$ for $N = 2$ is empty, as there are no intermediate vertices other than source vertex, which is denoted by h). So, in other words, $M'_{h,i\ldots j}$ can be replaced by M'_h where $(i\ldots j)$ represents source vertex as the most recent visited vertex. The reason for choosing the complement of most recent vertex is that we do not want to visit the same visited vertices again.

When $N \geq 3$, there are at least one most recent visited vertices other than the source vertex. So, it is required to not visit them again because we do not want any loop back to the visited vertices. So, it is required to compliment all the vertex masks of the visited vertices other than the source vertex and it is always going to be 1 less than the total number of visited vertices because source is counted as visited. Hence $M'i\ldots j = M'i \,\&\&M'i1 \,\&\&M'i2\&\&M'i3\ldots..\&\&M'j\ \forall i \ldots j$, source vertex $h \notin (i \ldots j)$.

The visited vertices are generated one after another in a sequential manner and are generated from the path trees at $(N - 1)$th iteration. Lastly, the resulting path tree of $M'_{i\ldots j}$ is logically AND by E_k at Nth level, because at that level we want to visit all the vertices from E_k excluding those which have been already visited $(M'_{i\ldots j})$. Hence, this is the proof for Theorem 1.

5.2 End Condition for the Algorithm

The end condition is not hard to determine. The algorithm stops when all the paths have been found and the condition which determines whether all the paths have been determined is the most recent path tree value of $E_{h,\, i\ldots j,\, k}$ from generalized formulae. If the path tree of all resulting $E_{h,\, i\ldots j,\, k}$ is $(0, 0, 0, 0)^T$ for all the vertices, that would tell that all the paths of various lengths have been found in the graph.

Theorem 2 *The value 0 for all indexes in any edge mask* $E_{h,i\ldots j,k}, \forall_h,\ h \in VL$, *with h as source vertex shows that there does not exist any un-counted path.*

Proof The vertex V_i which has been visited from a starting source vertex V_h are not included again by calculating logical AND with complement of M'_i. That means for any next iteration, the algorithm will calculate the logical AND between compliments of vertex mask (M_k) of all in visited vertices list. This implies that when there is 0 value at all the indexes at edge mask path tree ($E_{h,\, i\ldots j,\, k}$), and thus the algorithm cannot go any iteration further as there does not exist any new non-visited vertex that can be reached from current vertex. Hence, the value of k will also be 0 and we will not have any edge mask for k equals 0. So, it acts as end condition for the iteration.

5.3 Space Analysis of Proposed Algorithm

It can be seen from Fig. 6 that the algorithm requires exponential amount of space. For a simple graph G1, there were total of 84 edgepath vectors (4 in level-1, 16 in level-2, and 64 in level-3) generated in MBVT. In general, the total number of edgepath vectors of length equal to VL for a MBVT having N levels can be calculated from the following equation:

$$\#\text{of edgepaths} = \sum\nolimits_{i=1}^{N} (\text{VL})^i$$

where VL is the vector length (i.e., 4 for G1).

It is also seen in MBVT that a lot of computation is involved that results in zero edgepath vector (i.e., $E\ (0000)^T$). It is also seen that a vertex having a value 0 in an edgepath never appear in subsequent paths, so, it could be excluded from exploration to save space. For example, $E_1\ (0011)^T$ has value 0 for vertex 1 and vertex 2. To check all the paths generated from E_1, it is seen that edgepath vectors for E_{11} and E_{12} are zero and also their subsequent levels also results in zero edgepath vectors. So, this unnecessary computation could be avoided to enable faster generation of all paths and look-up during path search.

It is very important to present a suitable mechanism to make efficient use of space. We developed an algorithm that is another novel contribution to convert this exponential space requirement into linear space using indexing. Next section discusses generation of indexes and then conversion of these indexes to generate path labels.

6 Finding Shortest Paths

The shortest path is found from the MBVT described in Sect. 5. The MBVT is one-time process and has all the paths generated from each starting vertex. The addition or removal of any edge in the graph can be updated within the MBVT generated for all paths (discussed in Sect. 9.5). The approach to find shortest paths start from the top level (root or level-0) of MBVT and continues until the path is found or the leaf edgepath vector is reached. The root of the graph G1 has the edgepath vector E $(1111)^T$ at level-0 (see Fig. 7) and has three levels. Search of shortest path through each edgepath that was generated in MBVT is computationally expensive. As discussed in Sect. 5.3, zero edgepath vectors add computational and space complexity, so, we present only useful edgepath vectors in Fig. 7.

As discussed earlier, the MBVT requires exponential amount of space. So, this section also discusses our novel approach to convert exponential amount of space into linear amount of space. This is achieved through generation of indexes to keep track of paths. The index generation is discussed in next sub-section.

Multi-Level Path Trees

Level 0

E
1
1
1
1

Level 1 (1-length paths)

E1	E2	E3	E4
0	0	1	1
0	0	0	1
1	0	0	1
1	1	1	0

Index list up to Level-1
[3,4,8,9,12,13,14,15]

Level 2 (2-length paths)

E13	E14	E24	E31	E34	E41	E43
0	0	1	0	1	0	1
0	1	0	0	1	0	0
0	1	1	0	0	1	0
1	0	0	1	0	0	0

Index list up to Level-2
[3,4,8,9,12,13,14,15, 28,30,31,45,47,52,61,62,67,73]

Level 3 (3-length paths)

E134	E241	E243	E314
0	0	1	0
1	0	0	1
0	1	0	0
0	0	0	0

Fig. 7 Multilevel path trees for graph G1

6.1 Generation of Index List

The values at level-0 show that there are 1-length paths that exists from all the vertices, i.e., there is no isolated vertex. In order to generate index list, the index of 1's in all the edgepaths in level-1 are important to be known to generate subsequent level of MBVT. The following steps explain the generation of index list.

- *Step 1*: The index list at level-1 is formed by searching for the value of 1 in each edgepath vector. The index list is generated by scanning edgepaths in column-raster scan, i.e., E_1 is scanned first and the indexes 3 and 4 are stored in the list, followed by a scan of E_2 edgepath vector. The index list of level-1 is shown in Fig. 7.
- *Step 2*: Indexes of next level edgepath vectors are only included in index list if their logical operation results in non-zero bit vector. The advantage of storing indexes into a list is that it ensures efficient and quick search through the path tree.
- *Step 3*: It is very easy to generate vertical bit vector from index value (as shown in Fig. 7). For example, at level-1 the edgepath $E1$ is $(0011)^T$ and adds value 3 and 4 to index list. Similarly, at level-2 the edgepath E_{13} is $(0001)^T$ and its corresponding index value is 28 [first 16 corresponds to level-1 + 4 for E_{11} + 4 for E_{12} + 4 (because 1 is present at fourth bit of E_{13})]. E_{11} and E_{12} have zero-bit vectors and that is why their index value does not exist in index list. In this way, the indices are generated at each level of MBVT.
- *Step 4*: The highest index value for level-2 is 80 (because 16 for level-1 and 64 for level-2). The highest value of an index at level-3 will be 336, i.e., 80 for up to level-2 and 256 for level-3. So, the general formulae for highest number of an index at a given level L can be calculated by the following equation:

$$\text{Highest index\#} = \sum_{i=1}^{L} (\text{VL})^{i+1}$$

Using this formula, the highest # of index in level-3 is 1360 (i.e., 16 + 64 + 256 + 1024 = 1360). It is worth to note that the formulae above just give the highest possible value of index in the index list for a given level, whereas only those indexes are stored in index list where there was a 1 in the edgepath vector (see index list in Fig. 7).

Observation The MBVT is very sparse tree with only a few 1 s. So, storing only the values of 1 in index list would decrease the exponential space requirements to linear space requirements. The shortest paths are searched using the index list and the algorithm is explained in next sub-section.

6.2 Shortest Path Search Algorithm

The index list generated for MBVT can retrieve the edgepaths from the list values to search for any existing shortest path. The conversion from index list to edgepaths is very simple and is explained in this sub-section.

Conversion from Index List to Edgepaths The edgepaths E_k from index value are retrieved through simple mathematics. For example, consider an index value of 45 for graph having a Vector Length (VL) of 4. The conversion takes place in following steps:

- *Step 1*: Initially the index value is processed to retrieve the level of MBVT that this index value refers to. This is simply checked using the formulae defined to calculate highest index number, i.e., $\sum_{i=1}^{L}(\mathrm{VL})^{i+1}$.
- *Step 2*: The formulae when tested on index value 45, retrieves level-2 for this index value. This is calculated by checking for range of each level based on VL. The level-1 lies between 1 and 16 (VL^2), level-2 lies between 17 and $80 = 16 + 64$ ($\mathrm{VL}^2 + \mathrm{VL}^3$) and so on. Clearly, the index value falls into level-2; so, *45 is 29th place in level-2.*
- *Step 3*: Once, the information about the level of index value is known then it is very easy to compute intermediate path for this index value. Next, the formulae to generate intermediate path is explained as follows:

  1. *Value of k*: 29 modulus (%) VL gives k (i.e., 1).
  2. *Value of h*: $(29/\mathrm{VL}^{\mathrm{currentLevel}}) + 1$ gives h, i.e., 2. [value of current level is 2].
  3. *Value of intermediate path*: It is calculated as $[(29\%\mathrm{VL}^{\mathrm{currentLevel}})/\mathrm{VL}^{\mathrm{currentLevel\text{-}1}} + 1]$ gives 4. Here the value of current level is 2 and we recursively iterate until value of level is 1.

The outcome path for index value 45 is E_h, intermediate, k, i.e., E (2→4→1). Let us take another example with an index value of 126 that is explained in next sub-section (i.e., E_{1342} in Fig. 6).

6.3 Generalizability of our Index Conversion Algorithm

The generalizability of step 2 and step 3 above (Sect. 6.2) for any level of MBVT is explained by taking an example of index value 126 corresponding to edgepath vector E_{134} $(0100)^T$ for graph G1. In other words, this edgepath vector shows the path 1→3→4→2. The steps 2 and 3 should be able to retrieve this path and the working is described as follows:

- As mentioned in step 2, the first requirement is to calculate the level for this value. This is the edgepath vector of graph G1, so this has VL of 4. Using the formulae to find highest index # in a given level L (defined in Sect. 6.1), the highest level for index value 126 is 3. The index value 126 is 46th position in level-3 (see Fig. 6 to check graph).

- *Value of k*: this is calculated by computing the modulus of 46 with VL, and this gives 2. So, the $k = 2$ in this index case.
- *Value of h*: This is calculated by the formulae [(index_position_in_current_level/ $VL^{currentLevel}$) + 1], i.e., [(46/VL^3) + 1] is equals to 1. The value of h is calculated to be 1.
- *Value of intermediate path*: In this case of index value, the intermediate path contains two nodes (i.e., 3 and 4 for E_{1342}). In order to be able to find these two intermediate paths, our algorithm should be able iterate until a stopping condition is reached. The path is iterated until the value of currentlevel becomes 1 in the equation [(index_position_in_current_level % $VL^{currentLevel}$)/$VL^{currentLevel-1}$ + 1].
  - *Iteration 1*: The value of currentlevel variable is 3 for the index value 126 and the formulae is calculated as [((46%VL^3)/VL^2) + 1], where VL is 4 for graph G1. This iteration results in the intermediate path value of 3. The value of currentlevel is decrement by 1 after every iteration. So, the value of currentlevel becomes 2 after this iteration and would execute the formulae recursively until it becomes 1.
  - *Iteration 2*: The value of currentlevel is 2, so the formulae is calculated as [((46%VL^2)/VL^1) + 1], and this iteration results in 4. The value of currentlevel becomes 1 and the algorithm comes out of loop with two values as output, i.e., 3 and 4. This was our desired intermediate path.

The formulae described in step 2 and 3, was able to generate intermediate path for different levels. Hence, the algorithm is able to reproduce the path from the index value. The path is $E_{h,\text{ intermediate\_path},\, k}$ and this becomes E_{1342} from the values of h and k calculated above.

6.4 Explanation of Shortest Path Search with an Example

The strength of our MBVT approach is the tree traversal approach using the index lists. In a normal tree traversal approach, a shortest path from a vertex h to k (where $h, k \in$ VL) is searched within the multilevel path tree from E_h until first $\boldsymbol{k}$ appears.

- *Shortest Path Search from MBVT*: To find shortest path from $h = 1$ to $k = 2$ in graph G1 (see path tree in Fig. 6), level 1 is checked at index $h = 1$ to see if there is a value 1 at index 2 in edgepath vector E_1 $(0011)^T$. There is 0 at index value 2 in this edgepath and it means that there is no direct shortest path from 1 to 2. So, the next level is checked, i.e., level 2 within multilevel path tree which represents paths from E_h until we get 1 at index 2. As seen at this level we get 1 at index 2 in level 2 for $E_{1,4}$. So the shortest path is 1➔4➔2. The shortest path can be very easily looked up by traversing the multilevel tree level by level until we get 1 at the desired index when starting from source vertex bit vector.

```
ShortestPath (int Indexes, int VL, int source, int dest) {
For each value in Indexes:
Calculate currentlevel from the index
Calculate K from value % VL
 IF K equals dest THEN
   Calculate H from value / VL^currentlevel +1
    IF H equals source THEN
      Calculate intermediatePath (int VL, int currentlevel, int index)
      Print Shortest Path // i.e. H, intermediatePath and K
    ELSE break
 ELSE break
Read Next value from Indexes
END For
}
```

Fig. 8 Algorithm to search shortest paths from index values

- *Shortest Path Search from Index List*: The shortest path can be searched from the index list. For example, the path 1➔4➔2 can be searched from the index values. In this example, the path 1➔4➔2 can be expressed as E_{142}, which is equivalent of $E_{h,\ \mathrm{intermediate\_path},\ k}$. Here, the h is 1, intermediate path is 4 and k is 2. The shortest path can be checked, first of all, for the value of k using the formulae defined for conversion from index values. If the value of k is 2, then the value of h should be calculated for that index value. The value of intermediate path should only be explored if h and k have been obtained. The algorithm to find shortest path from index values is shown in Fig. 8. The algorithm takes, index list, source vertex, destination vertex, and vector length as arguments.

The details about the algorithm in Fig. 8 have already been discussed above in sub-sections B and C.

6.5 Graph Data Sets Used in This Study

There are three data sets that have been taken in this study to perform analysis (see Fig. 9). We called them graph 1 (G1), graph 2 (G2) and graph 3 (G3). All these graphs had different number of vertices and edges. These graphs were selected to

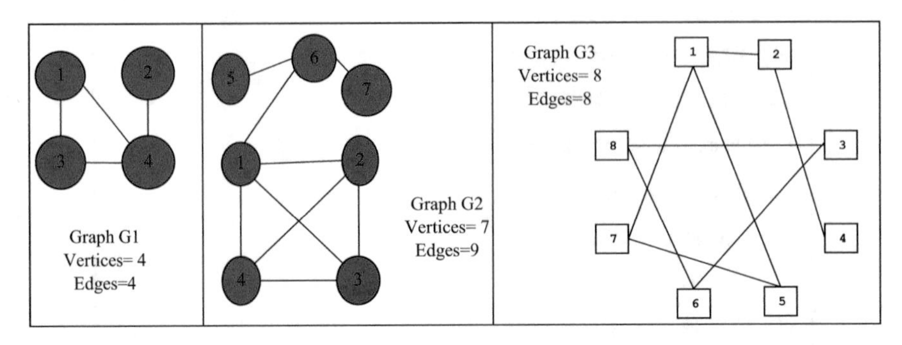

Fig. 9 Various graph data sets used in this study

study the execution time effect by taking simple graphs with different nodes and interconnecting edges.

The three graphs are selected based on a linear increase in number of nodes. These graphs are shown in Fig. 9. Another motivation was to test our algorithm on smaller graph to study and explore efficient methods that could be analyzed manually to validate the results. We tested our algorithm over graphs in which some of the nodes are not reachable (e.g., graph G3, nodes 3 and 4). It was also intended that if promising results are found then our next step would be to use bigger graphs and execute our algorithm using distributed processing. Some big social network graphs are also next in line to be explored using our proposed algorithm.

7 Results and Discussions

Multilevel bit vector tree (MBVT) algorithm requires exponential amount of space to store all the paths that are generated. This proposed approach also presents a way to convert exponential space requirement into linear space by storing paths in the form of indexes. The results and discussion in this section is presented using shortest path search using index list. The search for shortest path using index list is faster because very least comparison is needed. In our proposed work, MBVT was generated to find all the paths in a graph and index list was used to search for the shortest path.

This section presents discussion on time taken by our proposed algorithm (Allpath/MBVT) to search shortest path between source and destination vertices (selected at random during runtime). This section also compares results of shortest path search time (Fig. 10) and execution time (Fig. 11) taken by Allpath, Dijkstra and Floyd's algorithm for three graphs namely G1, G2, and G3. This section also compares results of shortest path search time (Fig. 10) and execution time (Fig. 11) taken by algorithms in Nano-seconds.

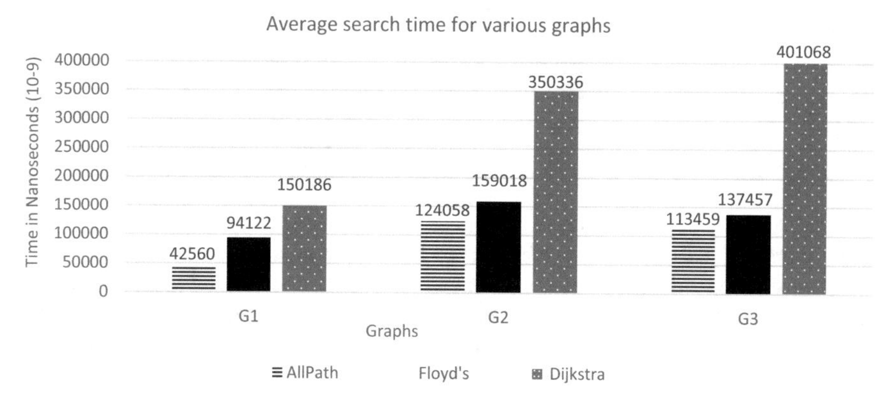

Fig. 10 Results on average search time for various graphs

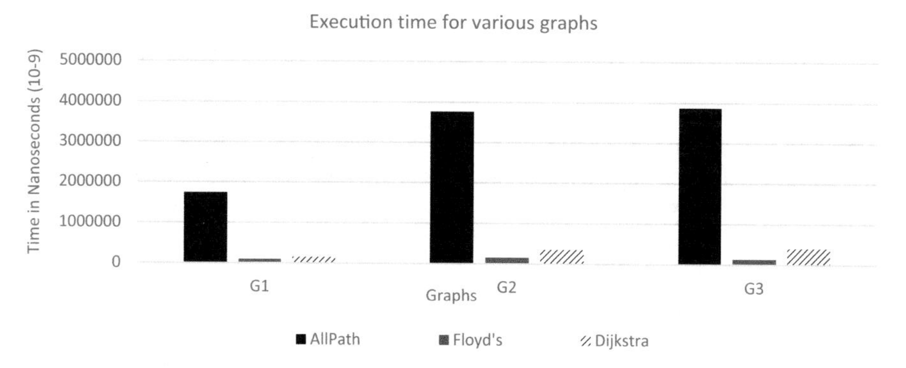

Fig. 11 Results on overall execution time for all three graphs

7.1 Experiment Details

The experiment was run on intel-core-i7 processor with main memory of 4 GB and CPU clock of 2.4 GHz. The algorithms are executed in java programming environment through Eclipse IDE. The experiment was run 100 times to avoid any researcher's bias to obtain more precise and accurate results.

7.2 Performance Results

The search time (efficiency) for finding shortest path from source to destination vertex was repeated 100 times and the average is plotted in graph shown in Fig. 10. The source and destination vertices were also selected at random during each experiment run. The execution time (Fig. 11) for all three algorithms was also repeated 100 times and their average is taken as final execution time. It is seen from

Table 1 Number of comparisons

Algorithms	Algorithm operations	Comparison for edge update
Dijkstra's (single source)	$O(k^2 \log r \log(k \log r))$	$O(k^2 \log r \log(k \log r))$
Floyd's	$O(r^3)$	$O(r^3)$
Allpath (at any level)	$O(m \text{ x VL})$	$O(\underline{n} \log_{VL} M)$

Fig. 10 that Allpath algorithm outperforms Floyd's and Dijkstra for all three graphs w.r.t search time. Allpath performed best while Dijkstra performed least w.r.t search time. Floyd's algorithm slightly underperformed Allpath. On the contrary in Fig. 11, Allpath performed exponential w.r.t overall execution time to generate multilevel path vectors. The execution time approximately becomes twice when number of vertices are doubled in a graph (Fig. 10).

7.3 Discussion of Results

The results of Allpath algorithm can be better understood by exploring its complexity. The result showed significant improvement in shortest path search time (Fig. 10). Therefore, the analysis of comparisons needed to find shortest paths is performed in Table 1. In this section, we also present theoretical discussion on path update in Allpath (multilevel) algorithm.

We present analysis of our Allpath (multilevel) algorithm in terms of number of comparisons with Dijkstra's algorithm (undirected edges and equal weights) [9], Floyd's algorithm [9]. The Table 1 shows worst-case comparisons between these algorithms.

Symbols Used to Analyze Complexity In Table 1, k is the tree width, r is number of nodes, n is number of edges, M is maximum number of bit vectors present and L is total number of levels in multilevel path tree. The analysis of the result is discussed in next section alongside advantages of index based solution to our MBVT approach. From the results it can be inferred that multilevel path tree algorithm is slower at tree generation step while it is faster when it comes to search or update an edge in a graph.

7.4 Allpath Complexity

Allpath Update Complexity: Path update in worst case assumes that if there are maximum possible number of bit vectors (M) at last level of vector length (VL) are present; then based on bit vectors at last level, our multilevel path tree algorithm has maximum of $\log_{VL} M$ levels (i.e., $L = \log_{VL} M$). For example, in a graph with VL = 4 and having maximum of 256 total # of bit vectors (M) at last level, then the total # of levels (L) are 4 (i.e., $\log_4 256$). The analysis of complexity has been presented in Table 1. If n edges have been updated at each level, then the upper bound of number of updates required at a particular level for the whole graph are ($n \log_{VL} M$).

Allpath Complexity: In a similar way, to calculate the complexity of the MBVT algorithm in a worst-case scenario is calculated using number of bit vectors and number of 1 s at a given level. Assuming there are m number of bit vectors and each bit vector has VL number of 1 s then there are ($m \times$ VL) number of bit vectors that are generated at next level. It is also worth noting that if $m \approx$ VL at each level then the algorithm runs in exponential time but it is one-time process and new edges can be dynamically added or removed without computing the whole tree again. The shortest path search algorithm described in Sect. 6.4 (Fig. 8) using indexes has resulted in shortest path calculation even faster in quadratic amount of time. We expect that this algorithm can further be improved by using distributed processing (subject to evaluations).

Allpath algorithm generates new bit vectors for subsequent level on each occurrence of 1. This makes Allpath algorithm exponential in execution. That is why the execution time taken by Allpath algorithm is more than other two algorithms. The advantages of our proposed algorithm despite exponential complexity are as follows:

- It is very convenient to be executed in distributed computing because bit vectors at root node can be processed independent of each other.
- Generation of multilevel path vectors is one-time process and results in speed gain for shortest path search.
- Path update is easy to accommodate without repeating whole process.

Multilevel tree algorithm has proven to be the superior algorithm (among existing ones) to find the shortest paths with forbidden paths [22] and without forbidden paths [10]. In [6], an algorithm to find multiple shortest paths (k-shortest paths) is presented [6],which (multiple shortest paths) our algorithm is also generating by generating all lengths of paths. Newman in [5] presented an algorithm to find all the collaboration of authors in scientific papers in various fields. Newman described his technique to find shortest path between two authors in his collaboration network through the use of Queue [14].

Our multilevel path algorithm also finds shortest path between two authors in relatively faster manner with the use of vertical data structures because vertical data structure is best fit for logical operations to perform. Restricted Shortest Path (RSP), $\in$-Approximation, backward-forward heuristic and Lagrangian based methods have major issues of large computational time [16] while our multilevel path algorithm's computation time is less expensive using the logical operations, which can further be reduced to *the factor of* $O(n \log_{VL} M)$ *by the use of indexes* to represent position of 1's in multilevel trees. When indexes are used then we need not to traverse throughout the bit vector to check the presence of 1's and this makes algorithm even more efficient by skipping unnecessary computations.

8 Threats to Validity

Throughout our study we tried to address various threats so that our proposed algorithm could be replicated. We chose source and destination vertices randomly to simulate real world selection. The efficiency results were obtained by repeating the experiment 100 times and then taking average of all the results. We recorded shortest-path search time for our algorithm and excluded any system output/print operations from our calculations.

There can still be few threats that can affect validity, e.g., size of graphs (as it is difficult to get a clear picture of vertical approach by taking small graphs). One-time processing of vertical approach is costly, but addition/removal of any path does not require re-computation from scratch. We expect that the efficiency results will improve if distributed processing is taken into consideration.

An additional threat is that we have compared the Allpath algorithm with just two existing approaches. However, this threat is addressed to some extent by the fact that Dijkstra's and Floyd's approaches have been found to be the most efficient shortest-path identification approaches. The fact that the average time taken by Allpath algorithm to search for shortest paths is lower compared to the average time taken by the Dijkstra's and Floyd's approaches is motivation for further exploring the Allpath algorithm.

9 Applications

Multilevel path trees need one-time execution to generate all the paths. The space requirement is exponential in nature but with the advancement in storage capacity like cloud computing, the data for very large graphs can be stored easily on cloud or even on personal hard drive. More importantly, once the multilevel path trees are generated, it is very convenient through our approach to traverse among them using simple tree traversal.

9.1 Social Networking Applications

The path tree generated in the form of multilevel path trees provides quick information updates about any singleton vertex from level-0 path tree. Singleton vertex represents an isolated node. This is of particular importance in social networks like Facebook in which a singleton vertex represents very recently joined user. So, in this case, recommendations for connecting to other friends in Facebook can be provided to the singleton vertex. At level 1 (1-length path), if the count of 1 in path tree E_k for some value k is not more than one, then for social networking graph like Twitter, it can be easily predicted that the vertex/user k is just a follower and is not been followed by anybody else.

9.2 Requirement Engineering

Another important contribution of this approach is towards the automation of certain processes in requirement engineering (RE). The RE phase gather requirements from multiple stakeholders and document them in software requirement specification (SRS) document [19–21]. The RE phase has certain activities where application of our approach is best suited. The RE phase in software development life cycle needs to analyze changes and their impact over subsequent requirements when requirements undergo a change due to evolving user needs.

The requirements could be converted into a graph based on semantic similarity between various requirements in an SRS. Once the requirements are converted into a graph (where nodes represent requirements and edges represent semantic similarity), the impact of a change in an SRS can be studied by exploring all the paths from a changed node to other nodes in the graph. This approach is very suitable to locate fault-prone areas within the requirements as well as to study the change impact analysis. There has been an ongoing research in which the authors of this paper are trying to implement semantic analysis algorithms over requirements artifacts to develop a graph that can be mined to report fault-prone areas within an SRS document.

9.3 Generic Application

At level 2 (2-length paths), if the count of 1 in path tree $E_{h,k}$ for some h and $k \in VL$, is one then the vertices h, k and index of 1 in that path tree represents the 2-path isomorphic vertices in graph. At level 3 (3-length paths), we can see that if $E_{h,j,k}$ is 1 at index h for some values of h, j, and $k \in VL$, then h, j and k vertices forms three clique. At level 4 representing 4-length paths, having 1 in path vector would make it contender for 1-plex and so on. This very quick analysis can help in making recommendation system for any social networking site.

Alternate recommendations can very easily and quickly be provided for routing, processor interconnected networks and social networking sites. The multilevel path trees are best suited to find diameter and edge-betweenness of a graph without explicitly defining additional metrics (details out of the scope of this paper).

9.4 Distributed Processing Applications

The use of vertical data structures ensures that our approach is easily applicable to distributed processing such as Hadoop to further speed up computations for very large graphs. The Allpath/MBVT algorithm explores the edgepaths vertically.

In distributed processing environment, the edgepaths at level-1 can be explored separately in multiple processors until all the paths have been explored from each source node. Moreover, our approach can also be explored in depth-first manner that makes it more adaptable and independent of any specific tree generation approach. Also, the edgepath generation process is independent to other edgepaths generated at the same level of MBVT. Hence, our proposed approach is most suitable for distributed processing environment.

9.5 Path Update

The path update for any graph using path tree approach is very easy to compute within human time. The reason lies in the fact that addition of new edge in the graph does not need to re-generate all paths from the beginning. Also, the edge addition would only need to update the index list. The new edge is added to the existing adjacency matrix. The newly generated bit vectors trees for the added edge in graph is updated in existing path trees' index list. The update involves addition of new path vectors at appropriate places as shown in Fig. 12.

The new edge between 1 and 2 is added into the multilevel path tree. Here, we update the indexes in path vectors at Level 1 at places corresponding to the vertices forming new edge (i.e., edge between 1 and 2). In this case, the indexes are 1 and 2 in $E1$ and $E2$ path vectors. The location of new addition is then updated in list

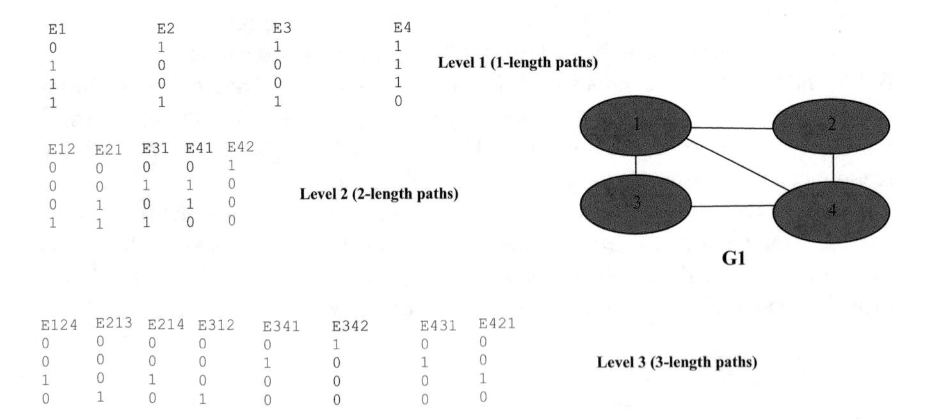

Fig. 12 Path update in multilevel path tree

data structure. Let us see the update operation in Fig. 12 for graph G1 upon the addition of edge between 1 and 2. The changes caused by the addition of new edge in the edgepaths of Fig. 12 are marked in red. The edgepath vectors that are newly generated because of the addition are colored in red completely at each level (Fig. 12) while those which are just updated are colored red at corresponding position of a change.

At level-1, only edgepath vector $E1$ and $E2$ are impacted but this addition has generated new paths at subsequent levels (i.e., level-2 and level-3). The algorithm updates the index list at higher levels for only those edge paths that are either generated at the higher level or contains added vertex value at the end of final path (in this case 1 and 2). At level-1, the impacted edgepath vectors are $E1$ and $E2$, so these are updated. For level-2, only $E1$ and $E2$ are further explored because are updated at level-1 and new paths exist because of the update. For example, edgepath vector $E342$ at level-3 contains 2 at the last position in its final path, so, it is only updated while based on updates at level-2, and new paths are generated at level-3 (labeled in red in Fig. 12). The existing MBVT tree is updated with either generation of new path vectors or with just updating the positions within the edge vectors corresponding to the new added edge (Fig. 12).

10 Conclusion and Future Work

This paper has shown that, when compared to existing techniques, our *vertical breadth-first multilevel path tree* approach can successfully reduce the number of comparisons required to identify shortest path. We have also described in this paper that our approach can perform more efficient path updates when compared to existing approaches when new edges are added or some edges are deleted from the graph.

The next step in our research is to implement and evaluate the Allpath/MBVT algorithm over a distributed processing environment. The one-time process of creating a multilevel path tree can be implemented using MapReduce in distributed processing. This is because each edgepath vector is independent of all other edgepath vector in a given multilevel path tree. Even though the vertical breadth-first multilevel path tree algorithm has shown encouraging results, there is scope for improvement, especially from an optimization point of view. Therefore, we are currently working on implementing the multilevel path tree algorithm using MapReduce. We expect that utilizing such a distributed processing technique (i.e., MapReduce) will yield better efficiency when our algorithm is applied on bigger graphs.

In a future study, we intend to replicate the study described in this paper, but over a distributed processing environment (using MapReduce). Therefore, Allpath, Dijkstra's, and Floyd's algorithm will be used to identify shortest paths in a graph, with all algorithms utilizing MapReduce paradigm. Additionally, we also intend to evaluate the scalability of our approach by testing it with bigger, more complex graphs.

References

1. Ittai, A., Shiri, C., Daniel, D., Goldberg, A. V., & Werneck, R. F. (2016). On dynamic approximate shortest paths for planar graphs with worst case costs. In *SODA 16 Proceddings of the Twenty-Seventh Annual ACM-SIAM Symposium on Discrete Algorithms*. Philadelphia: SIAM.
2. Cheng Nan, L. (April 2016). On the construction of all shortest node-disjoint paths in star networks. *Elsevier Information Processing Letters, 116*(4), 299–303.
3. Dorogovtsev, S. N. (2003). Real networks. In *Evolution of networks from biological nets to the internet and WWW* (pp. 31–73). Oxford, UK: Oxford University Press.
4. Newman, M. E., & Girvan, M. (2004). Finding and evaluating community structure in networks. *Physical Review E, 69*(2), 026113.
5. Newman, M. E. J. (2001). Scientific collaboration networks. II. Shortest paths, weighted networks and centrality. *Physical Review E, 64*, 016132-1–016132-7.
6. Hershberger, J., Maxel, M., & Suri, S. (2007). Finding the k shortest simple paths: A new algorithm and its implementation. *ACM Trans. Algorithms, 3*(4), 45.
7. Lucchese, C., Orlando, S., & Perego, R. (2006). Fast and memory efficient mining of frequent closed itemsets. *IEEE Transactions on Knowledge and Data Engineering, 18*(1), 21–36.
8. Akiba, T., Iwata, Y., & Yoshida, Y. (2013). Fast exact shortest-path distance queries on large networks by pruned landmark labeling. In *Proceedings of the 2013 ACM SIGMOD International Conference on Management of Data* (pp. 349–360). New York: ACM.
9. Goldberg, A. V., & Harrelson, C. (2005). Computing the shortest path: A search meets graph theory. In *Proceedings of the sixteenth annual ACM-SIAM symposium on discrete algorithms*. Philadelphia: SIAM.
10. Szeider, S. (2003). Finding paths in graphs avoiding forbidden transitions. *Discrete Applied Mathematics, 126*(2–3), 261–273.
11. Abadi, D. J., Marcus, A., Madden, S. R., & Hollenbach, K. (2007). Scalable semantic web data management using vertical partitioning. In *Proc. 33rd Int. Conf. Very Large Data Bases* (pp. 411–422).
12. Kang, U., & Faloutsos, C. (2013). Big graph mining: Algorithms and discoveries. *ACM SIGKDD Explorations Newsletter, 14*(2), 29–36.
13. Perrizo, W., Ding, Q., Khan, M., Denton, A., & Ding, Q. (2007). An efficient weighted nearest neighbour classifier using vertical data representation. *International Journal of Business Intelligence and Data Mining, 2*(1), 64.
14. Houque, S. R., Imam, S. M., Hossain, M. K., & Perrizo, W. Algorithm for shifting images in Peano mask trees. In *ICCIT, Islamic University of Technology, 28-30 December 2005*. ICCIT.
15. Zaki, M. J. (2014). Graph data. In *Data mining and analysis fundamental concepts and algorithms* (pp. 93–132). New York: Cambridge University Press.
16. Kuipers, F., Van, M. P., Korkmaz, T., & Krunz, M. (December 2002). An overview of cobstraint based path selection algorithms for QoS routing. *IEEE Communications Magazine, 40*(12), 50–55.
17. Spira, P. (2004). A new algorithm for finding all shortest paths in a graph of positive arcs in average time. *SIAM Journal on Computing, 2*(1), 28–32.
18. Johnson, D. B. (1973). A note on Dijkstra's shortest path algorithm. *Journal of the ACM, 20*(3), 385–388.
19. Singh, M., Anu, V., Walia, G. S., & Goswami, A. (2018). Validating requirements reviews by introducing fault-type level granularity. In *Proceedings of the 11th Innovations in Software Engineering Conference on - ISEC '18* (pp. 1–11).
20. Singh, M., Walia, G. S., & Goswami, A. (2017). Validation of inspection reviews over variable features set threshold. In *2017 International Conference on Machine Learning and Data Science (MLDS)* (pp. 128–135). IEEE.

21. Singh, M., Walia, G. S., & Goswami, A. (2017). An empirical investigation to overcome class-imbalance in inspection reviews. In *2017 International Conference on Machine Learning and Data Science (MLDS)* (pp. 128–135). IEEE.
22. Daniel, V., & Guy, D. (2005). The shortest path problem with forbidden paths. *European Journal of Operational Research, 165*(1), 97–107.

Workflow Provenance for Big Data: From Modelling to Reporting

Rayhan Ferdous, Banani Roy, Chanchal K. Roy, and Kevin A. Schneider

Abstract Scientific workflow management system (SWFMS) is one of the inherent parts of Big Data analytics systems. Analyses in such data intensive research using workflows are very costly. SWFMSs or workflows keep track of every bit of executions through logs, which later could be used on demand. For example, in the case of errors, security breaches, or even any conditions, we may need to trace back to the previous steps or look at the intermediate data elements. Such fashion of logging is known as workflow provenance. However, prominent workflows being domain specific and developed following different programming paradigms, their architectures, logging mechanisms, information in the logs, provenance queries, and so on differ significantly. So, provenance technology of one workflow from a certain domain is not easily applicable in another domain. Facing the lack of a general workflow provenance standard, we propose a programming model for automated workflow logging. The programming model is easy to implement and easily configurable by domain experts independent of workflow users. We implement our workflow programming model on Bioinformatics research—for evaluation and collect workflow logs from various scientific pipelines' executions. Then we focus on some fundamental provenance questions inspired by recent literature that can derive many other complex provenance questions. Finally, the end users are provided with discovered insights from the workflow provenance through online data visualization as a separate web service.

Keywords Scientific workflow management systems · Workflow provenance · Logs · Modular programming · Provenance programming model

R. Ferdous (✉) · B. Roy · C. K. Roy · K. A. Schneider
Department of Computer Science, University of Saskatchewan, Saskatoon, SK, Canada
e-mail: rayhan.ferdous@usask.ca; banani.roy@usask.ca; chanchal.roy@usask.ca; kevin.schneider@usask.ca

R. Alhajj et al. (eds.), *Data Management and Analysis*, Studies in Big Data 65,
https://doi.org/10.1007/978-3-030-32587-9_11

1 Introduction

In Big Data analytics, the whole analysis process always goes through Big Data analytics lifecycle [9, 12]. In each step of the lifecycle, a specific fashion of analysis is projected on the data which is/are derived from the previous step/s. Such fashion of analysis creates the necessity of using common data analysis tools over the whole process. Thus re-usability of data analysis tools becomes important. On the other hand, distributed and high performance computing technologies are necessary in data intensive research areas. They are provided through web services enabling collaboration. Better scientific workflow systems or simply workflows leverage all these features and provide data scientists with cutting edge and most updated data analytic services—to implement data intensive pipelines [6, 18, 19, 25].

Big Data analytics deals with unstructured data and has to produce comprehensive information about different datasets from different sources. Such comprehensive information is more valuable than information of any single dataset [9]. Data provenance is the way of associating subject data with related log data during an analysis process. Such logs can be used to regenerate data lineage. Lineage of data is necessary to answer any question associated with the data source, configuration related to its analysis, any error or anomaly, its changes over time, process based information related to the data and so on. Data provenance itself has many different categories [7, 8, 11, 14, 23]. Any workflow itself processes data through simple to complex pipelines. Such workflow process logs are called workflow provenance. In workflow provenance, the pipeline modules are considered as black boxes and internal operations are not taken into account. Data elements are both input and output of any module [2]. In case of any errors, unwanted behaviors of the analysis/security problems, or even to investigate particular data/process condition, the workflow cannot be just shut down/restarted. Data intensive task management does not allow such operations because only a single analysis run may need significant amount of time, memory, and processing power to finish. Thus, tracing back the problem or condition using the logs becomes necessary. Backtracking dataflow events and situations also become important for further deeper investigation [2, 13]. A workflow system offering workflow provenance enables such investigations. For example, the provenance information could be used to answer the questions—***'What particular parameter setting is responsible for a target error?', 'Which type of data element is most used for a particular module?', 'What is the source dataset of an intermediate data element?'*** and so on. So clearly, provenance analysis is the further analysis of data product that is derived from previous analyses and workflow runs. Big Data sources generating such provenance data create variety of (unstructured data) in those provenance data products. Thus workflow provenance itself becomes another Big Data problem.

Workflow systems are provided with a highly/loosely coupled provenance services [11]. Their logging mechanisms also vary significantly because of domain differences [11, 23]. In this era of Big Data analytics, we have already entered such a period where cross domain research and collaboration is taking place among researchers. Consequently, scientific systems like workflows also need to feature cross domain facilities and collaboration. The problem is, one workflow system which is best for a certain domain is not best for another. As already mentioned, different workflow systems' architectures differ significantly on different aspects. So, fusing any two workflows into one with their provenance features is not very easy. We focus only on workflow provenance and face the lack of a general and standard model for answering provenance questions. Working with any workflow also requires minimum amount of domain expertise. So, it is also necessary to separate all the concerns as much as possible while developing such a standard workflow model. For example, provenance logging configuration can be handled by data scientists and only workflow implementation can be handled by developers.

In order to overcome the above problems, in this paper, we propose a programming model for workflow provenance. We build the programming model solely based on object oriented programming model and inspired by existing novel workflow models [1, 2]. Thus it is easy to implement with less learning curve by any developer with minimum programming experience. We define different workflow components (e.g., data, module, condition, and dataflow) to offer various workflow features such as concise way of building pipelines and incorporating conditionals. The model is designed in a manner that enables automated logging of workflow provenance data [5]. The logging mechanism is not only fused with the programming model, but the log structure is also easily configurable by a domain expert without modifying the model. So, while implementing any pipeline with the model, there is no burden of log management. This is how we separate the concerns of logging and workflow development in our approach. Besides, necessary data analysis tools can be easily and independently implemented with our model by any developer of a certain domain. They can later be used just as a tool. In summary, our model offers and makes everyone related to a workflow system to work in a systematic procedure that makes use of the separation of concerns (SoC) design principle [17]. Furthermore, it can be extended to scalability for Big Data analytics with prominent technologies (e.g., Hadoop [22], Apache Spark [26], and so on). Any domain specific language (DSL) can be used on top of our programming model layer to facilitate further domain specific features. Then all the features of our programming model will be carried to that DSL automatically. The whole idea is illustrated as a layer based architecture in Fig. 1. Here, the OOP layer is the base layer of the whole system that can be further extended with any technology from the Extension. The programming model is built on the OOP model. Logging Configuration is in the same layer of the modelling but also independent from the proposed model. Any DSL could be built on the proposed model. Various tools could be presented at the top Tool layer. The workflow user directly uses the tools and model developer directly uses the OOP model to develop/extend the proposed programming model. Domain expert can independently configure logging configuration independent of any model developer or user.

Finally, to evaluate our provenance model, we will develop tools and pipelines from Bioinformatics. We gather a bunch of log data through simulations to use our proposed model—to implement workflow tools and pipelines. We also focus on the logs to discover important insights related to provenance. So, we target a number of provenance questions [3, 20] and analyze how much we can answer those questions

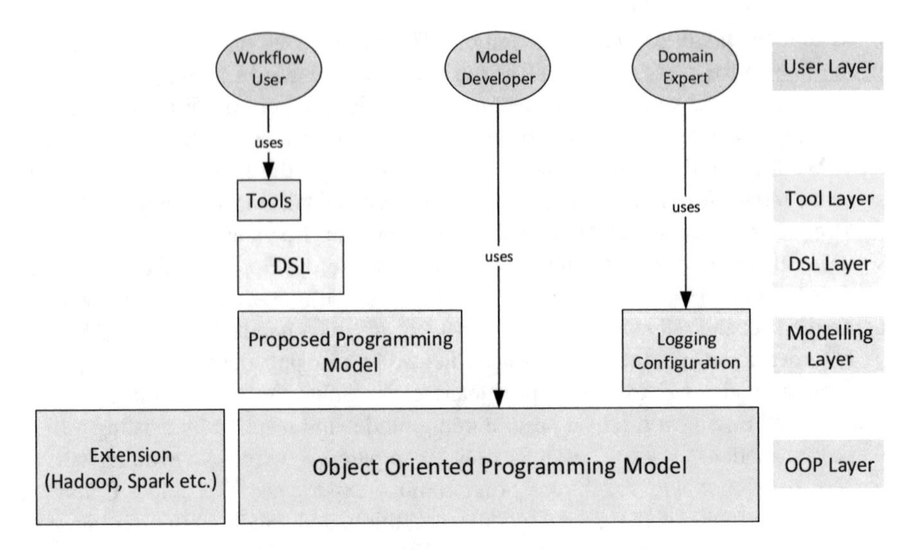

Fig. 1 A layer based architecture for our proposed programming model

from the logs that are further described in Sect. 2.2. A future work is to find out all the elementary provenance questions. By elementary provenance questions we indicate such provenance questions that are atomic/fundamental and can be used to derive any other provenance questions including advanced ones. Finally, all these findings can be provided to the end users in a meaningful way such as data visualization or reporting [9, 21]. We are developing a data provenance visualization service that will be offered as a web service. It will connect itself with the workflow system to facilitate online streaming log data analysis. SoC is again followed here and even only this visualization service can be further developed independently. Prominent machine learning tools and deep learning methods can be integrated with this visualization system to conduct big log data analytics. Consequently, all the components associated with the whole system will provide with distinct online services. The distinct services and their internal communication architecture are illustrated in Fig. 2. In this prototype of Fig. 2 the user directly uses the workflow system with all enabled features inside it and the online visualization service as well. The workflow process logs are saved in a database that are parsed through a parser. The logs can only be written in the database and the parser can only read from the log database. The visualization or reporting service reports the users using the online parser data based on their needs.

2 Research Methodology

Our work contains several phases. Each of the phases is divided into different sub-phases and covers versatile topics of research and development. Those phases are briefly described below.

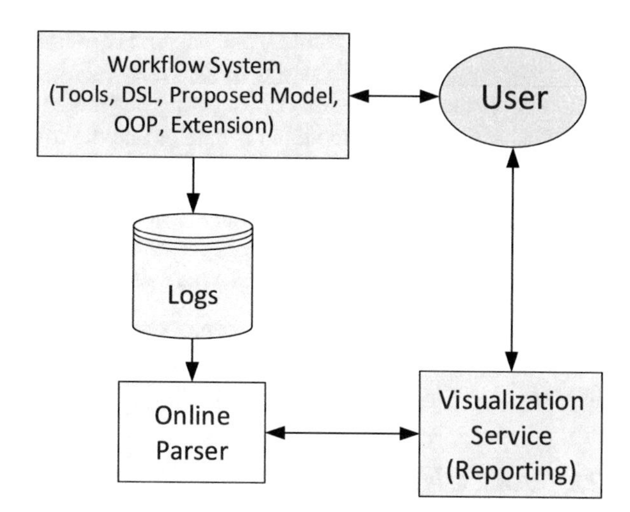

Fig. 2 System components services architecture

2.1 *Modelling Phase*

This phase covers the design and implementation of the programming model itself.

Designing Log Structure The structure of log is designed. This design can also vary. We primarily focus on plain text based logs. For certain reasons, other file formats can be useful. We will conduct a comparative study on which way is the best in a certain scenario.

Designing Programming Model We design the programming model and define certain workflow components, such as ***Data*** (that are classified into sub-categories), ***Module***, ***Dataflow***, ***User***, and ***Conditions*** at the moment and can be extended further.

Featuring Automated Logging The programming model is then integrated with the logging mechanism with latest logging technologies. We fully engineer the mechanism to make it automated.

Facilitating Data Management The logs are primarily saved as flat files and they can also be saved into database. We use NoSQL Database technology in this context. To enable online data streaming for any component, choose to use Apache Spark [26] and any related frameworks/technologies.

Implementation Phase Implementation phase relates to make the developers use the programming model for building workflows. Also a number of workflow tools are developed and pipelines from different angles are implemented.

Configuring Logs The logs are easily configured by any domain experts. Developers do not need to touch the configurations.

Implementing Analysis Tools Analysis tools are implemented by a group of tool developers (e.g., image processing tools, statistical tools, data cleansing tools, and so on). While converting their tools following our model, a migration of development happens. We design our model in a manner that the migration hassle is reduced and the task follows a similar pattern.

Layering with DSL A DSL can be layered upon our programming model. This way, all our model features are brought to the DSL layer. On top of it, the DSL provides more flexibility to develop workflows.

Designing Pipelines Pipelines and consequently complex workflows are designed and implemented using the DSL at this phase. This will generate log data for analysis.

2.2 Analysis Phase

This phase is about the generated logs and their analysis. The task of this phase is to discover as much provenance insights as we can and provide them to the end users in a standard way.

Parsing Logs Logs are parsed with our simple parser. These logs are semi-structured data because they are structured and also hold unstructured data.

Extracting Pipelines We leverage the power of Graph Database technology to re-extract the executed workflows and pipelines from previous phases. This way, all the features of Graph Database are integrated in our system.

Querying Provenance We focus on a number of provenance questions from different angles. They cover questions about data lineage, user-data, data-module or user-module patterns, errors and anomalies, information retrieval, and recommendation.

Workflow Provenance Questions:

- What are the inputs of a module in an execution?
- What are the parameter settings of a module in an execution?
- What are the outputs of a module in an execution?
- What is the type of a data element in a workflow?
- What is the directed acyclic graph (DAG) representation of a workflow?
- Who is the user of a workflow component (module/data)?
- What are all the properties of a workflow component (module/data/user)?
- What is the lineage DAG representation of a data element from root source to data product?
- What is the user-defined condition of a module for its true execution?
- What is the time series data for any workflow component (module/data/user) with respect to a certain property?
- What is the DAG representation of a workflow for an error?

- What are all the properties of a workflow component (module/data/user) for an error?
- What is the classification of related modules in a workflow system?
- What is the classification of related data elements in a workflow system?
- What are the module–module, data–data, user–user, module–data, module–user, and data–user usage patterns in a workflow system?
- What is the best visualization approach for a particular provenance question?

Reporting or Data Visualization Building a web service that can analyze online streaming log data from the log database of a workflow system is possible. The reporting can be done with data visualization techniques using modern technologies.

```
#import libraries
from ProvModel import Object, Module

#A module to double the input data

#Inherit Module
class Double(Module):
    #Define body
    def body(self):
        #P is a list of parameters
        #Get value of 1st parameter
        a = self.P[0].ref
        c = a + a
        #Return output as model object
        res = Object(c)
        return res


#A workflow to double a data value
#d1 -> Double -> d2

#Create a data object holding value 111
d1 = Object(111)
#Define a pre-built module
double = Double(d1)
#Run the module
#Output data in d2
d2 = double.run()
```

Listing 1 A pipeline implementation with our model

3 Implementation Details

The implementation of ProvMod is provided in Fig. 4. The user uses a workflow through the user interface. Through the user interface, they may use a DSL to implement their workflows that stands on the ProvMod model. ProvMod stands on Python Interpreter at the core. The logging configuration can be customized by a different user who is an expert in the domain. External tools can be integrated with ProvMod that can even be developed by other users. ProvMod also offers a number of tools as Library Tools. External Tools and Library Tools may have their own database facilities. The ProvMod, leveraging the power of Python Programming Language and Logging Configuration, saves the logs in a Graph Database that we implemented with Neo4j [24]. Through the user interface, the user may later submit a query through a query engine. The query engine uses Cypher Query Language to parse logs from the Graph Database. The query result is provided with D3 in a web browser. All the communication between each pair of components is done through RESTful Web Services [10]. We also emphasize using NoSQL database such as Cassandra [16] for Library Tools. An example of the pipeline in Fig. 3 is provided in Listing 1 code snippet (Fig. 4).

4 Experiments

We implement two different workflows from Bioinformatics described in Figs. 7 and 8. The first workflow is about counting DNA letters from a genetic dataset. We also count the length of the gene. Based on the nucleotide base counts, we can calculate the Entropy of the gene sequence. We also find out, which base is having the most and least probability of occurrence over the full sequence to get an understanding of the full sequence along with its entropy. In the second workflow, we run FastQC [4] over the datasets to generate FastQC results. Note, in the simulation, a collection of genetic data is used that is described in Fig. 5. The .fastq files are only valid inputs for FastQC and generate error otherwise. In the simulation, to generate user-oriented usage scenario, we choose a data randomly from the dataset to input through the workflows. Also, from the first workflow, only DNALetterCount is executed or DNALetterCount with Entropy is executed or DNALetterCount with Entropy and MaxMinProv tools are executed. Otherwise, FastQC is executed with random inputs. They are selected randomly. Between

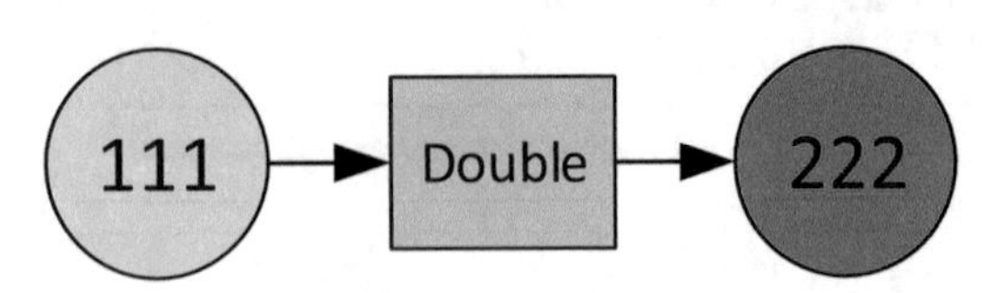

Fig. 3 A pipeline that doubles the input to output

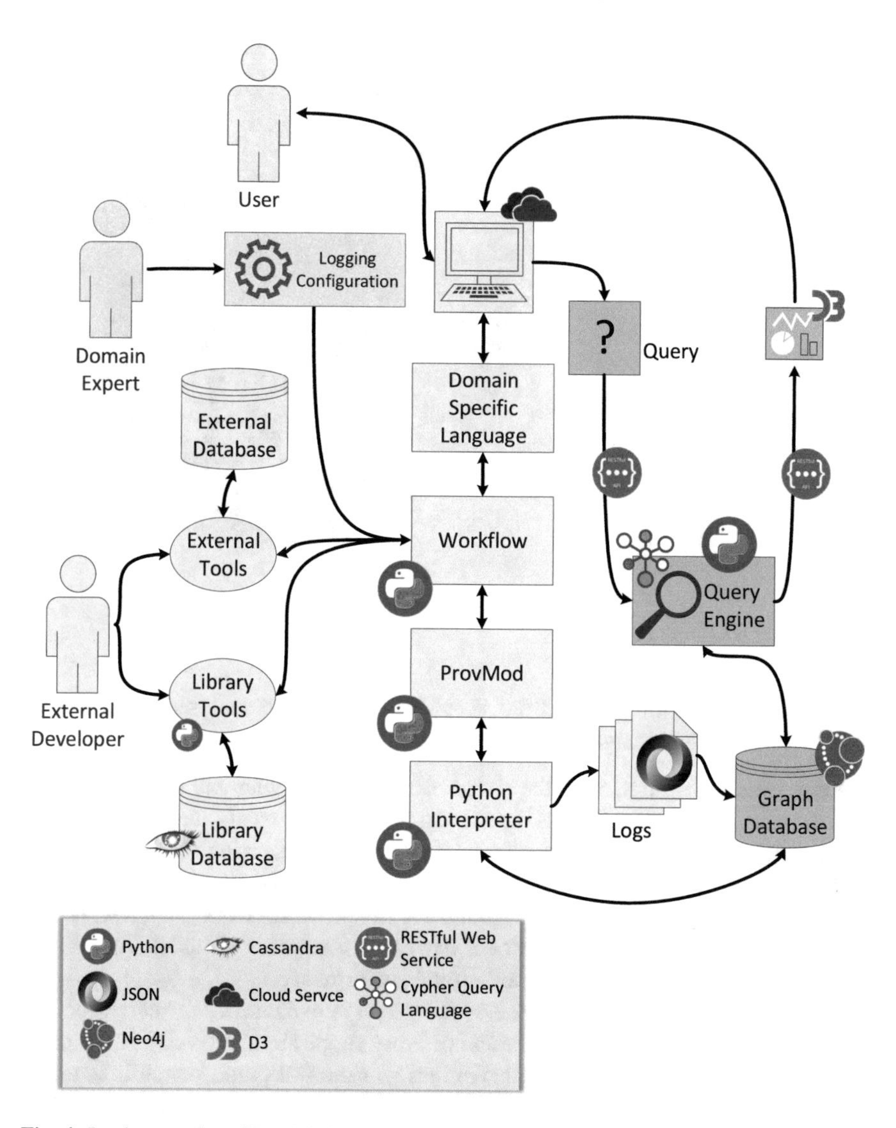

Fig. 4 Implementation of ProvMod and relation between other components of the whole workflow system that we propose

the executions, there is a random gap of 1–7 s. From the simulation, we create a provenance graph of around 20,000 nodes that contains logs about FastQC errors too. A portion with 300 nodes from the provenance graph is shown in Fig. 6 (Figs. 7 and 8).

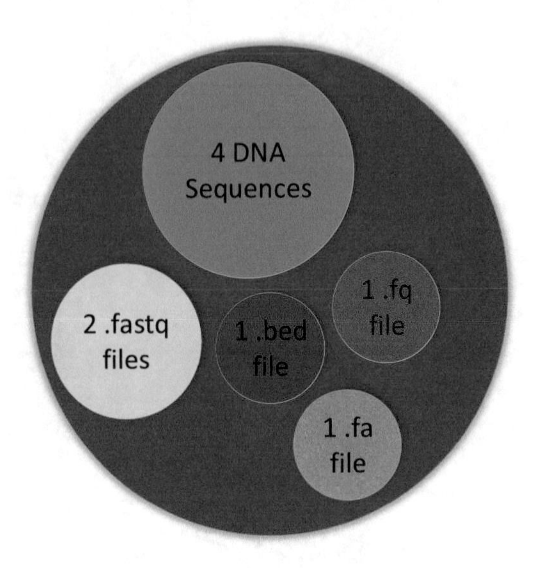

Fig. 5 Experimental dataset overview

5 Performance Analysis

We analyze several things about our ProvMod model. The analyses are described below with the found insights:

1. As our model is fused with the Graph Database, querying and adding nodes is always happening throughout the execution. It can be easily turned off, but we are eager to see how much performance overhead is occurring for that. In Fig. 9, we can see, when there are around 20,000 nodes in the simulated provenance graph, the tool execution time is around 2 s. In real-world workflows, a workflow may contain around 10 nodes or so, but never thousands of nodes for a single user. So, our ProvMod model shows good performance.
2. The query time will also increase as the graph is expanded. We search the full graph during the simulation at the end of every single simulation step and capture the time to collect the full graph. We find that the full graph search is returned within 1.5 s when there are around 20,000 nodes in the provenance graph in Fig. 10. This clarifies that our ProvMod model query is not time consuming and fast.
3. Finally, we compare the whole simulation with and without provenance and measure the performance overhead the ProvMod logging is actually creating that we present in Fig. 11. It becomes clear that, for such a huge graph with 20,000 nodes, the provenance creates an overhead of around 0.5 s in average.

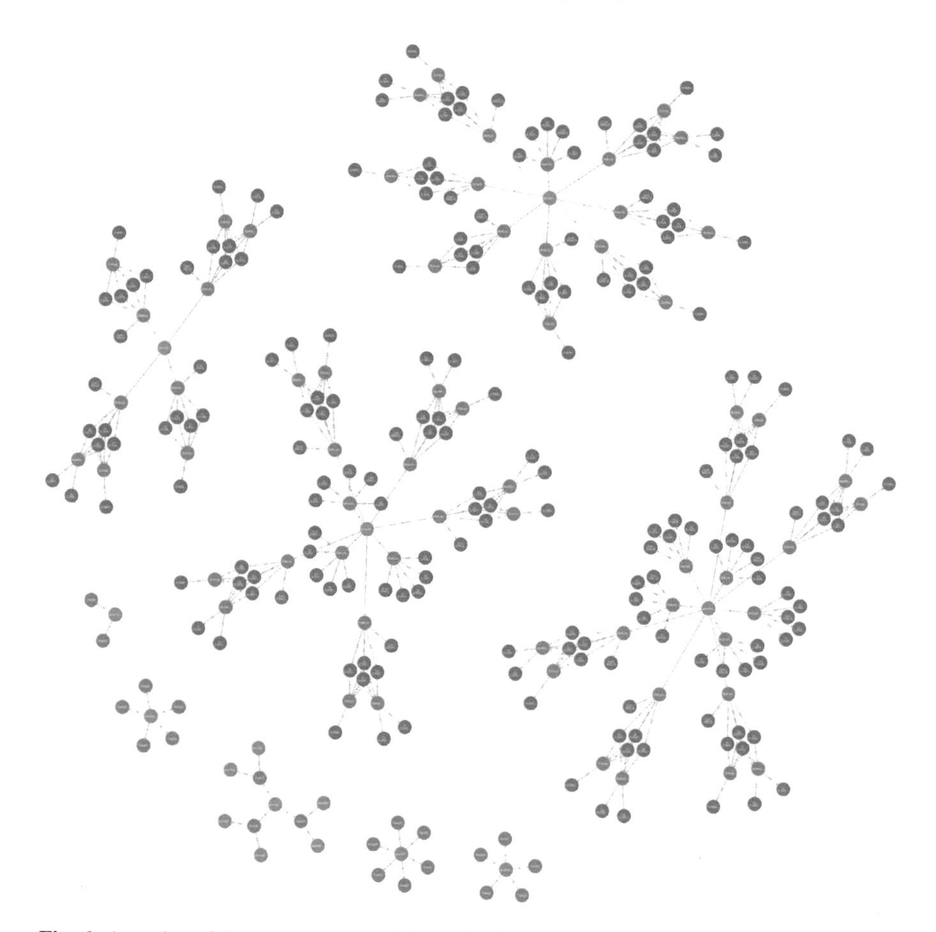

Fig. 6 A portion of the provenance graph from the simulation. This snapshot is taken from the big graph view of Kibana implementation. Different node types are represented with different colors with zoom in and out feature. The overall view is showing how big graphs can be used to capture provenance graph patterns

6 Related Works

Significant amount of research works were conducted on Big Data and that is still going on. Big Data being one of the most demanding technologies now flourished significantly. Dietrich et al. describe all the phases of Big Data analytics lifecycle in their book in details [12]. The survey of Chen et al. describes the challenges, open questions, analytics lifecycle, related important technologies, and impact of Big Data in their work [9]. Online data streaming as well as analysis is a crucial part in Big Data. Hadoop [22] and Spark [26] are two well-known technologies to achieve such requirement. The practice of Software Engineering is also very important for building a perfect system, specially when it involves different groups

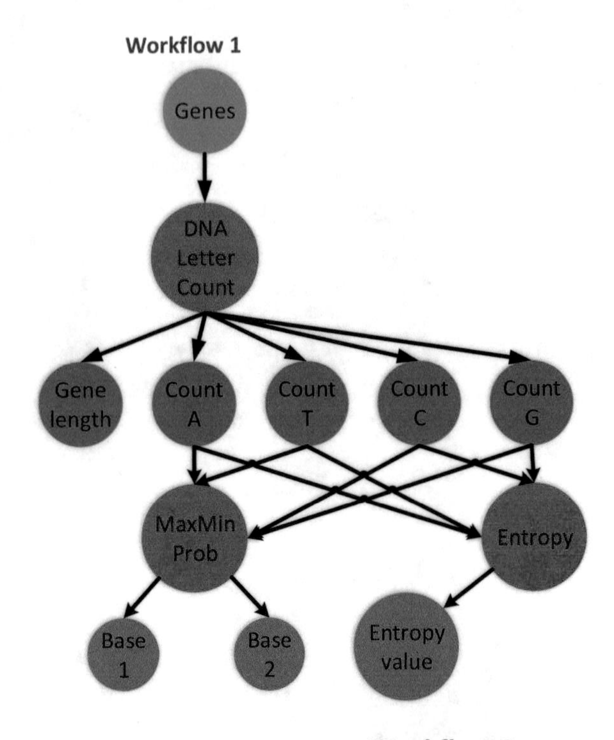

Fig. 7 First workflow for simulation

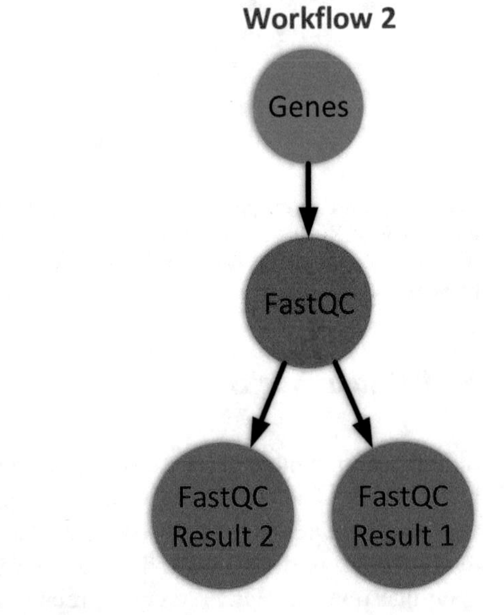

Fig. 8 Second workflow for simulation

of developers and experts. Separation of Concerns (SoC) is one of the design principles of Software Engineering [17]. While designing different services in our work, we tried to follow this principle.

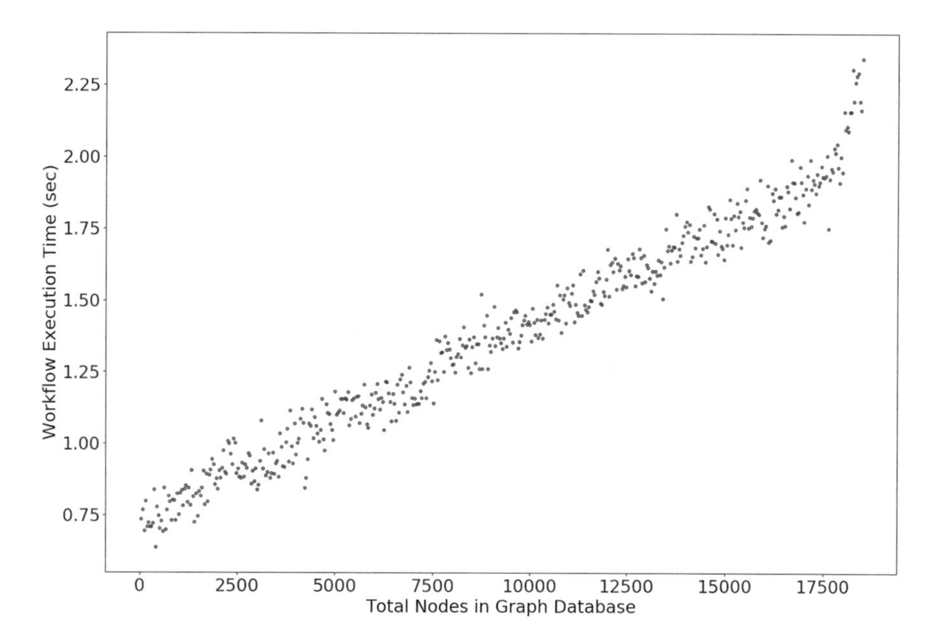

Fig. 9 Execution overhead of ProvMod

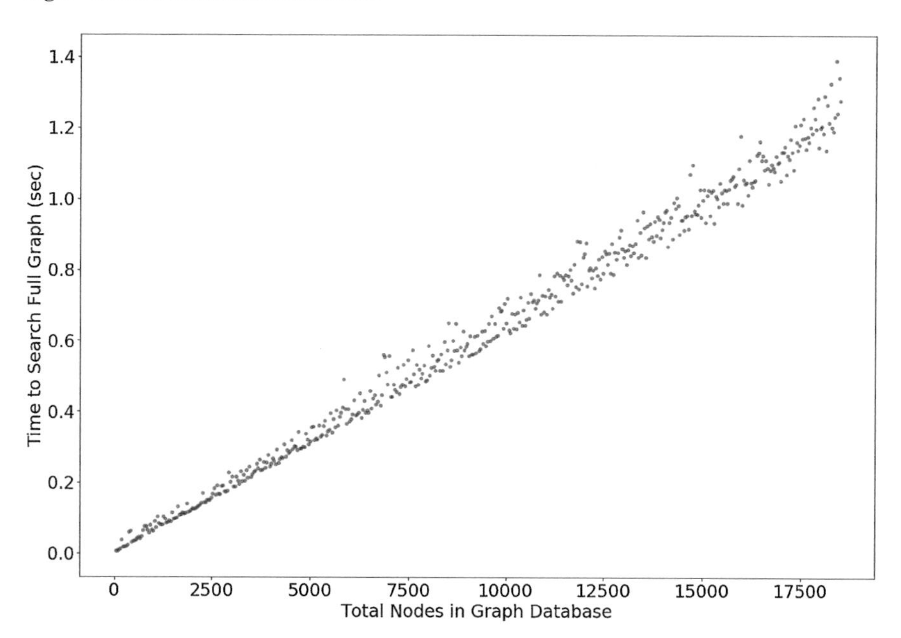

Fig. 10 Query overhead of ProvMod

Scientific workflow systems or workflows have created various research directions. Each of them focuses on different research problems. A good survey of this topic and future direction could be found in the work of Barker et al. [6]. Besides,

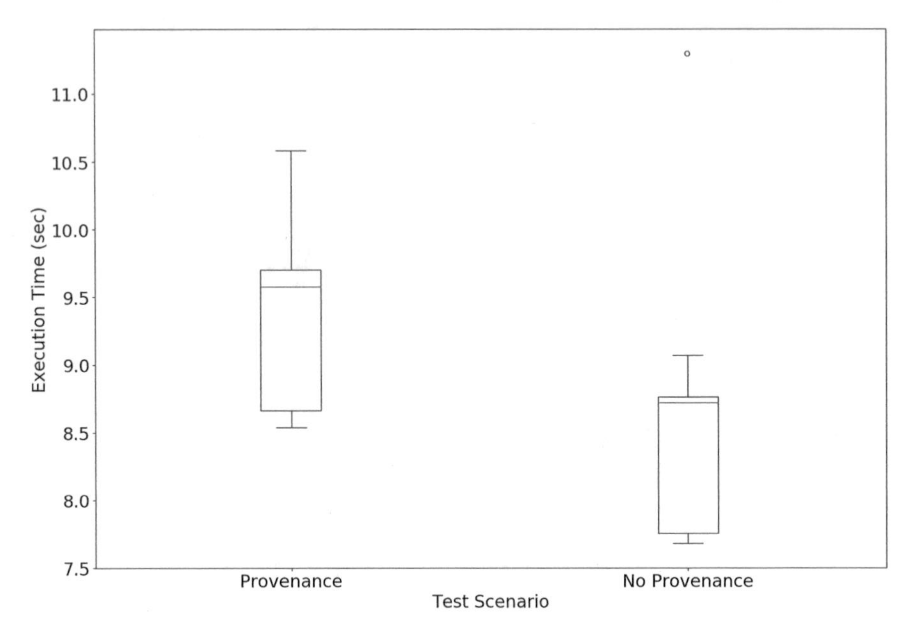

Fig. 11 Comparison of ProvMod execution time with and without provenance

all workflows are not same and workflows in Big Data analytics require integration of further data intensive tools and technologies. Liu et al. in their work survey on such data intensive workflows [18]. A scientific classification of workflow systems is presented by Yu et al. [25]. Kepler [19] and Galaxy [15] are two such examples of scientific workflows for general purpose to domain specific research works.

Workflow provenance, that is the central topic of our work, is a big issue. The problems, research angles, solutions, and implementations vary from domain to domain. A well classification for all these provenance related topics in workflow systems is described by Cruz et al. [11]. They demonstrate how provenance in workflows differs in different aspects. They also take into account a number of existing workflows and evaluate them with their taxonomy. The importance of automated provenance in workflows is presented by Barga et al. [5]. How provenance information could be gathered from only manipulating logs is presented in the work of Ghoshal et al. [13]. Many programming models were emerged for solving problems in workflow provenance. One such work is the work of Amsterdamer et al. [2] that differentiates between data provenance and workflow provenance very clearly. They also propose a method that leverages the fashion of data provenance for capturing workflow provenance. Another work is the work of Acer et al. [1] that proposes a graph based workflow provenance model to describe lineage of dataflow.

Workflow provenance has been separated from the concept of data provenance itself. Workflow provenance is the provenance of such data that were originated from workflow systems. Still provenance of workflows are data elements. To be successful in analyzing provenance of any data, studying the topic of data provenance becomes necessary. A survey of data provenance in e-science was done by Simmhan et al. [23]. Buenman et al. [7] characterize data provenance with respect to the question of 'Why' and 'Where'. Hartig et al. [14] present an approach of data provenance that extends previous approaches and suitable for data involved in web technologies. Buenman et al. [8] overview the concept of provenance in database technologies.

Querying is the final problem of provenance. A set of fundamental provenance questions may lead to an empirical research in this topic. Anand et al. [3] describe techniques for efficient querying of workflow provenance graphs. Missier et al. [20] present an approach for fine-grained lineage querying that is also efficient. Analytic provenance is another topic that was emerged from workflow provenance and involves data visualization, which is also another research domain. The importance of data visualization in workflow provenance could be understood from the work of Ragan et al. [21].

7 Conclusion and Future Works

We try to bring every related component starting from workflow design to end user reporting into one place. Our proposed approach is for any kind of workflow system. Bioinformatics is primarily selected for our study and system evaluations because this research topic covers versatile ranges of scientific domains and also ranges to Big Data research problem. Our research can lead to a general recommendation and standard for workflow provenance research. Data provenance research can be merged with this topic and overall provenance research can flourish. We also plan to find the elementary provenance questions that is applicable in all domains of Data Science.

References

1. Acar, U., Buneman, P., Cheney, J., Van Den Bussche, J., Kwasnikowska, N., & Vansummeren, S. A graph model of data and workflow provenance.
2. Amsterdamer, Y., Davidson, S. B., Deutch, D., Milo, T., Stoyanovich, J., & Tannen, V. (2011). Putting lipstick on pig: Enabling database-style workflow provenance. *Proceedings of the VLDB Endowment, 5*(4), 346–357.
3. Anand, M. K., Bowers, S., & Ludäscher, B. (2010). Techniques for efficiently querying scientific workflow provenance graphs. In *EDBT* (Vol. 10, pp. 287–298).
4. Andrews, S. (2015). Babraham Bioinformatics - Fastqc A Quality Control Tool For High Throughput Sequence Data.
5. Barga, R. S., & Digiampietri, L. A. (2006). Automatic generation of workflow provenance. In *International Provenance and Annotation Workshop* (pp. 1–9). Berlin: Springer.
6. Barker, A., & Van Hemert, J. (2007). Scientific workflow: A survey and research directions. In *International Conference on Parallel Processing and Applied Mathematics* (pp. 746–753). Berlin: Springer.

7. Buneman, P., Khanna, S., & Wang-Chiew, T. (2001). Why and where: A characterization of data provenance. In *International Conference on Database Theory* (pp. 316–330). Berlin: Springer.
8. Buneman, P., & Tan, W.-C. (2007). Provenance in databases. In *Proceedings of the 2007 ACM SIGMOD International Conference on Management of Data* (pp. 1171–1173). New York: ACM.
9. Chen, M., Mao, S., & Liu, Y. (2014). Big data: A survey. *Mobile Networks and Applications, 19*(2), 171–209.
10. Christensen, J. H. (2009). Using restful web-services and cloud computing to create next generation mobile applications. In *Proceedings of the 24th ACM SIGPLAN Conference Companion on Object Oriented Programming Systems Languages and Applications* (pp. 627–634). New York: ACM.
11. da Cruz, S. M. S., Campos, M. L. M., & Mattoso, M. (2009). Towards a taxonomy of provenance in scientific workflow management systems. In *2009 World Conference on Services-I* (pp. 259–266). Piscataway: IEEE.
12. Dietrich, D., Heller, B., & Yang, B. (2015). Data science & big data analytics: discovering, analyzing, visualizing and presenting data.
13. Ghoshal, D., & Plale, B. (2013). Provenance from log files: A big data problem. In *Proceedings of the Joint EDBT/ICDT 2013 Workshops* (pp. 290–297). New York: ACM.
14. Hartig, O. (2009). Provenance information in the web of data. In *LDOW*, 538.
15. Hillman-Jackson, J., Clements, D., Blankenberg, D., Taylor, J., Nekrutenko, A., & Team, G. (2012). Using galaxy to perform large-scale interactive data analyses. *Current Protocols in Bioinformatics*, 10-5.
16. Lakshman, A., & Malik, P. (2010). Cassandra: A decentralized structured storage system. *ACM SIGOPS Operating Systems Review, 44*(2), 35–40.
17. Laplante, P. A. (2007). *What Every Engineer Should Know About Software Engineering* (Boca Raton: CRC Press).
18. Liu, J., Pacitti, E., Valduriez, P., & Mattoso, M. (2015). A survey of data-intensive scientific workflow management. *Journal of Grid Computing, 13*(4), 457–493.
19. Ludäscher, B., Altintas, I., Berkley, C., Higgins, D., Jaeger, E., Jones, M., et al. (2006). Scientific workflow management and the kepler system. *Concurrency and Computation: Practice and Experience, 18*(10), 1039–1065.
20. Missier, P., Paton, N. W., & Belhajjame, K. (2010). Fine-grained and efficient lineage querying of collection-based workflow provenance. In *Proceedings of the 13th International Conference on Extending Database Technology* (pp. 299–310). New York: ACM.
21. Ragan, E. D., Endert, A., Sanyal, J., & Chen, J. (2016). Characterizing provenance in visualization and data analysis: An organizational framework of provenance types and purposes. *IEEE Transactions on Visualization and Computer Graphics, 22*(1), 31–40.
22. Shvachko, K., Kuang, H., Radia, S., & Chansler, R. (2010). The hadoop distributed file system. In *2010 IEEE 26th Symposium on Mass Storage Systems and Technologies (MSST)* (pp. 1–10). Piscataway: IEEE.
23. Simmhan, Y. L., Plale, B., & Gannon, D. (2005). A survey of data provenance in e-science. *ACM Sigmod Record, 34*(3), 31–36.
24. Webber, J. (2012). A programmatic introduction to neo4j. In *Proceedings of the 3rd Annual Conference on Systems, Programming, and Applications: Software for Humanity* (pp. 217–218). New York: ACM.
25. Yu, J., & Buyya, R. (2005). A taxonomy of scientific workflow systems for grid computing. *ACM Sigmod Record, 34*(3), 44–49.
26. Zaharia, M., Xin, R. S., Wendell, P., Das, T., Armbrust, M., Dave, A., et al. (2016). Apache spark: A unified engine for big data processing. *Communications of the ACM, 59*(11), 56–65.

A Perspective on "Working with Data" Curriculum Development

Emad A. Mohammed

Abstract In this paper, I am reporting a perspective on how to adapt current traditional courses in undergraduate engineering curricula to develop a curriculum for Data Science Specialization for Engineers at the undergraduate level. For engineers, to be able to handle data science related problems/projects at the undergrad level, their education needs to expose them more toward project-based learning scheme that covers all aspects of the data analytics lifecycle. However, given the robust and well-developed undergraduate engineering curricula and the limited resources, it would be beneficial to modify some of the courses offered at the undergraduate level to address the different aspects of data analytics lifecycle. I conclude this paper with a list of suggested/modified courses, their descriptions and objectives, tools and development platforms, challenges, project ideas, and teaching methodology. The list represents a seed for a curriculum proposal and a pilot project is needed to measure the effectiveness of the proposed curriculum.

Keywords Teaching Big Data · Data analytics curriculum · Data-centric curriculum · Curriculum development · Teaching methodologies

1 Introduction

Data analytics is a foundational topic for engineering, computer science, and business students, given its importance in subsequent coursework. Teaching is a multifaceted activity which involves planning for learning, organizing materials, prioritizing ideas, interacting with students, learning to "monitor and adjust," "communicate instruction" for students of various abilities, and learning how to accomplish goals.

E. A. Mohammed (✉)
Department of Software Engineering, Lakehead University, Thunder Bay, ON, Canada
e-mail: emohamme@lakeheadu.ca

R. Alhajj et al. (eds.), *Data Management and Analysis*, Studies in Big Data 65,
https://doi.org/10.1007/978-3-030-32587-9_12

In Winter-2015, I had the opportunity to co-design and deliver the first undergrad course at the University of Calgary "Engineering Large-Scale Analytics Systems," where the concepts of Big Data tools and analytics were discussed on the theoretical and practical characteristics. Since then, I developed more interests in teaching data analytics courses. In Spring 2017, I had another opportunity to co-lecture a graduate course "Hands-on Intelligent Systems Analytics." In this course, the concepts of deep learning, convolutional and recurrent neural networks, transfer learning, and domain to domain learning were explored.

In Fall 2017, I joined the Lakehead University in the Software Engineering Department. Since then, I taught different data analytics courses for graduate and undergraduate students, including in-database analytics, applied computational intelligence, data mining, and large-scale data analytics. I designed/updated the curricula of these courses based on other courses, personal experience, and data science career requirements.

I used different delivery "teaching" methods per course and assessed the performance of the student. Although there are many components to assess in these courses, I monitored the efforts of the students in their projects as an indicator of the success of my teaching methods. The project component of any courses requires the employment of many engineering skills, such as team and time management, deep understanding of the theoretical and practical parts of the course, and the most crucial part is how to validate and critically discuss the results of the projects.

Given the different nature of the projects at different course levels, I used different teaching methodologies to manage the project component of each course. My teaching methods are (1) Asking the students to bring their ideas, write proposals, formulate the engineering problem, design, and implement their solution "Reviewer," (2) Explaining some existing data science projects "Learning by example," ask the student to follow the guidelines of these projects, and adapt the guidelines to their projects, (3) Acting as the team leader for all the projects by explaining and giving concrete examples of what is needed and how to solve similar situations.

The average project performance per group per course showed that adopting the "Learning by example," teaching method showed slightly better results than the other two methods. In the next run of the courses, I will use a mixture of the last two methods. Furthermore, I concluded that Big Data analytics course might not be offered as an elective course in the fourth year, as students are ready to graduate and have no additional capacity to learn new concepts, this is in addition to their degree project workload. For graduate students, it was almost the same thing, and they need more support and interactions. It is better to have a data science program or track that should contain several courses to prepare the students for data science job requirements, which is described in Fig. 1.

A dedicated high availability distributed and parallel processing infrastructure is needed for research and educational purposes. The infrastructure will allow the students to practice data science project with real-life use-cases and build usable data products. The significant problems with this conclusion are (1) limited resources, e.g., faculty and infrastructure, (2) compliance with the student learning outcomes

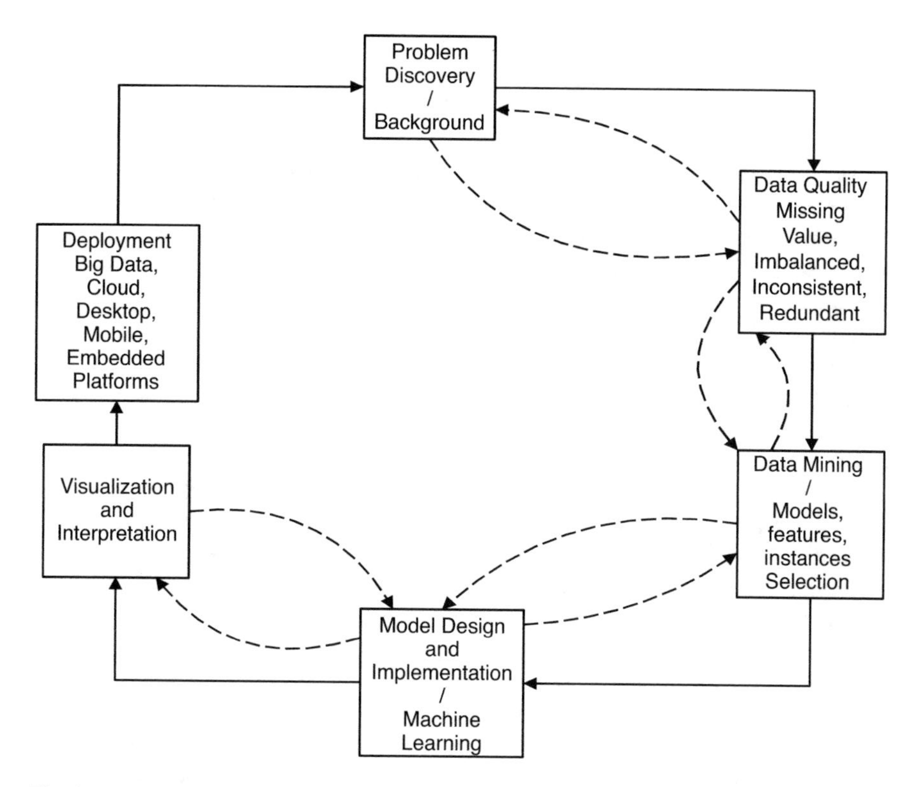

Fig. 1 Data analytics life cycle

(SLOs). The SLOs must comply with the departmental rules and accreditation bodies. In this paper, I propose some changes to the traditional courses curricula and make them prerequisites to each other in a specific order that can guarantee specific sequence of topics and hands-on practice toward a data scientist career. The course topics can be tailored without violating any departmental or accreditation rules.

In the following sections, I briefly describe my viewpoint about data analytics curriculum development. I further list the suggested courses with objectives, challenges, development tools, and platform, and the suggested teaching methodology per course.

2 Toward Knowledge Discovery Curriculum

Big Data [1] is the technical term that describes massive volumes of data with many varieties (images, text, video, speech) and high value (utility). The analysis of Big Data is primarily different from traditional databases because of its characteristics.

However, from the data mining perspective, the same algorithms can be used to extract useful patterns regardless of the size of the database, given that an algorithm can be implemented in a way that suits the distributed nature of a Big Data application. This fact represents a strategy to address a "*working with data*" curriculum that may include both traditional and Big databases.

A data scientist career requires engineers to be skilled in many tasks [2] including problem domain understanding, data collection and preparation, data analysis using statistical models, interpreting, visualizing, and communicating the results. One crucial step to realize the efforts of a data science project is to deploy the data solution/product to a suitable platform and make it available.

Project-based courses were implemented into undergraduate engineering curricula and were approved to be very beneficial to improve the undergraduate engineers understanding of complicated engineering courses [3, 4]. However, given the nature of the data science project, it seems to be challenging to offer project-based courses that focus only the course material without relying on the students to understand other parts of the projects by themselves. The data science projects are usually offered at the final year of the undergraduate engineering program and require substantial independent work which might not be feasible given the other course workloads including the fourth-year degree project.

An alternative solution is to develop a set of courses that must be offered in sequence from the freshman to graduation level. Each course may address one specific requirement/skill for a data science career through one substantial project. In the next section, a graphical representation of the required data scientist career skills is presented and discussed. This exploration is mandatory to highlight the tasks and activities related to the analysis of data and hence develop a detailed proposal of a "*working with data*" curriculum to address these specific tasks and activities including development tools, development platform, challenges, and project ideas.

2.1 Data Analytics Lifecycle Driven Curriculum

The data analytics lifecycle illustrated in Fig. 1 is a structured way of visualizing the activities involved in a data science project and the iterative nature of these activities. The data analytics lifecycle starts by defining the problem domain and interviewing domain experts to collect project requirements and goals. The data scientist must have a clear understanding of the problem domain (business scope) or regularly consult with a domain expert. In a limited resources data science project, data scientist depends on themselves to understand a specific problem domain. However, the elicited project requirements and goals must be verified by an external reviewer to make sure of the project consistency. The requirements elicitation based on the domain knowledge task is followed by data sources identification and collection. The collected datasets must be refined and reviewed against the domain knowledge to make sure that the collected data will help in identifying the required business goals.

Data preprocessing is a mandatory step to enhance the quality of the datasets being used to extract useful information [5]. The preprocessing may include many steps, such as missing value imputation, noise removal, normalization, etc. [5]. Data collection may include a variety of data sources to increase the probability of finding hidden patterns and correlations within the data.

The next step of the data analytics lifecycle is to find suitable statistical data mining techniques that can help in to identify relevant information with the datasets. Although there are several guidelines [6] on how to select and train machine learning models, the nature of the dataset will impose ad hoc strategy to select the relevant features and instances to be able to reveal the hidden pattern in the data with the highest accuracy.

Big data projects impose several considerations that need to be addressed to ensure the feasibility of the implementation of machine learning algorithms. Due to the characteristics of Big Data, the machine learning algorithms must be iterative and distributed among physical computing nodes. Many Big Data applications are required to provide real-time/high throughput analysis, which imposes another challenge on how to guarantee the timing performance of the distributed machine learning algorithms.

Several tools can be used to address the above issues related to the distributed machine learning algorithms implementation such as Hadoop [7], Spark [8], and H2O [9]. Although these tools are open source and widely available, there are significant challenges to leverage the power of these tools such as the steep learning curves and the limitation of the technical support of the open-source tools.

Data visualization is an essential step in any data science project. Visualization techniques can be used in almost all data mining and machine learning process to communicate visual information about the data and the insights discovered. While several development tools (programming framework) such as Python [10] and R packages [11] provide a variety of data visualization and plotting packages, they require significant programming efforts (Lines of Code) to produce the different visualization graphs that are required extensively especially at the exploratory phase of the data science project. Several commercial and open-source packages are developed to address these concerns such as Data Science Studio [12], QlikView [13], and Tableau [14].

The final step in the data analytics lifecycle is to deploy the data product in a suitable production environment. Many deployment environments/infrastructures are available nowadays and can be used as a production and test environment for the data product. Some data analytics projects may require a distributed deployment environment such as WindowsAzure [15], Bluemix [16], Domino [17], and Ubuntu JUJU [18]. Other applications, especially real-time applications, require embedded deployment environment. The Raspberry Pi embedded system [19] can be a suitable environment for real-time data products.

The data science firms, when announcing for a job position, they typically list all the skills described by the data analytics life cycle in the job posting [20]. The firms expect to receive applications from experienced engineers, and they interview them for the list of data science projects they did previously.

The engineering programs must prepare students for the current job market. The curriculum must be modified to reflect the readiness of the undergraduate students for such data science jobs. The curriculum modifications will be integrated during the course time, and no extra hours are needed. The negative impact is minimal as the core theoretical part of the original courses will be covered, and the project/assignment material will be designed targeting the data science part of the course. In the following section, a "*working with data*" curriculum is illustrated to address the challenging today's job market in a data science career.

2.2 Proposed Coursework of Working with Data Curriculum

Data warehouse infrastructures are intended for historical data storage for supporting enterprise decision-making strategies. However, these infrastructures did not leverage sophisticated analysis beyond reporting of statistical information. This is because of the lack of trained and specialized engineers who can design, implement, and deploy such data products for decision-making purposes. Figure 1 describes the data analytics lifecycle and states the required skills at each stage. This figure can be utilized to efficiently develop a curriculum in data analytics to serve as in-depth training for engineers to help them develop data analytics skills based on hands-on experience with real-life projects. Table 1 shows a layout of a "*working with data*" curriculum. Table 1 describes eight courses that may be used in sequence and each course can be a prerequisite for the next one.

In the "Database Integrity and Management" course, the students learn how to design a database that can preserve the integrity of the data and make it more useful to extract patterns. In this course, the concept of how the database characteristics can affect the data quality and how to improve the database characteristics to improve the data quality are addressed.

The "Data Mining" course is dedicated to exploring and preprocessing the data in the database framework. The concepts of in-database analytics and how this can improve database performance are addressed. Furthermore, the different preprocessing and noise removal steps are addressed in-depth.

The "Applied Computational Intelligence" course focuses on machine learning and search algorithms. Many algorithms and concepts are discussed in this course. The major topics include A_* search algorithm [21], support vector machine [22], neural network, and model parameters tuning [22]. This course covers varieties of the theoretical and practical aspects of the machine learning techniques.

The "Visualization" course covers many topics on how to select and implement the optimal visualization graphs based on the type of the datasets being processed. Different graph characteristics are discussed and covered in detail. The goal is to create automatic scripts to generate these graphs to help speeding up the exploratory phase of the data science projects.

The "Big Data Tools" course is devoted to describing and exploring the various Big Data ecosystems and how to use them to design and implement Big Data

Table 1 Proposed "working with data" curriculum courses

Course/duration hours)	Objective	Challenges	Development tools	Development platform	Project ideas	Teaching method	Project activities
Database integrity and management/36 h	To improve data quality	How to address Schema Refinement, data warehouse, indexing and security from the perspective of data quality	SQL NoSQL R Python	PCs	Kaggle UCI data	Team leader	Assignments/ projects
Data mining/36 h	To think about data	How to build a map between data types, types of learning and models for different tasks (feature selection, dimensionality reduction, instance selection, models selection)	Data Science Studio R Python	PCs	Kaggle UCI data	Team leader	Quizzes/projects
Applied computational intelligence/36 h	To work with data	How to train and validate a model in an adaptive way for different types of learning	Data Science Studio R Python	PCs	Kaggle UCI data	Learning by example	Assignments/ projects
Visualization/36 h	To support design decisions and actionable insights	How to select variables to visualize	QlikView Tableau	PCs	Kaggle UCI data	Learning by example	Discussion/ projects/ presentations

(continued)

Table 1 (continued)

Course/duration hours)	Objective	Challenges	Development tools	Development platform	Project ideas	Teaching method	Project activities
Big data tools/36 h	To use technology	How to provide technical support for naive user to a variety of tools	R Python	Hadoop, Spark, H2O On distributed platforms (CPUs and GPUs)	Motivate the student to bring their ideas	Reviewer	Assignments/ projects
Unstructured data processing/36 h	To extract features from images, sound, natural language	How to define the required features (Background Knowledge)	R Python	Hadoop, Spark, H2O On distributed platforms (CPUs and GPUs)	Motivate the student to bring their ideas	Reviewer	Assignments/ projects
Deep learning (this course can be part of the Applied Computational Intelligence)/36 h	To prepare the data (especially nonimage data) To use pre-trained models to learn and experiment with Convolutional NN To learn and experiment with Recurrent NN	How to provide resources and technical support	R Python	Hadoop, Spark, H2O On distributed platforms (CPUs and GPUs)	Motivate the student to bring their ideas	Reviewer	Projects/ presentation
Deployment platforms/36 h	To have hands-on practice with different deployment platforms	How to provide resources and technical support	Ubuntu JUJU Embedded OS	Hadoop Cluster, Bluemix, Azure, Domino, Data Science Studio, Raspberry Pi	Motivate the student to bring their ideas	Reviewer	Projects/ presentation

application. This course covers characteristics of Big Data, benefits of Big Data analytics to various industry domains, programming paradigms and middleware technologies for scalable data analysis, algorithms that enable Big Data analytics, application of Big Data algorithms in selected application domains.

Big data analytics platforms and frameworks such as Hadoop, MapReduce, Spark, and H2O, will be discussed. The students will be introduced to various machine learning algorithms with examples using the Spark and H2O frameworks. The students will be introduced to data storage, batch and real-time analysis, and interactive querying frameworks.

The "Unstructured Data Processing" course is dedicated to processing unstructured data such as free text, speech, and images and extracting useful, structured information to be used by the machine learning algorithms. One main characteristic of the Big Data is the variety of the input format that represents a bottleneck in the analytics pipeline. The major topics include free-text information extraction and representation, speech noise removal and features extraction, and image preprocessing, enhancement and feature extraction.

The "Deep Learning" course is a natural extension of the "Applied Computational Intelligence" course. The course provides hands-on practice on different types and topology of deep neural networks such as convolutional neural network (DNN) and recurrent neural network (RNN). A major topic of this course is how to implement and test different types of deep learning real-life applications, including speech and image classification.

The final step of the data analytics lifecycle is to deploy the data product on a suitable platform for production and testing purposes. For this purpose, the "Deployment Platform" course is designed to cover various data product platforms such as Windows Azure, Bluemix, and Dominos. These platforms are cloud-based and require deployment tools such as Ubuntu JUJU that can help in remote configuration of different cloud-based platforms. Dedicated platforms with embedded operating systems are also available as a deployment platform for data products such as the Raspberry Pi systems.

The above courses are all project-based course. Many open-data platforms are existed to support these courses including project ideas and datasets such as the Kaggle competition website [23] that provides real-life machine learning problems and the University of California, Irvine Machine Learning Repository [24].

Recent IT job market shows high demands for data scientists who can create actionable insights from the massive datasets exist in a modern data warehouse. The change in IT job market, in turn, mandates the need for proper data science education at the university level.

Traditional courses offered by electrical and computer departments are not meeting the needs of those seeking training. The current curricula in most electrical and computer engineering are focused on the electrical and computer engineering applied roots and on developing field specific techniques for a particular analysis to help to study and to illustrate the related theoretical properties.

Given the high weight on the theoretical part and the hand-crafted tutorial/lab, the current curricula should be adapted to allow the training in today's era in information technology and produce the market-ready university graduate in the data science field. In today's IT job market, engineers must be trained using multiple disciplinary data science curricula that should not only have engineering training but also have extensive hands-on practice analyzing data to produce end-to-end solutions to real-world problems.

In this book chapter, I share a general personal perspective and offer detailed recommendations derived from my successful experience (at the University of Calgary and Lakehead University) developing and teaching undergraduate, graduate-level, introductory data science courses centered entirely on real-life projects, and case studies at the university level.

The "*working with data*" curriculum comes with many challenges including how to implement any modifications to existing courses without affecting course integrity and accreditation requirements, how to provide a suitable infrastructure for the curriculum, and how to provide continuous technical support for the students. Although it is quite hard to find one concrete solution to address these challenges, I firmly believe that an implementation of this curriculum will boost the undergraduate engineering data science skills and prepare them to the future job market.

2.3 *Performance Measurement and Evaluation*

An essential part of any new or modified curriculum is to collect enough data and measure different quality attributes and compare the attributes against the goals of the curriculum. Currently, I am in the process of collecting and analyzing the outcome of the first time applying the modification to the traditional courses (Database Integrity and Management, Data Mining, Big Data Tools, and Unstructured Data Processing). For the analysis to be indicative, I will collect the same measures for the next year as well. The measures can be categorized into two groups, i.e., controlled and uncontrolled. The controlled measures are identified by the set of student learning outcomes (SLOs) that are linked specific, measurable set of graduate attributes indicators (GAIs). The controlled measures can be assessed using different methods such as exams and projects. The challenges measures are the free measures that measure how students benefited from the modification in the curriculum. The free measures may include the number of students that have jobs in the data science field and the number of students who have started their own data science company.

3 Conclusion and Future Work

Data science career has become one of the most desirable professions in today's market. However, the optimal curricula to train undergraduate engineers have not been prepared in a robust format to addresses the different data analytics lifecycle for educators to use it as guidelines for courses development. This paper addresses the challenges of training undergraduate engineering students for a data science career. This paper illustrates a useful curriculum to prepare undergraduate engineering students for data collection and preprocessing, data mining and machine learning theories, operational requirements of a data product including visualization and deployment options. The proposed curriculum is a project-based curriculum that leverages student skills and makes them comfortable when *"working with data"* in different real-life projects.

The goal is to provide an improved educational experience that emphasizes the different skills that an undergraduate engineer must have to be able to design, implement, and deploy a data product. Training an engineer to design and implement a data science project requires a considerable effort toward a "*working with data*" skills. The proposed curriculum presents a seed toward having a structured data science track in undergraduate engineering curricula.

The future work of this paper will focus on a pilot project to collect surveys from different stack-holders including students and program directors on the feasibility of "*working with data*" curriculum for further improvement and feedback and eventually a concrete implementation of the proposed curriculum.

References

1. LaValle, S., Lesser, E., Shockley, R., Hopkins, M. S., & Kruschwitz, N. (2013). Big data, analytics and the path from insights to value. *MIT Sloan Management Review, 21*, 20–31.
2. Stanton, J. M., et al. (2011). Education for eScience professionals: Job analysis, curriculum guidance, and program considerations. *Journal of Education for Library and Information Science, 52*(2), 79–94.
3. Macías, J., et al. Enhancing project-based learning in software engineering lab teaching through an E-portfolio approach. *IEEE Transactions on Education, 55*(4), 502–507.
4. Hadim, H. A., & Esche, S. K. (2002). Enhancing the engineering curriculum through project-based learning. In *Frontiers in education, 2002. FIE 2002. 32nd Annual* (Vol. 2, p. F3F). IEEE.
5. García, S., Luengo, J., & Herrera, F. (2016). *Data preprocessing in data mining*. New York: Springer.
6. Abdulrahman, S. M., Brazdil, P., van Rijn, J. N., & Vanschoren, J. (2018). Speeding up algorithm selection using average ranking and active testing by introducing runtime. *Machine Learning, 107*(1), 79–108.
7. White, T. (2012). *Hadoop: The definitive guide*. Sebastopol, CA: O'Reilly Media.
8. Shanahan, J. G., & Dai, L. (2015). Large scale distributed data science using apache spark. In *Proceedings of the 21th ACM SIGKDD international conference on knowledge discovery and data mining* (pp. 2323–2324). New York: ACM.
9. H2O.ai. Retrieved from https://www.h2o.ai/
10. *Welcome to Python.org*. Retrieved from https://www.python.org/
11. R: The R Project for Statistical Computing. Retrieved from https://www.r-project.org/
12. Dataiku | Collaborative Data Science Platform. Retrieved from https://www.dataiku.com/
13. Qlik: Data Analytics for Modern Business Intelligence. Retrieved from https://www.qlik.com/us/
14. @tableau. (2018). Tableau Reader.

15. Microsoft Azure Cloud Computing Platform & Services. Retrieved from https://azure.microsoft.com/en-ca/
16. IBM Cloud. Retrieved from https://www.ibm.com/cloud
17. @dominodatalab. *What is Domino?* Domino Data Lab. Retrieved from https://www.dominodatalab.com/
18. Canonical. (2018). Juju | Cloud | Ubuntu.
19. Raspberry PI board. Retrieved from https://www.raspberrypi.org/
20. Data Scientist | Job Post | LinkedIn. Retrieved from https://www.linkedin.com/jobs/view/592290132/
21. @redblobgames. (2018). Introduction to A_*. Retrieved from https://www.redblobgames.com/pathfinding/a-star/introduction.html
22. Kamber, M., Han, J., & Pei, J. (2012). *Data mining: Concepts and techniques*. Amsterdam: Elsevier.
23. Competitions | Kaggle. Retrieved from https://www.kaggle.com/competitions
24. UCI Machine Learning Repository. Retrieved from https://archive.ics.uci.edu/ml/index.php

Approaches for Early Detection of Glaucoma Using Retinal Images: A Performance Analysis

Abdullah Sarhan, Jon Rokne, and Reda Alhajj

Abstract Sight is one of the most important senses for humans, as it allows them to see and explore their surroundings. Multiple ocular diseases damaging sight have been detected over the years such as glaucoma and diabetic retinopathy. Glaucoma is a group of diseases that can lead to blindness if left untreated. No cure for glaucoma exists apart from early detection and treatment by an ophthalmologist. Retinal images provide vital information about an eye's health. On the basis of advancements in retinal images technology it is possible to develop systems that can analyze these images for better diagnosis. To test the efficiency of some of the developed techniques, we obtained the code for four different approaches and did a performance analysis using four public datasets. We investigated the results along with the analysis time. The outcomes of the study are

- approaches for glaucoma detection;
- behavior of glaucoma related approaches on retinal images with different ocular diseases;
- challenges faced when analyzing retinal images; and
- glaucoma risk factors.

Keywords Glaucoma · Retinal images · Machine learning · Performance analysis · Blindness

A. Sarhan (✉) · J. Rokne
Department of Computer Science, University of Calgary, Calgary, AB, Canada
e-mail: asarhan@ucalgary.ca; rokne@ucalgary.ca

R. Alhajj
Department of Computer Science, University of Calgary, Calgary, AB, Canada

Department of Computer Engineering, Istanbul Medipol University, Istanbul, Turkey
e-mail: alhajj@ucalgary.ca

R. Alhajj et al. (eds.), *Data Management and Analysis*, Studies in Big Data 65,
https://doi.org/10.1007/978-3-030-32587-9_13

1 Background

A study by Lancet Global Health indicates that as of 2015 there are around 444 million people living with visual impairments; 39 million were blind, 216 million people had moderate to severe visual impairment, and 189 million have mild visual impairment [5]. In the Canadian context, as of 2018 there are 5.59 million having an eye condition that could lead to sight loss. Glaucoma is one of the most common condition occurring to these people [18].

Treating blindness and compensating for individuals' lost ability to find meaningful work is a significant cost to both individuals and society. For example, in Canada blindness-related costs and compensations are as of 2016 on the order of C$ 19 billion per annum, and it is believed that they will increase to C$ 25 billion per annum by 2024. Approximately 80% of these cases can be treated if diagnosed early [45–53].

Glaucoma is the world's second leading condition of irreversible vision after cataracts, accounting for 12% of annual cases of blindness [19]. It is estimated that the number of people, between the age of 40–80, affected by glaucoma will increase from 64.3 million to 80 million by 2020 and to 111.8 million by 2040 [53]. Furthermore, 2.4% of all individuals and 4.7% of those over 70 are at risk of developing the condition [37].

The term glaucoma refers to a condition caused by group of diseases that leads to the degeneration of retinal ganglion cells (RGCs). The death of RGCs lead to (i) structural changes to the optic nerve head and the nerve fiber layer, and (ii) simultaneous functional failure of the visual field [34, 37]. These two effects of glaucoma cause peripheral vision loss, and, if left untreated, eventually blindness. One of the main indicators of glaucoma is increased intra ocular pressure (IOP) causing more pressure on the optic nerve head which damages the RGCs and thus causes structural changes to the optic nerve head area. These structural changes affect the area of the cup shown in Fig. 1. Glaucoma starts with undetectable visual loss that increases over time, as shown in Fig. 2. The black regions in the image appear gradually and not suddenly and the individual will not notice any changes until advanced visual loss occurs.

There are multiple types of glaucoma and each has its own characteristics in terms of severity, complexity, and occurrences between different ethnic groups [33, 42, 55]. The various types are generally classified as primary open-angle glaucoma (POAG), angle-closure glaucoma (ACG), normal-tension glaucoma (NTG), primary congenital glaucoma (PCG), pseudo-exfoliative glaucoma (XFG), uveitic glaucoma (UG), traumatic glaucoma (TG), pigmentary glaucoma (PG), and neo-vascular glaucoma (VG). The two most frequently occurring type are primary open-angle and angle-closure glaucoma and they are more dangerous and harder to detect than the remaining cases [19]. However, in this paper we analyze glaucomatous retinal images regardless of its type.

Multiple approaches have been developed for glaucoma detection. Some of them rely solely on calculating the cup disc ratio (CDR) through segmenting the disc and

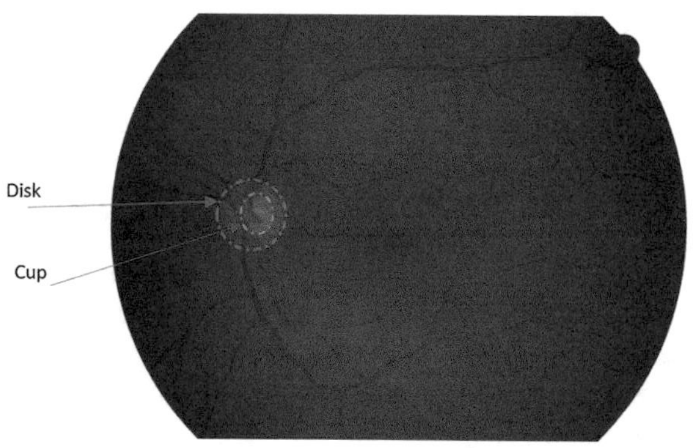

Fig. 1 Optic disc and cup in a retinal image

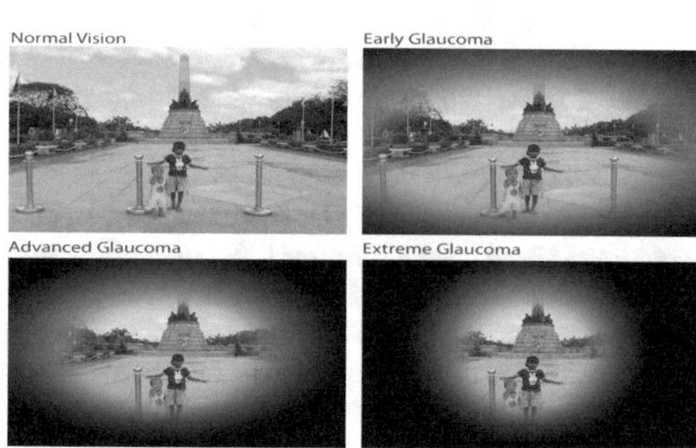

Fig. 2 Progression of glaucoma

the cup, while others use feature extraction techniques. To test the efficiency of some of the developed techniques, we obtained the code of four different approaches and did a performance analysis using four distinct public datasets. Some of the datasets included are related to other ocular diseases. Doing this allowed us to study the behavior of the tested approaches on retinal images with different ocular diseases such as diabetic retinopathy (DR). We investigate the outcome of these approaches along with the analysis time. This paper summarizes the findings concerning these approaches.

The rest of the paper is organized as follows. Section 2 discusses some of the factors that have been discovered and which may be used by clinics when diagnosing for glaucoma. Section 3 then provides insights on how we conducted our analysis. Section 4 highlights the approaches tested. Section 5 shows the output of each of the tested approached on the adopted datasets along with the limitations discovered for each of the approach. Section 6 offers a conclusion of the analysis done. Finally, Appendix "Detailed Evaluation" lists a detailed description of the features handled by each approach.

2 Risk Factors

Studies have been conducted to discover factors that can help in the early diagnosis of glaucoma. Advances have led to the discovery of factors with both strong and low correlations with glaucoma. The most critical factor is the IOP, with a high IOP indicating that someone has a risk of contracting glaucoma. Another important factor is age; in particular, studies have shown that the risk of glaucoma increases with age [36]. Ethnicity is another factor that has been reported by many scientists. For example, African Americans have a greater glaucoma risk than Caucasian Americans [33, 54]. Another study shows that East Asian has the highest number of people with glaucoma: around 60% of all cases. In addition, Asians with Japanese ancestry are at higher risk of having normal-tension glaucoma than others [52]. Further, Mongolians and Burmese are more targeted by ACG than POAG [7, 49]; this also applies on East Asians [26]. [52] predicts that most of the glaucoma cases will be in Asia and Africa by 2040.

Other factors have been indicated to affect IOP, such as caffeine [3, 8], weight lifting [55], tight neck ties [51], cigarettes [35], alcohol [29], body mass index [22], tooth loss [39, 41], yoga postures [20], tears [46], sleeping postures [27], Vitamin D [31], metabolic syndrome [32], diabetes [33, 38], and diet [28]. [24] also showed that there is a correlation between serum ferritin levels and glaucoma. Furthermore, [21] demonstrated that a correlation exists between glaucoma and diabetic retinopathy (which is a condition found in people with diabetes).

Indicators of various kinds might be used to help in the early diagnosis of glaucoma, thereby decreasing the number of people who become blind by applying an early treatment. However, so far the discovered risk factors do not reliably indicate glaucoma (reliability varies from case to case). Because of this they have not been adopted in clinics except for age, ethnicity, and heredity. More studies therefore need to be performed to verify the reliability of these factors and thus make a decision on whether or not to use them while diagnosing a patient. Questions related to ethnicity, age, and heredity are the main questions asked for patients in clinics nowadays. However, IOP levels and CDR are the main two indicators used for glaucoma [56]. These two indicators are not sufficient to detect all cases of glaucoma and many people are left untreated and thus become blind or partially blind [25].

3 Methodology

In order to test the efficiency of some of the techniques developed, we obtained the code for four different approaches and ran them on multiple dataset using a windows 10 machine with a core i5 processor and 8 GB RAM. We summarize the findings by showing the characteristics of the tested approaches, classification outputs, and their weaknesses. Section 4 discuss the tested approaches and Sect. 5 highlights the results achieved by each of one of them.

Only a few datasets are available online for glaucoma. The most well-known are ORIGA, Drishti, HRF, and RIMOne. However, the ORIGA dataset has been taken down by its publisher, and we therefore could not use it. RIMOne is another glaucoma-based dataset that contains partial images, mainly showing the area of the optic disc. Drishti and HRF are among those related to glaucoma, where a ground truth for glaucoma detection is available. They are the only datasets that show the whole fundus image. Moreover, the Drishti dataset contains a ground truth for the disc region annotated by four experts. Therefore, we used the HRF and Drishti datasets, with a total of 130 images for our analysis. A list of available retinal datasets can be found in Table 1.

To compare the performance of these approaches to fundus images with other ocular diseases, we decided to use DRIONS and DiaretDb1 datasets. However, since no ground truth for glaucoma is available for these datasets we decided to show the number of images that these approaches failed to analyze. By failing we mean that the application was unable to provide a classification of results. Another reason for selecting these two datasets is that the DRIONS and DiaretDB1 contain more noise (PPA and Exudates respectively) than glaucoma related datasets. The total number of images used in this study is 329. 130 images are from the glaucoma datasets and 199 from the other datasets.

4 Tested Approaches

Four approaches have been tested in this study. The performance of these approaches is tested on different type of datasets. In this section we introduce these approaches and their performance will be reported in Sect. 5.

4.1 Vascular Displacement

A vascular displacement in the optic disc region is one of the indications of glaucoma. The proposed approach relies on detecting the center of blood vessels in four different regions in the disc and then measuring the distance to a reference point [12]. These four regions are called inferior, superior, nasal, and temporal (collectively denoted by the ISNT region), as shown in Fig. 3. Figure 3 depicts a left eye. The right eye has the same regions, with the temporal and nasal sections switched. The approach proposed here measures the displacement of vessels in each region with respect to a reference point which should be the cup edge farthest from the nasal region. First the disc region is segmented and then the vessel displacement is measured. Furthermore, a graphical user interface (GUI) was provided by the application, as shown in Fig. 4.

The analysis steps are shown in Fig. 5. A user should first select an image and then the option "detect cup region." This option identifies the region of interest

Table 1 Available retinal datasets

Dataset	Images			Resolution	Condition				Availability	SGT[a]			
	N[b]	C[c]	T[d]		GL[e]	DR[f]	CA[g]	AMD[h]		V[i]	D[j]	M[k]	
HEI-MED	115	54	169	2196*1958		✓			R[l]				[23]
ARIA	51	52	113	768*576		✓	✓		P[m]	✓			[57]
HRF	15	15	30	3504*2336	✓				P				[14]
GLDB	17	103	120	1504*1000	✓				P				[30]
IOSTAR			54	1024*1024					P	✓	✓		[1]
RC			250	2595*1944					P			✓	[1]
EOPTHA	47	35	82	2544*1696, 2048*1300		✓			P				[14]
ROC		100	100	768*576		✓			P				[44]
SHIFA	19	92	111	1936*1296					R				[2]
Retinal Dataset	300	301	601	2592*1224	✓		✓		P				[11]
Arriage et al.	36	62	98	720*576	✓				R				[12]
CHASEDB			28	768*576					P	✓			[10]
Drishti	31	70		2049*1757	✓				P		✓		[48]
STARE			397	700*605					P	✓			[50]
DRIVE	33	7				✓			P				[17]
DIARETDB0	20	110	130	1500*1152		✓			P				[15]
DIARETDB1	5	89	94	1500*1152		✓			P				[16]
MESSIDOR	540	660	1200	2240*1488		✓			P				[13]
DRIONs			110	600*400					P		✓		[6]
RIMOnev2	255	200	455	394*380	✓				P		✓		[43]
RIMOnev3	85	74	159	2144*1424	✓				P		✓		[40]

[a] Segmentation ground truth
[b] Normal
[c] Condition
[d] Total
[e] Glaucoma
[f] Diabetic retinopathy
[g] Cataract
[h] Age-related macular degeneration
[i] Vessels
[j] Disc
[k] Microaneurysm
[l] Requested
[m] Publicly available

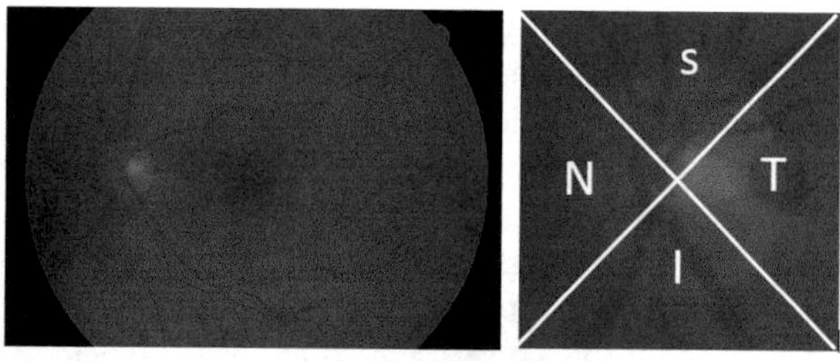

Fig. 3 ISNT regions in the optic disc for a left eye

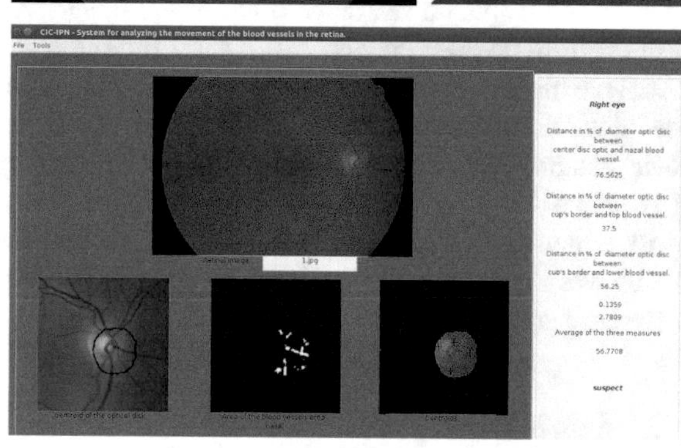

Fig. 4 Vascular displacement application graphical interface

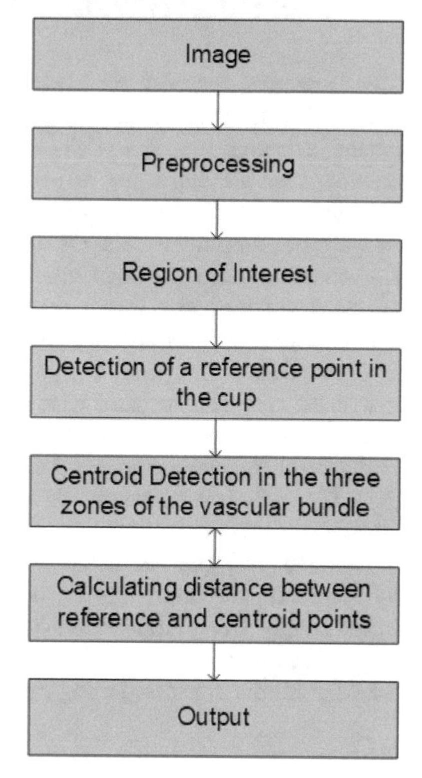

Fig. 5 Analysis process for the vascular displacement approach

(ROI) using Fourier transformation and p-tile thresholding. The main purpose of the ROI is to limit the analysis steps for blood vessels and thus to identify only the region of the optic disc. Before identifying the ROI, some preprocessing steps are applied including image normalization and adjusting the dimensions. After the preprocessing steps are finished, the green channel is extracted to identify the ROI. This is the brightest region, identified using p-tile thresholding and Fourier transformation. The output image is then displayed to the user. Subsequently, the user should display a reference point in the image, which should be the cup edge farthest from the nasal region. After selecting the reference point, the menu option "Analyze displacement" should be selected. This option is responsible for detecting the centroid in the three zones (nasal, superior, and inferior) and then calculating their distance from the reference point. The average distance is then calculated; if it is above 45, then this person is suspected of having glaucoma. This threshold is identified by a domain expert. To analyze the performance of this approach which was implemented using MATLAB, we tested it on 130 images obtained from difference sources.

4.2 *CDR Calculation Using Self-Organizing Maps (SOM)*

This is another approach for glaucoma detection; it computes the cup disc ratio (CDR) [47]. If the CDR is >0.3, then the fundus image belongs to a glaucomatous person. The approach first works by extracting the disc using the edge detection method, then the cup using self-organizing maps, from the fundus image. C++ language was used to develop the proposed methodology along with the famous image processing library, the OpenCV library. To run the analyses, image masks are needed to detect the boundaries of the image. However, these masks were not provided, and we had to create them programmatically. To this end, we used visual studio to write the C++ code for generating the masks.

Figure 6 shows the general steps performed for the classification. First, an image is selected, and then the green channel is extracted. Green channels are used for the detection of blood vessels due to the high contrast between the vessels and their background. A Gaussian matched filter is then used to highlight blood vessels, and the OTSU filter is used to improve the representation of the vessels. Morphological closing is applied to remove blood vessels using the output of the OTSU filter and the original green channel image. A Sobel filter is applied to extract edges, followed by increasing the brightness of the detected edges using adaptive thresholding. Subsequently, Hough transform is used to extract the optic disc from the extracted edges. The disc is then fed to the self-organizing map to extract the cup, after which the CDR ratio is calculated using Eq. 1.

$$\mathrm{CDR} = \frac{\text{Cup Diameter}}{\text{Disc Diameter}} \tag{1}$$

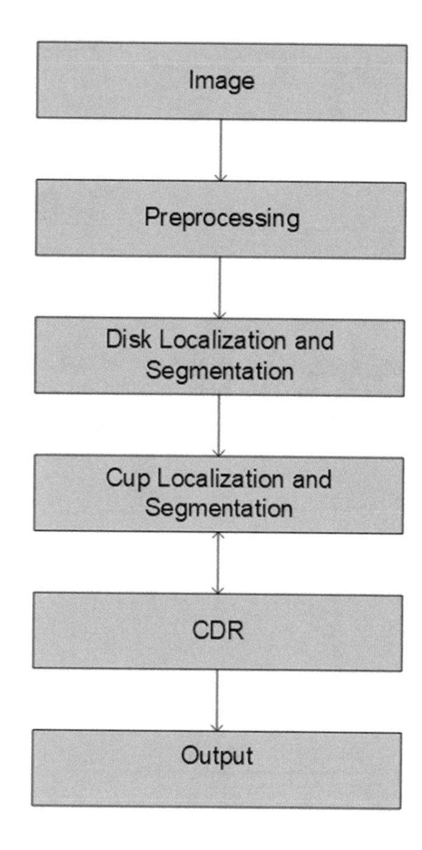

Fig. 6 Analysis process for the approach using self-organizing map

The output of the application is the CDR, which indicates the severity of glaucoma, and an image marking the extracted cup and disc. Since we did not have validated CDRs for the images, we only measured the accuracy of the classification by considering CDR >0.3 as glaucomatous. However, since the author of this approach indicated that 0.7 is a good indicator for glaucoma, we decided to study the performance using both ratios, 0.3 and 0.7.

4.3 *Feature Extraction Using Histogram of Oriented Gradients*

This approach differs from the previously discussed ones [4]. Instead of segmenting different objects from the fundus images, it extracts features and then uses them to classify an image. A histogram of oriented gradients (HOG) feature extraction approach is adopted here with a GUI interface (Fig. 7). A HOG is a feature descriptor used for object detection. The aim is to extract the most important features from an image and ignore extraneous information. However, choosing the important features differs from one application to another. The feature vector created by the HOG is of size n, where n = Imagewidth * Imageheight * 3. In the present study, two

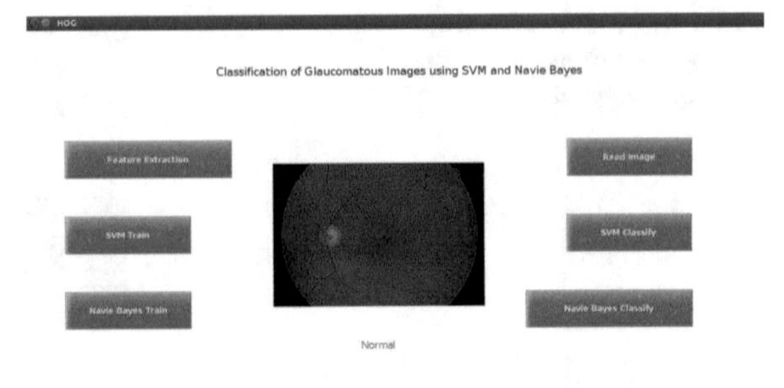

Fig. 7 HOG application graphical interface

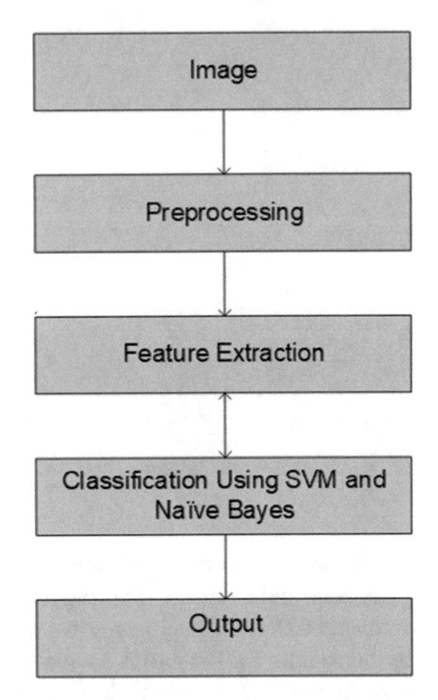

Fig. 8 Analysis process for the approach using HOG

classifiers were used and then the accuracy of each one was measured separately for glaucoma detection. The analysis steps involved in this methodology are shown in Fig. 8.

This approach requires training the SVM and Naive Bayes classifiers on the extracted features before being able to predict the status of new images. To this end, we split the data randomly between training and testing datasets. The training dataset consisted of 26 normal and 26 suspect fundus images selected randomly from the datasets HRF and Drishti.

Each image in the training dataset was resized to [512 512], the green channel was extracted, and then adaptive histogram equalization (AHE) was applied to fix the contrast. Subsequently, image boundaries were identified using a Gabor filter, and the features were extracted using HOG. The extracted HOG features were then used to calculate six different values: mean, variance, entropy, skewness, kurtosis, and energy. The sets of these features were utilized to train the classifiers. Finally, the test images were fed to the application and accuracy was measured.

4.4 *CDR with Ellipse Fitting*

This is another approach that uses the CDR to detect glaucoma [9]. A ratio >0.3, is considered to be glaucomatous. As the ratio increases, the patient is increasingly suspected of having glaucoma. A least square ellipse fitting approach is applied for both disc and cup segmentation. First the disc is segmented and then the same steps are used for cup segmentation. Figure 9 shows the steps followed in this approach.

No training process is required for this approach. The image is first selected and then some preprocessing steps are done, including image adjustment and channel extraction. The green channel is used in the rest of the analysis for vessel, disc, and cup segmentation. To create fundus image boundary's mask, the green channel is used. Pixels with an RGB value >5 are set to 255; otherwise, they are kept. This is because pixels <5 are considered to be black. After creating the image mask, edge

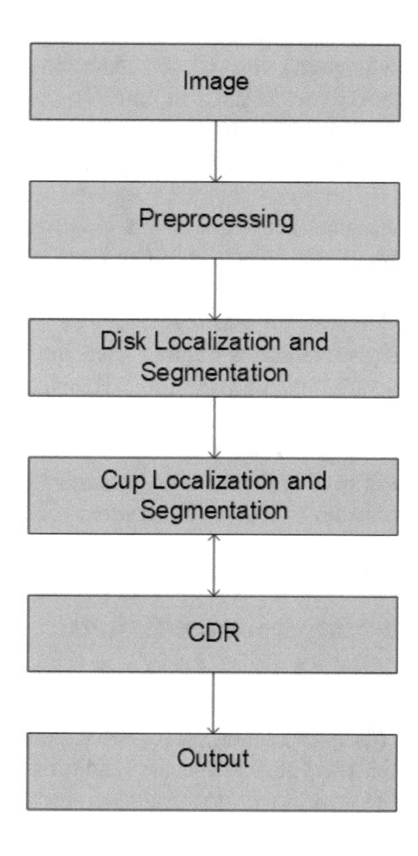

Fig. 9 Analysis process for the approach using ellipse fitting for disc and cup segmentation

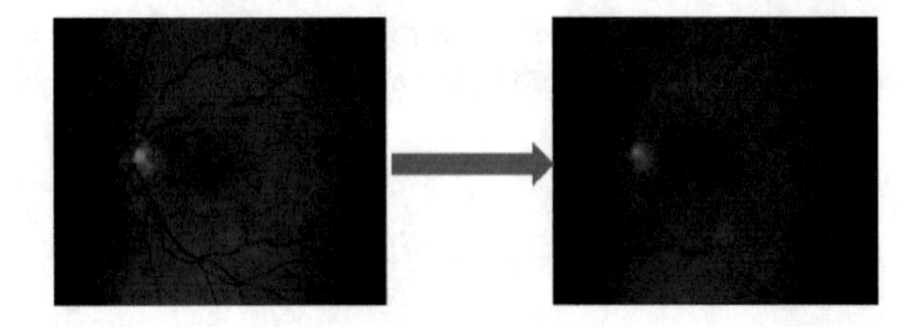

Fig. 10 Vessel free image using the green channel

detection is performed. To this end, the green channel is used and 100 is subtracted from each of its values because edges usually have higher intensities greater than 100, as described by the authors of this approach. However, this may change from one image to another depending on the intensity. This approach led to failure in edge detection in more than 60% of the images tested in the present study.

Unlike the previous approaches, filters were used to detect disc boundaries. The boundary function uses eight filters to detect the boundaries of the disc. First, an image with same size as the original one is created, and then eight filters are used separately to detect a matched region. This approach is called template matching. Each filter has its own template which is used to detect the region. We should note that the output of every filter is an image with the same size as the original one. Combining the output of these filters creates a region that is used for detecting and segmenting the optic disc. Morphological operations with circular average filters is used to detect the disc. Initially, the diameter was set to nine in this study, but this caused the failure of all the images, so we changed it to three, which yielded better results. However, it did not reach the expected results, and accuracy remained low.

The green channel was used to segment the optic disc. Image normalization was performed, and then a Gaussian filter was applied. A least square ellipse filter was then utilized to better segment the boundaries, and the segmented disc was used to extract the cup by following the same steps but using different thresholds. However, for cup segmentation, vessel removal was done beforehand. For vessel segmentation, the author used the average value of the neighboring pixels using a threshold of [100 100]. This means that the value of pixels in this boundary is the average of their neighbors (see Fig. 10). However, this approach affects the information stored in the neighboring pixels which may be needed later on. After segmenting the cup and disc, the ratio is calculated, and the classification is made. If the ratio >0.3, then the fundus is classified as glaucomatous; otherwise, it is normal.

5 Experimental Results

This section demonstrates the performance output for each of the adopted approaches along with related confusion matrix. Confusion matrices are one of the ways to evaluate the output of specific approach by comparing the output of the system with the available ground truth of the dataset used. Moreover, we also show the number of failed images grouped by the dataset. By failing we refer to the app not being able to produce any output (neither glaucomatous nor normal). Table 2 shows the accuracy, sensitivity, specificity, and time for each of the tested approached when using the glaucoma related datasets (Drishti and HRF). Table 10 shows a detailed breakdown of the features handled by each of the four approaches.

For the vascular displacement approach, the application failed to analyze 11 out of 130 images. To measure the analysis time taken per image we modified the code to calculate and visualize the time. Table 3 shows the confusion matrix for the discussed approach with an average of 5.5 s/image. We eliminated those images that the application failed to analyze. Table 4 shows the distribution of the images which the application failed to analyze.

The accuracy achieved by this approach is 52%, which is low. This is because of multiple reasons such the improper detection of blood vessels in each ISNT region, and thus failure to detect the centroid properly. This leads to improper calculation of the distance between centroids and the reference point. Another reason is that the approach does not detect disc boundaries properly because of noise such as peripapillary atrophy (PPA) and image edges. Furthermore, another limitation is that when there are many blood vessels in the detected disc regions, the application fails to calculate the centroids. Therefore, even if the disc region is detected, the accuracy of the application relies also on vessel detection, centroids, and selected reference points, which makes the process more vulnerable to failure. Finally, the

Table 2 Performance analysis output for the tested approaches

		Accuracy (%)			Sensitivity (%)			Specificity (%)			
		HRF	Drishti	Total	HRF	Drishti	Total	HRF	Drishti	Total	Time(s)
Vascular displacement		39	36.2	52.1	43.8	85.2	72	33	38.6	37.7	5.5
CDR using SOM	0.7	53.3	64.1	61.5	57.1	73.4	71.8	52.2	42.9	47.1	3.5
	0.3	50	65.2	61.5	50	67.8	63.2	0	20	20	3.5
Feature extraction using HOG		NA			NA			NA			NA
CDR with ellipse fitting		53.6	32.8	39.6	0	83.3	83.3	53.6	26.9	36.2	14

Table 3 Confusion matrix for the vascular displacement approach

	Predicted			
	Positive		Negative	
Observed	HRF	Drishti	HRF	Drishti
Positive	7	29	8	35
Negative	9	5	4	22

Table 4 Failed images/dataset when applying the vascular displacement approach

	Number of failed images
HRF	2
Drishti	9
DRIONS	5
DIARETDB1	18

application sometimes fails to properly detect whether the image is of the right or the left eye.

Recall that the application first selects an ROI which is then used for the calculating displacement. In some of the images, the ROI was not detected properly because of the types of noise in those pictures. Several types of noise can affect the selection of the ROI, such as exudates and bright regions. For example, Fig. 11 shows a fundus that contains a bright region. This causes the application to consider this bright region as the ROI instead of the true ROI shown in the same figure. The application ignores the actual disc area and considers this noise region as the disc region for the analysis which misleads the results. Changing the threshold of the p-tile algorithm that is responsible for detecting the ROI does not change the result, as the developed algorithm still goes towards the noise region rather than the disk, and then fails to detect the centroids. Another factor is image low resolution which the approach proposed here does not handle. A further reason for failure is not handling the edge of the discs properly when applying the morphological operation, such as the one in Fig. 12. This causes the algorithm responsible for detecting the disc to move towards the region of the arrows as they are the sharpest edges. These edges are because of the threshold used in the morphological operation. Modifying the threshold solves this problem in some images but not for others. We developed a way to bypass this issue by trimming the end of the image and then re-sizing the image; however, it still does not resolve the issue. Having these sharp edges in Fig. 12 prevents the edge function from detecting the proper edges in the image; thus, the Circular Hough Transformation function fails, leading to improper detection of the disc boundaries. Failing to detect the optic disc region leads to receiving NaN values for the points used by the Kass Snake algorithm, leading to improper identification of the disc contour.

One of the advantages of this approach is its fast computation, with an average analysis time of 5.5s. Another advantage is that it takes into consideration whether the image is of the left or the right eye. Moreover, it detects blood vessels in each

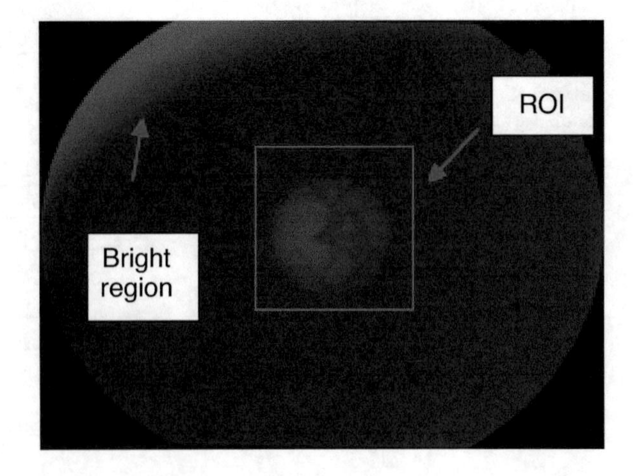

Fig. 11 Fundus image with bright regions

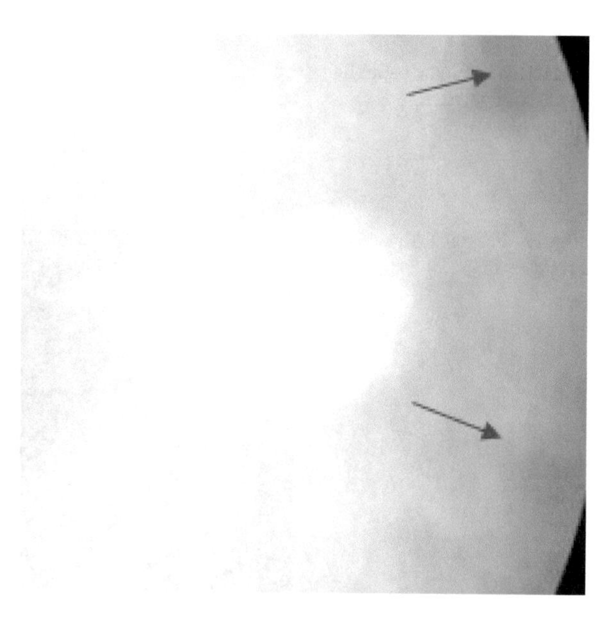

Fig. 12 Image showing improper handling of edges

Table 5 Confusion matrix for the approach using self-organizing maps with CDR 0.7

	Predicted			
	Positive		Negative	
Observed	HRF	Drishti	HRF	Drishti
Positive	4	47	11	16
Negative	3	17	12	12

Table 6 Confusion matrix for the approach using self-organizing maps with CDR 0.3

	Predicted			
	Positive		Negative	
Observed	HRF	Drishti	HRF	Drishti
Positive	15	59	0	4
Negative	15	28	0	1

region but not all of them. The weaknesses of the approach must be managed to obtain proper results; these weaknesses include difficulty with managing low-resolution images, handling negative values, automatically detecting the farthest reference point from the nasal area, properly detecting the disc region, vessel segmentation, and improving the detection of the centroids.

Recall that for the approach using SOM we measured the performance using two CDR: 0.3 and 0.7. Tables 5 and 6 shows the confusion matrix for CDR values 0.7 and 0.3 respectively. Moreover, Table 7 shows the distribution of the images which the application failed to analyze.

The system failed to analyze 8 images for similar reasons as the ones discussed for the vascular displacement approach. The system was not able to handle bright regions either. However, it was more sensitive to bright regions than the vascular approach, such as the one in Fig. 13. Furthermore, the system did not fail to extract

Table 7 Failed images/dataset when applying the SOM approach

	Number of failed images
HRF	0
Drishti	8
DRIONS	39
DIARETDB1	16

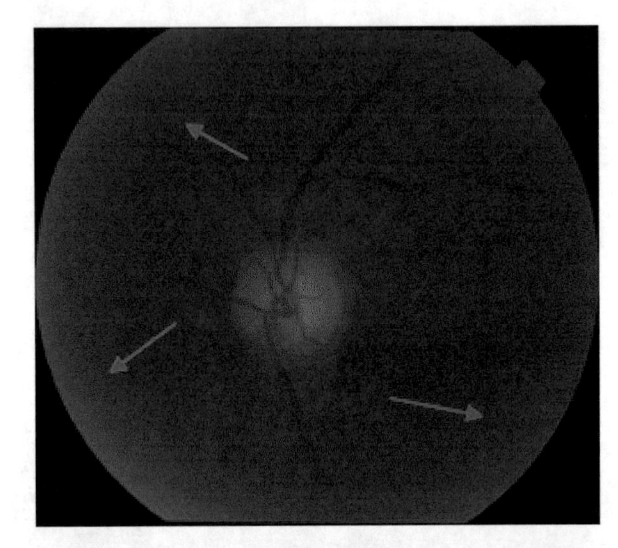

Fig. 13 Fundus images with bright regions

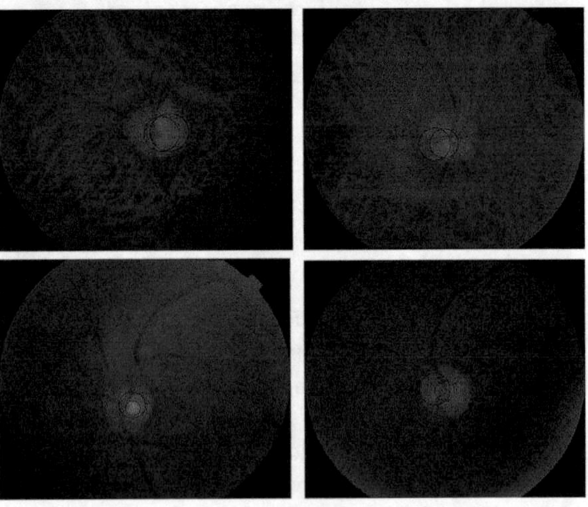

Fig. 14 Improper detection of the optic disc

the cup/disc, but it did fail to extract it accurately in most of the cases. This is highly dependent on the model used and the proper extraction of the disc region. Out of 122 images, the system failed to properly detect the disc regions in 91 images (see Fig. 14). We did not check for the cup regions as we do not have the ground truth. Even when building our own weights for the model using the training method provided in the code, the results were less accurate, so we decided to use their model. This was mainly because of the ANN structure used, in which only one layer and 26 connected nodes were used. Moreover, it is known that self-organizing maps may differ from one image to another; thus, a more robust ANN model needs to be constructed to obtain better results.

One of the advantages of this approach is its fast computation, with an average analysis time of 3.5s which is less than that of the vascular. Another advantage is the ability to extract blood vessels from a retinal image. However, the results, for glaucoma detection, achieved by the SOM approach are not good. This may be related to multiple reasons, such as improper selection of weights for the organizing map, pixel intensities, noise, and thresholds used. It should also be noted that the application failed to calculate the CDR for 8 images because of the improper handling of brightness in other places in the images, which is a similar issue to the one seen in the vascular displacement approach.

While running the analysis for the approach using HOG, we realized that the Gabor filter failed to detect the edges of multiple images with different intensities. This was because of the threshold used to detect image boundaries. The way the Gabor filter works is that it checks for specific changes of frequencies over n iterations using different angles and then combines the output of all iterations in a single image. Figures 15 and 16 presents the Gabor filter output for two different images. It is clear that the edges were not properly detected in Fig. 16. However, changing the threshold of the intensity led to the output shown in Fig. 17. Thus, the performance of the Gabor filter is highly dependent on the specified thresholds.

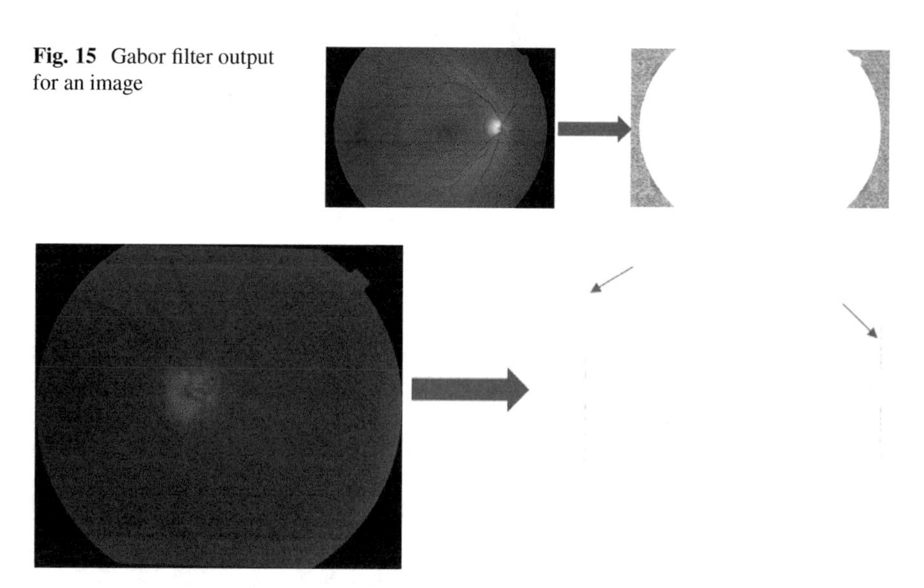

Fig. 15 Gabor filter output for an image

Fig. 16 Gabor filter output for an image

Fig. 17 Gabor filter output for Fig. 16

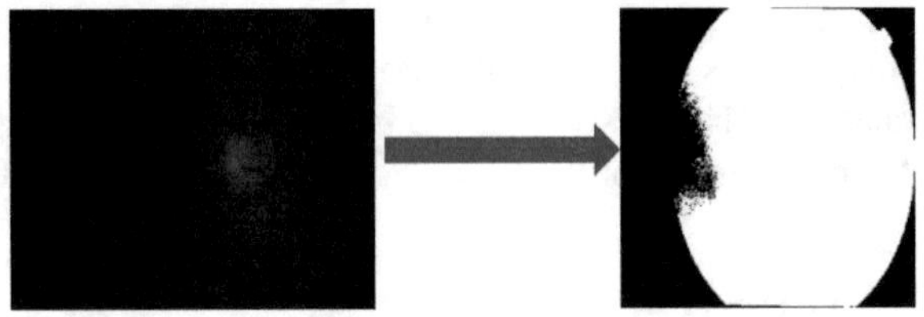

Fig. 18 Image mask generated for an image with dark regions

For some images, this threshold may work, but for others it may not. Therefore, an adaptive approach is highly preferred here.

To examine the accuracy of this approach, we tested it on the dataset used for other the approaches. However, after testing it on 50 images, we realized that it always gave the output as "normal." Moreover, the application only yields proper results if one of the trained images is selected for testing. This indicates that overfitting is occurring here and thus that the output is unreliable. Therefore, no confusion matrix was made for this approach. In general, HOG provides global information about the image. A way to avoid this is to divide the image into sub-images, to extract an HOG vector for each one, and then to combine all vectors at the end and feed those to a classifier. A further weakness is that HOG does not use noise handling.

The fourth approach adopted in this study is by calculating the CDR using ellipse fitting. Recall that for creating image masks pixels with an RGB value >5 are set to 255. However, this is not always accurate. For example, Fig. 18 shows an image with dark regions and how its related mask was created. Table 8 provides the confusion matrix, which shows the performance of this approach on image classification. Moreover, Table 9 shows the distribution of the images which the

Table 8 Confusion matrix for the approach using ellipse fitting for cup extraction with CDR threshold 0.3

	Predicted			
	Positive		Negative	
Observed	HRF	Drishti	HRF	Drishti
Positive	0	5	13	38
Negative	0	1	15	14

Table 9 Failed images/dataset when applying the ellipse fitting approach

	Number of failed images
HRF	2
Drishti	42
DRIONS	4
DIARETDB1	50

application failed to analyze. The average time needed to analyze one image is 14s, which is considered be acceptable. However, This approach performed the worst when compared to the vascular and HOG approaches.

This approach failed to compute results for 44 cases. This is because the application could not properly detect the optic disc region, as it is unable to handle noise such as PPA and exudates. Moreover, the same issue appeared with this approach as with the previous ones, where bright regions at the edges of the fundus image were considered as the optical disc. Moreover, the filters and templates used misled the location of the optic disc. For example, the boundary detection methods sometimes failed to detect to disc boundaries when multiple edges were identified, as seen in Fig. 19. This was because of bright regions. In other cases, the application failed to detect the disc region mainly because of the intensity of the image, as shown in Figs. 20 and 18. We should mention that this approach failed to properly detect the optic disc region in more than 95% of the cases, and the output of the CDR is therefore not reliable. In summary, multiple factors affect the segmentation of the disc, such as vessels, PPA, bright/dark regions, pixel intensity, and edge sharpness. It is also worth mentioning that we experimented with many thresholds to perform the analysis for this approach. However, these thresholds did not lead to good results, which indicates that the approach may be biased towards the set of 30 images originally used by the authors who developed it. We even tried changing thresholds for edge and boundary detection, but realized that this did not solve the issue as well.

For images that were analyzed successfully, an accuracy of around 39.3% was achieved. However, as previously mentioned, in most of the cases the disc region was not segmented properly, as shown in Fig. 21. Figure 21 demonstrates the analysis process for a fundus image by showing the related outputted image at each step. The arrow indicates the image showing the final disc (pink) and cup (black) segmentation. It is clear that the detected disc region is wrong, and thus the computed CDR should not be valid. There are multiple reasons for this, such as the threshold being used, the application not handling noise, and the use of the ellipse fitting approach.

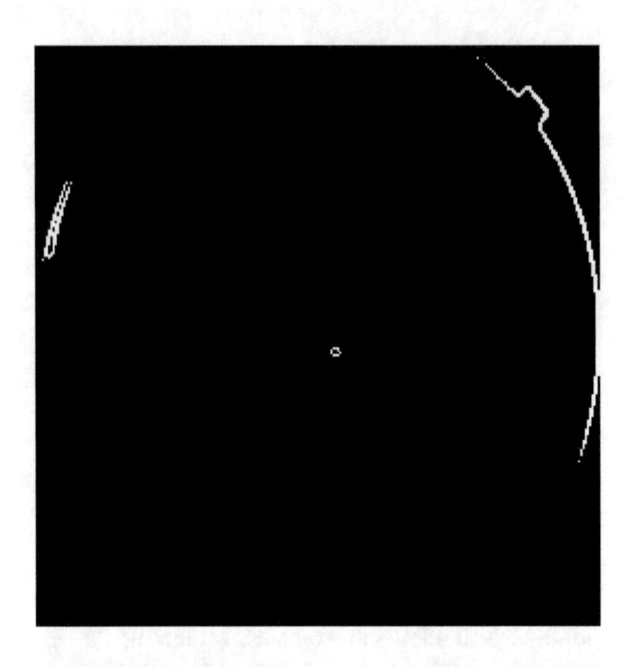

Fig. 19 Multiple separate edges detected for a fundus image

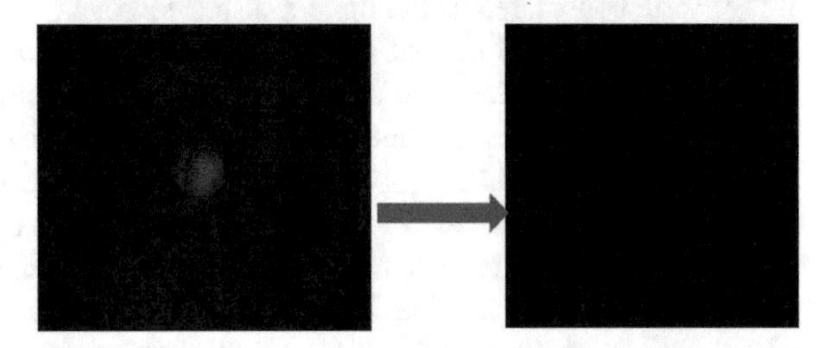

Fig. 20 Edges for a fundus image with dark regions

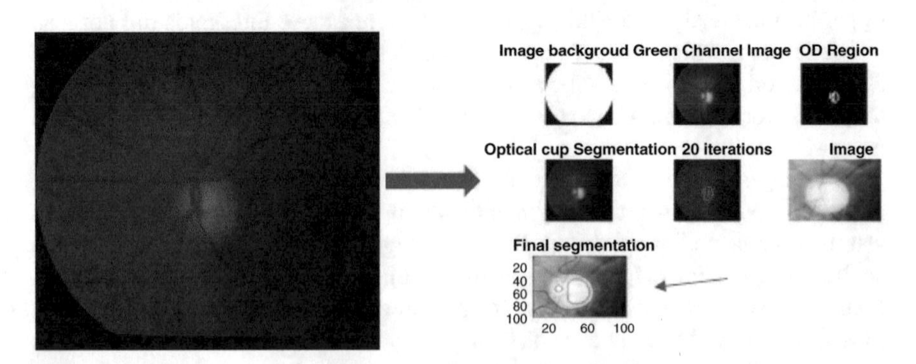

Fig. 21 Output generated by the ellipse fitting approach

6 Conclusion

Glaucoma is a dangerous eye disease and the second leading cause of blindness after cataracts. Approximately 80% of cases are left undetected and thus lead to vision loss. This is mainly because the diagnosis of glaucoma is dependent on the optometrists/ophthalmologist, whose expertise may vary. Automated techniques that consolidate these individuals' expertise along with discovering new features not previously realized are thus greatly needed. In this paper we have discussed different approaches applied for glaucoma diagnosis. These approaches vary between segmentation and feature extraction. We have demonstrated that some approaches rely on extracting features from a specific region of an image after undertaking segmentation while others extract features from an entire image. Multiple approaches for the detection of glaucoma have been developed from fundus images. However, the accuracy of these approaches varies from one dataset to another.

In this paper, we examine the performance of four different approaches for which we were able to obtain the code. We found that most of the tested approaches failed to detect noise in the images, such as bright/dark regions and exudates. Moreover, performance relies highly on image intensity as low ones are not analyzed. Further, adopted edge detection approaches do not handle noise and thus affect the real segmentation of the disc and cup. Another limitation is that the number of blood vessels and their distribution affect the segmentation of the disc. All of this affects the overall results for proper classification. Therefore, these issues must be addressed to obtain good results. Feature extraction is one of the techniques used in the tested approaches, but it is not done efficiently and thus additional work needs to be done. The approach involving vascular displacement analysis performed the best in terms of proper classification of glaucoma. Although the self-organizing maps performed well when the ratio was 0.7, it is not good enough since the aim is to detect glaucoma early and not in the advanced stages. Moreover, this approach failed to properly detect disc regions in many of the images (check Fig. 14). Further, all these approaches (except HOG) relied on proper segmentation of the disc which was not done properly. Furthermore, the specificity reported in all approaches (except the HOG) is very low.

One of the main challenges in research related to glaucoma is the very limited availability of datasets. Thus, developing data repositories for glaucoma research would be a very important contribution for people working in this field. Moreover, researchers can develop ensemble based approaches which may improve the detection of glaucoma cases by ophthalmologists. For instance, researchers can include patient's life-style, retinal images from both eyes along with clinical data when developing their approach which may help in improving the diagnostic accuracy of the developed approach. We believe developing such an approach will have positive impact on people by decreasing blindness and on economy by decreasing the expenses of late treatments.

Appendix: Detailed Evaluation

See Table 10.

Table 10 Features handled by the tested approaches

Characteristics	Approaches			
	CDR with ellipse fitting	Feature extraction using HOG	CDR calculation using self-organizing maps	Vascular displacement
Handling images of any size	✓	✓	✓	✓
Able to detect thick blood vessels	✓	X	✓	✓
Able to detect thin blood vessels	✓	X	X	X
Fast analysis	✓	✓	✓	✓
Using ROI instead of analyzing all images	✓	X	✓	✓
Size adjustment	✓	✓	✓	✓
Image normalization	X	X	X	✓
Adaptive thresholding for increasing pixel intensity	X	X	✓	X
Using image boundaries for analysis only	✓	✓	✓	✓
Contrast adjustment	X	✓	X	X
Ability to handle bright regions for segmentation	X	NA	X	X
Image boundaries detected as candidate disc edges	✓	NA	✓	✓
Not handling images with low intensities	✓	X	✓	✓
Not handling noises such as PPA and exudates for segmenting	✓	NA	✓	✓
Vessel centroids in the ISN regions are t accurate	NA	NA	NA	✓
Disc boundaries are not detected properly	✓	NA	✓	✓
Unautomated approach	X	X	X	✓
Inaccurate generated weights for self-organizing maps	NA	NA	✓	NA
Taking into consideration eye location (left/right)				
Overfitting	X	✓	X	X
Using HOG for whole image	NA	✓	NA	NA

(continued)

Table 10 (continued)

Characteristics	Approaches CDR with ellipse fitting	Feature extraction using HOG	CDR calculation using self-organizing maps	Vascular displacement
Relying on many thresholds, which may make it biased to the dataset used	✓	✓	✓	✓
Inaccurate energy formula used	NA	✓	NA	NA
Removing vessels affects information of other pixels	✓	NA	X	X
Not handling dark regions	✓	NA	✓	✓
Identifying multiple regions as disc edges	✓	NA	X	✓
Disc detection relies on high intensities	✓	NA	✓	✓
Template-based approach	✓	X	✓	X
Improper separation between foreground and background	✓	NA	X	X
Using adaptive thresholding to enhance pixel brightness when segmenting for vessels	✓	NA	X	X
Segment Disc	✓	X	✓	✓
Segment Cup	✓	X	✓	X
Vessels Distribution affects the analysis	✓	X	✓	✓

References

1. Abbasi-Sureshjani, S., Smit-Ockeloen, I., Zhang, J., & Romeny, B. T. H. (2015). Biologically-inspired supervised vasculature segmentation in SLO retinal fundus images. In *International Conference Image Analysis and Recognition* (pp. 325–334). Berlin: Springer.
2. Abdullah, M., Fraz, M. M., & Barman, S. A. (2016). Localization and segmentation of optic disc in retinal images using circular Hough transform and grow-cut algorithm. In: *PeerJ, 4*, e2003.
3. Avisar, R., Avisar, E., & Weinberger, D. (2002). Effect of coffee consumption on intraocular pressure. *Annals of Pharmacotherapy, 36*(6), 992–995.
4. Balasubramanian, T., Krishnan, S., Mohanakrishnan, M., Rao, K. R., Kumar, C. V., & Nirmala, K. (2016, December). HOG feature based SVM classification of glaucomatous fundus image with extraction of blood vessels. In *2016 IEEE Annual India Conference (INDICON)* (pp. 1–4). Piscataway: IEEE.
5. Bourne, R. R., Flaxman, S. R., Braithwaite, T., Cicinelli, M. V., Das, A., Jonas, J. B., et al. (2017). Magnitude, temporal trends, and projections of the global prevalence of blindness and distance and near vision impairment: A systematic review and meta-analysis. *The Lancet Global Health, 5*(9), e888–e897.
6. Carmona, E. J., Rincón, M., García-Feijoó, J., & Martínez-de-la-Casa, J. M. (2008). Identification of the optic nerve head with genetic algorithms. *Artificial Intelligence in Medicine, 43*(3), 243–259.

7. Casson, R. J., Newland, H. S., Muecke, J., McGovern, S., Abraham, L., Shein, W. K., et al. (2007). Prevalence of glaucoma in rural Myanmar: The Meiktila Eye Study. *British Journal of Ophthalmology, 91*(6), 710–714.
8. Chandrasekaran, S., Rochtchina, E., & Mitchell, P. (2005). Effects of caffeine on intraocular pressure: The Blue Mountains Eye Study. *Journal of Glaucoma, 14*(6), 504–507.
9. *Cup/Disk Segmentation using Ellipse Fitting*. https://goo.gl/KQeUdL. Accessed 1 December 2017.
10. [dataset] *CHASEDB. CHASE DB*. https://goo.gl/vsvZWt. Accessed 28 October 2018.
11. [dataset] Retinal Dataset. *RetinalDataset*. https://goo.gl/XdyfDr. Accessed 20 October 2018.
12. De La Fuente-Arriaga, J. A., Felipe-Riverón, E. M., & Garduño-Calderón, E. (2014). Application of vascular bundle displacement in the optic disc for glaucoma detection using fundus images. *Computers in Biology and Medicine, 47*, 27–35.
13. Decencière, E., Zhang, X., Cazuguel, G., Lay, B., Cochener, B., Trone, C., et al. (2014). Feedback on a publicly distributed image database: The Messidor database. *Image Analysis & Stereology, 33*(3), 231–234.
14. Decencière, E., Cazuguel, G., Zhang, X., Thibault, G., Klein, J. C., Meyer, F., et al. (2013). TeleOphta: Machine learning and image processing methods for teleophthalmology. *Irbm, 34*(2), 196–203.
15. *DIARETDB0*. https://goo.gl/aq8re7. Accessed 8 September 2017.
16. *DIARETDB1*. https://goo.gl/r87R8r. Accessed 8 September 2017.
17. *DRIVE-DB*. https://goo.gl/ywPjXa. Accessed 8 September 2017.
18. CNIB Foundation. *Facts About Vision Loss*. https://goo.gl/qRCgvZ. Accessed September 2018.
19. Fu, H., Xu, Y., Lin, S., Zhang, X., Wong, D. W. K., Liu, J., et al. (2017). Segmentation and quantification for angle-closure glaucoma assessment in anterior segment OCT. *IEEE Transactions on Medical Imaging, 36*(9), 1930–1938.
20. Gallardo, M. J., Aggarwal, N., Cavanagh, H. D., & Whitson, J. T. (2006). Progression of glaucoma associated with the Sirsasana (headstand) yoga posture. *Advances in Therapy, 23*(6), 921–925.
21. Gangwani, R. A., McGhee, S. M., Lai, J. S., Chan, C. K., & Wong, D. (2016). Detection of glaucoma and its association with diabetic retinopathy in a diabetic retinopathy screening program. *Journal of Glaucoma, 25*(1), 101–105.
22. Gasser, P., Stümpfig, D., Schötzau, A., Ackermann-Liebrich, U., & Flammer, J. (1999). Body mass index in glaucoma. *Journal of Glaucoma, 8*(1), 8–11.
23. Giancardo, L., Meriaudeau, F., Karnowski, T. P., Li, Y., Garg, S., Tobin Jr, K. W., et al. (2012). Exudate-based diabetic macular edema detection in fundus images using publicly available datasets. *Medical Image Analysis, 16*(1), 216–226.
24. Gye, H. J., Kim, J. M., Yoo, C., Shim, S. H., Won, Y. S., Sung, K. C., et al. (2016). Relationship between high serum ferritin level and glaucoma in a South Korean population: The Kangbuk Samsung health study. *British Journal of Ophthalmology, 100*(12), 1703–1707.
25. Haleem, M. S., Han, L., Van Hemert, J., & Li, B. (2013). Automatic extraction of retinal features from colour retinal images for glaucoma diagnosis: A review. *Computerized Medical Imaging and Graphics, 37*(7–8), 581–596.
26. He, M., Foster, P. J., Johnson, G. J., & Khaw, P. T. (2006). Angle-closure glaucoma in East Asian and European people. Different diseases? *Eye, 20*(1), 3–12.
27. Hecht, I., Achiron, A., Man, V., & Burgansky-Eliash, Z. (2017). Modifiable factors in the management of glaucoma: A systematic review of current evidence. *Graefe's Archive for Clinical and Experimental Ophthalmology, 255*(4), 789–796.
28. Kang, J. H., Pasquale, L. R., Willett, W. C., Rosner, B. A., Egan, K. M., Faberowski, N., et al. (2004). Dietary fat consumption and primary open-angle glaucoma. *The American Journal of Clinical Nutrition, 79*(5), 755–764.
29. Kang, J. H., Willett, W. C., Rosner, B. A., Hankinson, S. E., & Pasquale, L. R. (2007). Prospective study of alcohol consumption and the risk of primary open-angle glaucoma. *Ophthalmic Epidemiology, 14*(3), 141–147.

30. Khalil, T., Akram, M. U., Khalid, S., & Jameel, A. (2017). Improved automated detection of glaucoma from fundus image using hybrid structural and textural features. *IET Image Processing, 11*(9), 693–700.
31. Kim, H. T., Kim, J. M., Kim, J. H., Lee, M. Y., Won, Y. S., Lee, J. Y., et al. (2016). The relationship between vitamin D and glaucoma: A Kangbuk Samsung Health Study. *Korean Journal of Ophthalmology, 30*(6), 426–433.
32. Kim, M., Jeoung, J. W., Park, K. H., Oh, W. H., Choi, H. J., & Kim, D. M. (2014). Metabolic syndrome as a risk factor in normal-tension glaucoma. *Acta Ophthalmologica, 92*(8), e637–e643.
33. Ko, F., Boland, M. V., Gupta, P., Gadkaree, S. K., Vitale, S., Guallar, E., et al. (2016). Diabetes, triglyceride levels, and other risk factors for glaucoma in the national health and nutrition examination survey 2005–2008. *Investigative Ophthalmology & Visual Science, 57*(4), 2152–2157.
34. Kumar, B. N., Chauhan, R. P., & Dahiya, N. (2016, January). Detection of Glaucoma using image processing techniques: A review. *2016 International Conference on Microelectronics, Computing and Communications (MicroCom)* (pp. 1–6). Piscataway: IEEE.
35. Lee, A. J., Rochtchina, E., Wang, J. J., Healey, P. R., & Mitchell, P. (2003). Does smoking affect intraocular pressure? Findings from the Blue Mountains Eye Study. *Journal of Glaucoma, 12*(3), 209–212.
36. Mitchell, P., Smith, W., Attebo, K., & Healey, P. R. (1996). Prevalence of open-angle glaucoma in Australia: The Blue Mountains Eye Study. *Ophthalmology, 103*(10), 1661–1669.
37. Mookiah, M. R. K., Acharya, U. R., Lim, C. M., Petznick, A., & Suri, J. S. (2012). Data mining technique for automated diagnosis of glaucoma using higher order spectra and wavelet energy features. *Knowledge-Based Systems, 33*, 73–82.
38. Muñoz-Negrete, F. J., Contreras, I., Oblanca, N., Pinazo-Durán, M. D., & Rebolleda, G. (2015). Diagnostic accuracy of nonmydriatic fundus photography for the detection of glaucoma in diabetic patients. *BioMed Research International, 2015*.
39. Pasquale, L. R., Hyman, L., Wiggs, J. L., Rosner, B. A., Joshipura, K., McEvoy, M., et al. (2016). Prospective study of oral health and risk of primary open-angle glaucoma in men: Data from the Health Professionals Follow-up Study. *Ophthalmology, 123*(11), 2318–2327.
40. Pena-Betancor, C., Gonzalez-Hernandez, M., Fumero-Batista, F., Sigut, J., Medina-Mesa, E., Alayon, S., et al. (2015). Estimation of the relative amount of hemoglobin in the cup and neuroretinal rim using stereoscopic color fundus images. *Investigative Ophthalmology & Visual Science, 56*(3), 1562–1568.
41. Polla, D., Astafurov, K., Elhawy, E., Hyman, L., Hou, W., & Danias, J. (2017). A pilot study to evaluate the oral microbiome and dental health in primary open-angle glaucoma. *Journal of Glaucoma, 26*(4), 320–327.
42. Raychaudhuri, A., Lahiri, S. K., Bandyopadhyay, M., Foster, P. J., Reeves, B. C., & Johnson, G. J. (2005). A population based survey of the prevalence and types of glaucoma in rural West Bengal: The West Bengal Glaucoma Study. *British Journal of Ophthalmology, 89*(12), 1559–1564.
43. *RIMONE-DB*. https://goo.gl/i8sQkR. Accessed 8 September 2017.
44. *ROC-DB*. https://goo.gl/E3sqJR. Accessed 8 September 2017.
45. Sarhan, A., Rokne, J., & Alhajj, R. (2019). Glaucoma detection using image processing techniques: A literature review. *Computerized Medical Imaging and Graphics, 78*, 101657.
46. Sánchez, J. B. D. C., Morillo-Rojas, M. D., Galbis-Estrada, C., & Pinazo-Duran, M. D. (2017). Determination of inmune response and inflammation mediators in tears: Changes in dry eye and glaucoma as compared to healthy controls. *Archivos de la Sociedad Española de Oftalmologia (English Edition), 92*(5), 210–217.
47. Sharma, S. (2015). *A Project Report on Biomedical Imaging for Eye Care*. Birla Institute of Technology and Science Pilani.
48. Sivaswamy, J., Krishnadas, S. R., Joshi, G. D., Jain, M., & Tabish, A. U. S. (2014). Drishti-GS: Retinal image dataset for optic nerve head (ONH) segmentation. In: *2014 IEEE 11th International Symposium on Biomedical Imaging (ISBI)* (pp. 53–56). Piscataway: IEEE.

49. Song, W., Shan, L., Cheng, F., Fan, P., Zhang, L., Qu, W., et al. (2011). Prevalence of glaucoma in a rural northern China adult population: a population-based survey in Kailu County, Inner Mongolia. *Ophthalmology, 118*(10), 1982–1988.
50. *STARE-DB*. https://goo.gl/zU6NyT. Accessed 11 September 2017.
51. Teng, C., Gurses-Ozden, R., Liebmann, J. M., Tello, C., & Ritch, R. (2003). Effect of a tight necktie on intraocular pressure. *British Journal of Ophthalmology, 87*(8), 946–948.
52. Tham, Y. C., Li, X., Wong, T. Y., Quigley, H. A., Aung, T., & Cheng, C. Y. (2014). Global prevalence of glaucoma and projections of glaucoma burden through 2040: A systematic review and meta-analysis. *Ophthalmology, 121*(11), 2081–2090.
53. Thienes, B. (2016). Canadian Association of Optometrists Pre-Budget Submission. Canadian Association of Optometrists.
54. Tielsch, J. M., Katz, J., Singh, K., Quigley, H. A., Gottsch, J. D., Javitt, J., et al. (1991). A population-based evaluation of glaucoma screening: The Baltimore Eye Survey. *American Journal of Epidemiology, 134*(10), 1102–1110.
55. Vieira, G. M., Oliveira, H. B., de Andrade, D. T., Bottaro, M., & Ritch, R. (2006). Intraocular pressure variation during weight lifting. *Archives of Ophthalmology, 124*(9), 1251–1254.
56. Zhang, L., Xu, L., & Yang, H. (2009). Risk factors and the progress of primary open-angle glaucoma. *Chinese Journal of Ophthalmology, 45*(4), 380–384.
57. Zheng, Y., Hijazi, M. H. A., & Coenen, F. (2011). Automated grading of age-related macular degeneration by an image mining approach. *Investigative Ophthalmology & Visual Science, 52*(14), 6568–6568.

Binary Thermal Exchange Optimization for Feature Selection

Mohammad Taradeh and Majdi Mafarja

Abstract A Feature Selection (FS) is a preprocessing step that becomes a mandatory when dealing with data a large set of features. FS process is known to be a NP-hard optimization problem. Therefore, metaheuristics algorithms proved their ability to tackle this problem as in other optimization problems. The Thermal Exchange Optimization (TEO) is a recent population-based metaheuristic algorithm that is based on Newton's law of cooling. In this paper, a binary version of TEO algorithm (called BTEO) as a search strategy was used in a wrapper feature selection method for the first time in literature. Both K-Nearest Neighborhood (KNN) and Decision Tree (DT) classifiers were used in the evaluation process. Eighteen well-known UCI datasets were utilized to assess the performance of the proposed approach. To prove the efficiency of proposed approach, three popular wrapper FS methods that use nature inspired algorithms (i.e., Genetic Algorithm (GA), Particle Swarm Optimizer (PSO), and Grey Wolf Optimizer (GWO)) as search strategies, were used for comparison purposes, and the results demonstrate the effectiveness of the proposed approach in solving different feature selection tasks.

Keywords Feature selection · Thermal exchange optimization · Metaheuristic · TEO · BTEO

1 Introduction

Data mining is an automatic or a semiautomatic process of extracting and discovering implicit, unknown, and potentially useful patterns and information from massive data stored and captured from data repositories (web, database, data warehousing). Data mining tasks are usually divided into two categories: predictive and descriptive. The objective of the predictive tasks is to predict or classify the value of a

M. Taradeh (✉) · M. Mafarja
Department of Computer Science, Birzeit University, Birzeit, Palestine
e-mail: mmafarja@birzeit.edu

R. Alhajj et al. (eds.), *Data Management and Analysis*, Studies in Big Data 65,
https://doi.org/10.1007/978-3-030-32587-9_14

target feature or class, based on the values of other features (i.e., independent or conditional features). An example of the prediction task is to predict if a new patient has a heart attack disease or not based on some clinical tests. Descriptive tasks aim to find clusters, correlations, and trends in the implicit relationships hidden in the underlying data.

With the advanced data collection tools, and since the collected data is not specified for the data mining purposes, it may contain out of range data (e.g., Salary $= -1500$), impossible data combination (e.g., Salary = 100 and Employed = False), missing values, redundant samples, irrelevant features (e.g., Personal ID), etc. Applying data mining on such data can produce massive and misleading results. Thus, data preprocessing is necessary in order to clean the data for use in any machine learning model. The main purpose of the preprocessing step is to clean and transform raw data into a suitable format that improves the performance of data mining tasks. Data preprocessing includes collecting the data from multiple data sources and cleaning the noisy, irrelevant, and duplicate objects (Observations). Data preprocessing often is the most time-consuming task in the KDD process. One of the most important preprocessing techniques is dimensionality reduction (DR). DR aims to reduce the number of features in a dataset to the minimum, in order to improve the performance of the different data mining tasks (e.g., classification, clustering, association rule mining, etc.). One of the tools in DR is Feature Selection (FS).

Feature selection (FS) is an essential preprocessing step that aims to deduct the irrelevant and redundant features. This elimination improves the performance of the learning algorithm (e.g., classification) [18]. FS methods can be classified in many ways, the most common one is classifying FS into [9]: filters, wrappers, embedded, and hybrid models. While filters consider the correlations and the dependency between dependent and independent features to decide about the best feature subsets, wrappers consider a learning algorithm to act as an evaluator in the search process [16]. Embedded methods perform FS during the machine learning algorithm modeling (i.e., C4.5 Decision Tree), and hybrid methods perform FS by combining filter and wrapper methods. First, a filter can be used to reduce the search space, filters might propose a set of subset candidates, and then a wrapper is involved to choose the best candidate according to the classifier accuracy [1, 7].

Searching for the best feature subset of all features in a dataset is a challenging problem. One possible solution is to generate all possible subsets from the available features, this approach is called complete search. If a dataset contains N features, then, 2^N possible feature subsets should be evaluated, and evaluating all possible subsets is a time-consuming task. Thus, employing a complete search approach is impractical with a feature selection problem, especially for high dimensional datasets. Another option is to use a random search approach. Due to the randomness nature of this option, in few cases, it may find the best subset very fast, but in the worst case, it may perform like the complete search without finding the best subset. Metaheuristic search algorithms come within a moderate state, where they use a piece of heuristic information to guide the search towards the global optimum solution (best subset).

Metaheuristic algorithm attracted the attention of many researchers in the FS field. Nature inspired metaheuristic algorithms are proven to be the most successful algorithms for solving various types of optimization problems. They are of three types according to the source of inspiration: evolutionary-based (e.g., Genetic algorithm (GA) [8]), swarm-based intelligence (e.g., Particle Swarm Optimization (PSO) [2]), and physics-based algorithms (e.g., simulated annealing (SA) [15]). Many physics-based algorithms were proposed in the recent years: Water Evaporation Optimization (WEO) [11], Charged System Search (CSS) [14], Gravitational Search Algorithm (GSA) [31]. Recently, Thermal Exchange Optimization (TEO) algorithm was proposed by Kaveh and Dadras in 2017 [12]. The main inspiration of this algorithm was Newton's law of cooling.

In recent years, many metaheuristics based FS methods were proposed. SA algorithm was used as a local search algorithm to enhance the exploitation ability of GA in hybrid FS approach in [19, 26] and Whale Optimization algorithms as well in [21]. Similar to the SA algorithm, Record Travel algorithm and Great Deluge algorithm were proposed to tackle FS selection problem in [20]. Population-based algorithms have proved their ability to converge towards the global optimum solution. This important property was proven by the superior performance of the FS methods that use such algorithms. Recently, Mafarja and Mirjalili proposed two FS approaches based on Whale Optimization Algorithm [22] and Antlion Optimization Algorithm [25]. A novel FS approach that based on GSA was proposed in [29], and improved GSA based FS approaches were proposed in [30] and [33].

In FS, a feature is either selected or not. So FS is considered as a binary optimization problem. Thus, binary version of the SI algorithms should be designed when tackling this problem. Many studies that use recent and classical metaheuristics algorithms to tackle binary optimization problems and especially FS can be found in the literature [5, 21–23, 27].

The objective of this paper is to propose a new FS method that uses TEO algorithm as a search method to find the minimal number of features while trying to increase the classification accuracy. It is worth mentioning that this is the first time in literature that TEO is used for FS problem. The original TEO algorithm was designed to deal with the continuous optimization problems, hence, to be used with FS, a binary version of this algorithm should be designed. For this purpose, a transfer function (TF) will be used.

The rest of the paper is organized as follows: In Sect. 2 we discuss the theoretical background of TEO algorithm. The proposed approach is described in Sect. 3. Section 4 shows the experimental results with some discussions. Finally, conclusions and future work are provided in Sect. 5.

2 Thermal Exchange Optimization

Thermal Exchange Optimization algorithm (TEO) was proposed in 2017 [12], and an improved TEO version (ITEO) is proposed in 2018 [13]. The main inspiration of this algorithm is Newton's law of cooling [6].

Newton's Law of Cooling states that: "The iron was laid not in a calm air, but in a wind that blew uniformly upon it, that the air heated by the iron might be always carried off by the wind and the cold air succeed it alternately; for thus equal parts of air were heated in equal times, and received a degree of heat proportional to the heat of the iron" [6]. In other words, an object rate of heat loss is proportional to the difference in temperature between the object and its surrounding environment.

TEO algorithm divides the solutions into two groups: a group of agents (solutions) representing the cooling objects, while the other group supposes to represent the surrounding environment. However, the temperature of each agent represents its position. The TEO algorithm Pseudo code is illustrated in Algorithm 1. Suppose there is a search space with D dimensions and with N objects. The TEO running steps can be summarized as follows.

TEO starts by initializing the temperature for all objects as follows:

$$T_i^0 = T_{min} + rand() \times (T_{max} - T_{min}) \tag{1}$$

where T_i^0 is the initial solution position, T_{max} and T_{min} are the upper and lower bounds of the problem, respectively. Where, $rand()$ is a random value to spread the agents in the search space achieving the exploration step. TEO, after that, computes the performance for all agents by the objective function.

The performance for all agents is computed via the objective function (Fitness value). TEO sorts the agents according to their performance, the better at first position, and so one. Then, in the update Thermal Memory (TM), a number of best so far solutions are added to the population, and in the same time the same number of worst solutions are removed from the population. The sorted agents are divided into two equivalent groups: cooling group and environment group based on their performance, where agent $T_{(N/2)+1}$ is considered as the colling object for the environment object T_1 and vice versa.

TEO assumes that the environmental objects lose the heat as the epochs goes with time. So the temperature for ith environment objects is consumed over the time as follows:

$$T_i^{env} = (1 - (c1 + c2 \times (1 - t)) \times rand()) \times T_i^{*env} \tag{2}$$

Where $c1$ and $c2$ are controlling constants between [0, 1]. t is the fraction of the elapsed time $iteration/\#iterations$ and T_i^{*env} is the previous temperature of the ith agent.

The new temperature for each colling object is updated by Eq. (3):

$$T_i^{new} = T_i^{env} + (T_i^{old} - T_i^{env}) \times \exp(-\beta t) \tag{3}$$

where $\beta = \frac{agentfitness}{worstfitness}$.

The previously mentioned steps are repeated until a termination condition is satisfied, either by achieving a satisfied fitness value or by consuming the whole iterations.

Each metaheuristic algorithm should have the ability to escape from falling in the local optimum. TEO presented a random distribution variable pro between [0, 1] to change one random dimension for each cooling object. The parameter tuning study in [12] proved that $pro = 0.3$ reducing the TEO computational cost. Algorithm 1 is the pseudo code for TEO:

Algorithm 1 Pseudo codes of the TEO algorithm

```
n=10
Iterations=100
i=1
agents[] = Random()
while i <= Iterations do
   Evaluate(agents) ;
   agent ⇐ Sort(agents) ;
   CollingObjects= { };
   EnvironmentObjects= { };
   for i = 0 to n/2 do
      CollingObjects.Add(agents[i])
   end for
   for i = (n/2 + 1) to n do
      EnvironmentObjects.Add(agents[i])
   end for
   for each agent in agents do
      CalculateBeta(agent);
   end for
   UpdateThermalMemory();
   UpdateTemperature(EnvironmentObjects);
   UpdateTemperature(CollingObjects);
   i = i + 1
end while
```

3 Binary TEO for Feature Selection

The current TEO algorithm is used to solve continuous problems. However, feature selection is a binary problem. A feature is either selected or not. Thus, TEO cannot be applied to feature selection problems. In this section, we will introduce the use of the Binary version of TEO algorithm (called BTEO) as a search strategy in a wrapper feature selection method for the first time in literature.

In BTEO, each feature subset represents a position which contains a set of items, each item is a single feature in the dataset. If there is a dataset with N feature, then there are 2^N possible feature subsets (positions) in the search space. A good feature subset can be considered according to two factors: the (minimal) number of features included in this subset and the (maximal) classification accuracy that can be obtained by using it. Therefore, we combined these two factors in the fitness function (see Eq. (4)).

$$Fitness = \alpha\gamma_R(D) + \beta\frac{|R|}{|N|} \tag{4}$$

where $\gamma_R(D)$ represent the classification error rate of the k-NN classier, $|R|$ is the number of selected features and $|N|$ is the number of original features in the dataset, α and β are the weights of the classification error rate and cardinality of the subset, $\alpha \in [0, 1]$ and $\beta = (1 - \alpha)$ adopted from [22]. TEO was originally proposed for continuous optimization problems. Due to the nature of the FS problem, a binary version of TEO should be introduced. According to [28], the simplest and most efficient way to convert an algorithm from continuous to binary is to use a transfer function (TF). In general, TFs are used to generate the probability of changing an element of a position to 0 or 1 based on a continuous value of that element in the step vector (temperature in TEO). In this work, we used the transfer function presented in Eq. (5) that was recommended to be used with a similar SI algorithm (i.e., BGSA) in [32]. See Fig. 1 that represents the employed $tanh$ TF.

$$TF(v_d^i(t)) = |tanh(v_d^i(t))| \tag{5}$$

where $v_d^i(t)$ is the value of the ith element in dth dimension in tth iteration.

The result $TF(v_d^i(t))$, obtained from Eq. (5) is then used to convert a position's element to 0 or 1 according to Eq. (6).

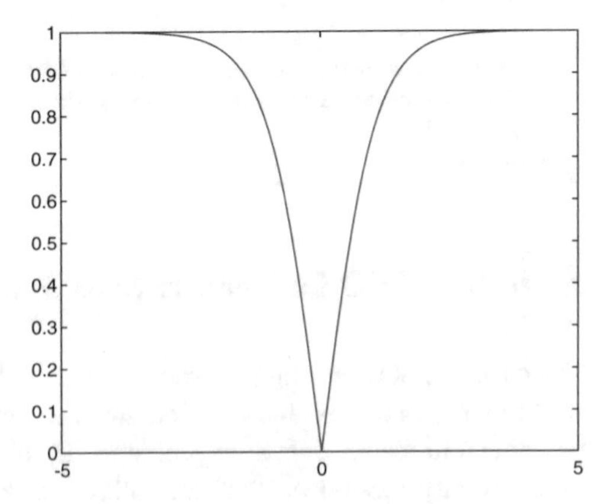

Fig. 1 Tanh transfer function

$$X(t+1) = \begin{cases} \neg X_t & r < TF(v_k^i(t)) \\ X_t & r \geq TF(v_k^i(t)) \end{cases} \tag{6}$$

where r is a random number in the range (0, 1).

4 Experimental Results

This section outlines the results of the proposed approach. The results of the BTEO approach will be analyzed and compared with the state-of-the-art approaches (i.e., GWO, PSO, and GA) in the second phase.

The performance of the proposed algorithm is further proved by comparing with the other available approaches in the literature. The performance comparison between the proposed approach and the latest approaches from the literature consists of the classification accuracy. A statistical test is also carried out to determine whether there is a significant difference between the compared approaches. The Wilcoxon rank-sum test is used to make sure about the significance of the results. Wilcoxon can be used to calculate the null hypotheses for two populations having the same continuous distribution. The p-value that is less than 0.05 could be considered as strong evidence against the null hypothesis.

4.1 Setup of Experiments

In all experiments, a PC with Intel Core i7, and 8 GB RAM was used. All the algorithms are performed on the same configurations and settings as illustrated in Table 1. Since the experiments focus on stochastic algorithms, we reported the average of the results for 30 runs on each dataset. Please note that the **bold** numbers in all subsequent tables denote the best values. Many researchers have recommended that $K = 5$ in KNN is the proper value to be used with the adopted datasets in this

Table 1 Experimental setup

Config. name	Value
Number of runs	30
Number of iterations	200
Number of agents	20
a (for GWO)	From 2 to 0
ω (for PSO)	From 2 to 0
GA selection	Roulette wheel selection
Mutation probability (in GA)	50%
Crossover probability (in GA)	50%
K for KNN	5

paper [21, 24, 32]. Moreover, K should be an odd value to avoid ties and the need for the majority voting. K is usually chosen based on the nature of the dataset. Where in this work we have eighteen dataset with different natures. One can think of a special K for each dataset. But in feature selection, the dataset is dynamically changing after each iteration. Because removing some features from a dataset might produce another different dataset. CART DT is used in this research.

To investigate the efficiency of the proposed approaches, eighteen different datasets from UCI repository [17] were used. The used datasets are with different properties (e.g., number of features, number of instances, and number of classes), and from various kinds of real-life problems. Table 2 reports a brief description (including the number of features and instances for each one) of the utilized datasets.

Since the proposed approaches are wrapper-based, two classifiers (i.e., KNN and DT) were used to measure the fitness of each feature subset. The value of k parameter (number of neighbors) has a major effect on the overall classification accuracy of the KNN classifier. Therefore, many researchers have recommended that $K = 5$ is the proper value for these datasets [3, 3, 4, 21, 24, 32].

4.2 Evaluation Criteria

Three performance indicators are used for comparative purposes: classification accuracy, number of selected features, and the fitness values.

Table 2 List of datasets used in the experiment

Dataset	No.of features	No.of instances
Breastcancer	9	699
BreastEW	30	569
Exactly	13	1000
Exactly2	13	1000
HeartEW	13	270
Lymphography	18	148
M-of-n	13	1000
PenglungEW	325	73
SonarEW	60	208
SpectEW	22	267
CongressEW	16	435
IonosphereEW	34	351
KrvskpEW	36	3196
Tic-tac-toe	9	958
Vote	16	300
WaveformEW	40	5000
WineEW	13	178
Zoo	16	101

- *Average classification accuracy*: this indicator measures how accurate is the classifier in predicting the right class using the selected subset of features. The average accuracy is calculated based on Eq. (7):

$$AvgAccuracy = \frac{1}{M}\sum_{j=1}^{M}\frac{1}{N}\sum_{i=1}^{N}(C_i == L_i) \quad (7)$$

where M is the number of runs for an algorithm to find the final subset of features, N is the number of dataset instances, C_i is the predicted class, and L_i is the actual class in the labeled data.
- *Average fitness*: This indicator is a composition from a classifier error rate (KNN or DT) and the features reduction rate. This indicator is used as an objective function in the optimization algorithm to identify the goodness of the selected feature subset. The average fitness value for each run is calculated as in Eq. (8):

$$AvgFitness = \frac{1}{M}\sum_{j=1}^{M} Fit_*^i \quad (8)$$

where M is the number of runs, and Fit_*^i is the fitness of the best solution resulted from run i.
- *Average selection size*: This indicator represents the performance of an algorithm in terms of selection size when solving the FS problem. This indicator is calculated as in Eq. (9):

$$AvgSize = \frac{1}{m}\sum_{i=1}^{M}\frac{d_i^*}{D} \quad (9)$$

where M is the number of runs, d_i^* is the number of selected features (turned on values) in the binary solution vector from the i-th run, and D is the total number of features in the original dataset.

4.3 Results and Discussion

In this section, we will present a comparative analysis of the TEO-based approaches, i.e., TEO and ITEO. An aggregated summary of results for both TEO and ITEO are presented in Tables 3 and 4. The aim of this comparison is to assess the TEO's feasibility in solving binary problems. The performance of the proposed approach is assessed on both KNN and DT classifiers. The proposed approach is then compared with the state-of-the-art FS algorithms that were implemented for

Table 3 Summary of ITEO accuracy measures using KNN and DT

	KNN				DT			
Benchmark	Average	Min	Max	StdDev	Average	Min	Max	StdDev
Breastcancer	0.98	0.98	0.98	0	0.966	0.966	0.966	0
BreastEW	0.98	0.975	0.986	0.003	0.97	0.965	0.975	0.003
CongressEW	0.955	0.945	0.968	0.004	0.962	0.959	0.963	0.002
Exactly	0.955	0.864	1	0.038	0.958	0.862	1	0.049
Exactly2	0.768	0.766	0.77	0.002	0.769	0.764	0.774	0.004
HeartEW	0.853	0.844	0.859	0.005	0.851	0.844	0.852	0.002
IonosphereEW	0.871	0.863	0.88	0.004	0.932	0.926	0.937	0.003
KrvskpEW	0.963	0.955	0.972	0.005	0.986	0.981	0.992	0.003
Lymphography	0.863	0.849	0.89	0.012	0.842	0.822	0.849	0.008
M-of-n	0.994	0.956	1	0.01	0.97	0.97	0.97	0
penglungEW	0.859	0.853	0.882	0.012	0.718	0.706	0.765	0.017
SonarEW	0.873	0.854	0.893	0.01	0.831	0.816	0.845	0.007
SpectEW	0.882	0.872	0.887	0.004	0.875	0.865	0.88	0.005
Tic-tac-toe	0.802	0.802	0.802	0	0.854	0.854	0.854	0
Vote	0.949	0.94	0.96	0.006	0.953	0.953	0.953	0
WaveformEW	0.785	0.777	0.797	0.004	0.754	0.747	0.762	0.004
WineEW	0.999	0.989	1	0.003	0.989	0.989	0.989	0
Zoo	0.969	0.959	0.98	0.01	0.971	0.959	0.98	0.01

Table 4 Summary of TEO accuracy measures using KNN and DT

	KNN				DT			
Benchmark	Average	Min	Max	StdDev	Average	Min	Mix	StdDev
Breastcancer	0.98	0.98	0.98	0	0.966	0.966	0.966	0
BreastEW	0.966	0.961	0.972	0.003	0.97	0.968	0.972	0.002
CongressEW	0.966	0.963	0.972	0.003	0.968	0.968	0.968	0
Exactly	0.932	0.85	1	0.044	0.956	0.894	0.972	0.022
Exactly2	0.765	0.758	0.768	0.003	0.763	0.758	0.764	0.002
HeartEW	0.888	0.881	0.889	0.002	0.854	0.844	0.859	0.004
IonosphereEW	0.888	0.88	0.903	0.005	0.946	0.937	0.954	0.005
KrvskpEW	0.965	0.955	0.976	0.004	0.983	0.977	0.987	0.003
Lymphography	0.888	0.863	0.904	0.012	0.868	0.849	0.89	0.017
M-of-n	0.988	0.96	1	0.012	0.99	0.99	0.99	0
penglungEW	0.821	0.794	0.853	0.012	0.694	0.676	0.735	0.017
SonarEW	0.877	0.854	0.903	0.01	0.873	0.854	0.884	0.008
SpectEW	0.859	0.85	0.872	0.006	0.877	0.872	0.887	0.004
Tic-tac-toe	0.795	0.795	0.795	0	0.829	0.829	0.829	0
Vote	0.96	0.953	0.967	0.005	0.973	0.973	0.973	0
WaveformEW	0.79	0.781	0.804	0.005	0.751	0.745	0.757	0.003
WineEW	0.988	0.977	0.989	0.003	0.964	0.955	0.966	0.005
Zoo	0.959	0.939	0.959	0.004	0.918	0.918	0.918	0

Table 5 Comparison between TEO and ITEO in terms of classification accuracy

Dataset	KNN		DT	
	TEO	ITEO	TEO	ITEO
Breastcancer	**0.980**	**0.980**	**0.966**	**0.966**
BreastEW	**0.980**	0.966	0.970	**0.970**
CongressEW	0.955	**0.966**	0.962	**0.968**
Exactly	**0.955**	0.932	**0.958**	0.956
Exactly2	**0.768**	0.765	**0.769**	0.763
HeartEW	0.853	**0.888**	0.851	**0.854**
IonosphereEW	0.871	**0.888**	0.932	**0.946**
KrvskpEW	0.963	**0.965**	**0.986**	0.983
Lymphography	0.863	**0.888**	0.842	**0.868**
M-of-n	**0.994**	0.988	0.970	**0.990**
penglungEW	**0.859**	0.821	**0.718**	0.694
SonarEW	0.873	**0.877**	0.831	**0.873**
SpectEW	**0.882**	0.859	0.875	**0.877**
Tic-tac-toe	**0.802**	0.795	**0.854**	0.829
Vote	0.949	**0.960**	0.953	**0.973**
WaveformEW	0.785	**0.790**	**0.754**	0.751
WineEW	**0.999**	0.988	**0.989**	0.964
Zoo	**0.969**	0.959	**0.971**	0.918

comparison purposes. Finally, a comparison between the proposed approach and a set of popular FS approaches in literature is conducted.

- Table 5 shows the average classification accuracy for TEO and ITEO using both classifiers, i.e., KNN and DT. The table shows that there is no big difference in the performance between the two algorithms. Where ITEO and TEO performed with better accuracy—for KNN—(Fig. 2) in 44% and 50% of the datasets, respectively. For DT, the situation is almost the same (see Fig. 3), where ITEO and TEO performed with better accuracy in 50% and 44% of the datasets, respectively.
- Table 6 shows the average fitness values for TEO and ITEO. The table shows that ITEO's average fitness values—for KNN—are better than TEO in 55.5% of the datasets. While both algorithms almost near to the same for DT classifier were ITEO and TEO performed better average fitness is 44% and 50% of the datasets, respectively.
- Table 7 shows the average feature selection rates for TEO and ITEO. It is clear that TEO's performance in reducing the number of features is better than TEO, where the ability to select the relevant feature was better than TEO in 61.1% of the datasets for both KNN and DT.

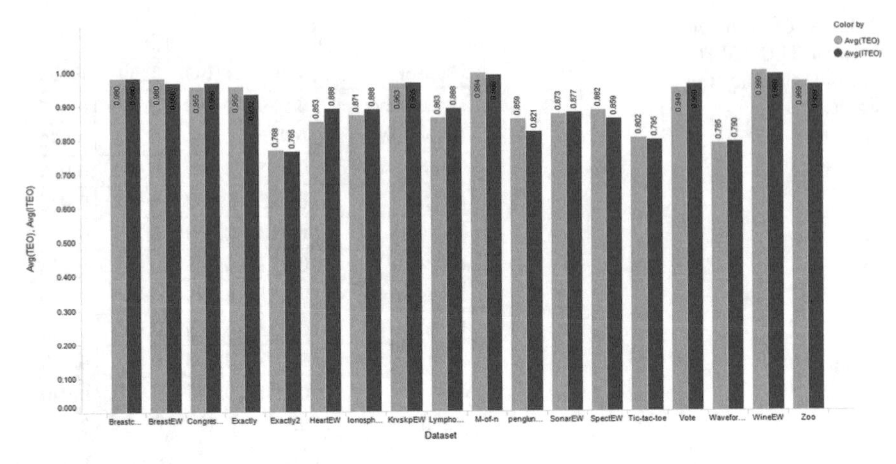

Fig. 2 Comparison between TEO and ITEO in terms of accuracy for KNN

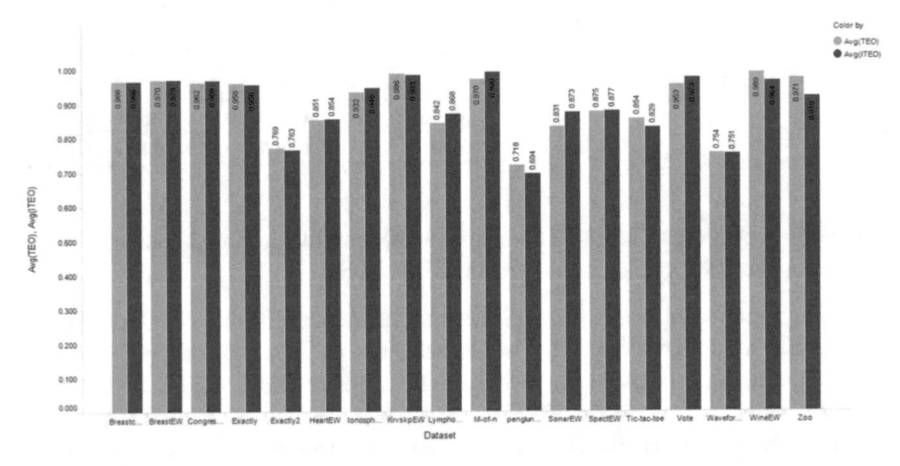

Fig. 3 Comparison between TEO and ITEO in terms of accuracy for DT

- Figures 4 and 5 show a comparison between ITEO and TEO in terms for convergence speed for both KNN and DT classifiers, respectively. The figures show that there is no big difference in convergence speed between the algorithms when KNN is used. While DT is used, ITEO is faster than TEO in convergence with the local optimum.

The comparison between ITEO and TEO proved that the improved ITEO is better than TEO in solving the feature selection problem. The conclusion was based on the three evaluation criteria in addition to the stability analysis and the convergence speed.

Table 6 Comparison between TEO and ITEO in terms of average fitness values

	KNN		DT	
Dataset	TEO	ITEO	TEO	ITEO
Breastcancer	0.024	**0.029**	**0.038**	**0.038**
BreastEW	0.025	**0.039**	**0.035**	0.035
CongressEW	**0.048**	0.037	**0.042**	0.035
Exactly	0.050	**0.073**	0.047	**0.049**
Exactly2	0.235	**0.238**	0.233	**0.238**
HeartEW	**0.151**	0.117	**0.150**	0.148
IonosphereEW	**0.131**	0.115	**0.073**	0.059
KrvskpEW	**0.042**	0.040	0.020	**0.024**
Lymphography	**0.141**	0.116	**0.160**	0.135
M-of-n	0.011	**0.017**	**0.035**	0.016
penglungEW	0.144	**0.182**	0.284	**0.308**
SonarEW	**0.131**	0.127	**0.172**	0.131
SpectEW	0.122	**0.144**	**0.128**	0.127
Tic-tac-toe	0.208	**0.214**	0.155	**0.178**
Vote	**0.053**	0.043	**0.049**	0.030
WaveformEW	**0.219**	0.213	0.249	**0.252**
WineEW	0.006	**0.017**	0.015	**0.040**
Zoo	0.036	**0.048**	0.033	**0.085**

Table 7 Comparison between TEO and ITEO in terms of number of selected features

	KNN		DT	
Dataset	TEO	ITEO	TEO	ITEO
Breastcancer	3.000	**7.000**	**3.000**	**3.000**
BreastEW	**16.567**	16.333	13.233	**14.467**
CongressEW	**6.333**	6.033	**6.567**	5.267
Exactly	6.633	**6.767**	6.500	**6.767**
Exactly2	6.033	**6.133**	**5.733**	4.567
HeartEW	5.867	**8.233**	3.867	**4.567**
IonosphereEW	**13.033**	13.000	15.933	**17.033**
KrvskpEW	**19.967**	18.500	**23.667**	23.233
Lymphography	8.633	**8.933**	**6.600**	5.867
M-of-n	6.600	**6.767**	6.700	**6.767**
penglungEW	**149.367**	147.367	150.967	**152.967**
SonarEW	27.933	**28.433**	26.733	**29.867**
SpectEW	**10.967**	9.833	9.167	**10.000**
Tic-tac-toe	**9.000**	**9.000**	**8.000**	7.000
Vote	4.033	**5.800**	4.400	**5.600**
WaveformEW	**22.533**	**22.533**	**21.267**	21.233
WineEW	**6.500**	6.433	4.567	**4.933**
Zoo	7.100	**10.067**	**6.600**	5.800

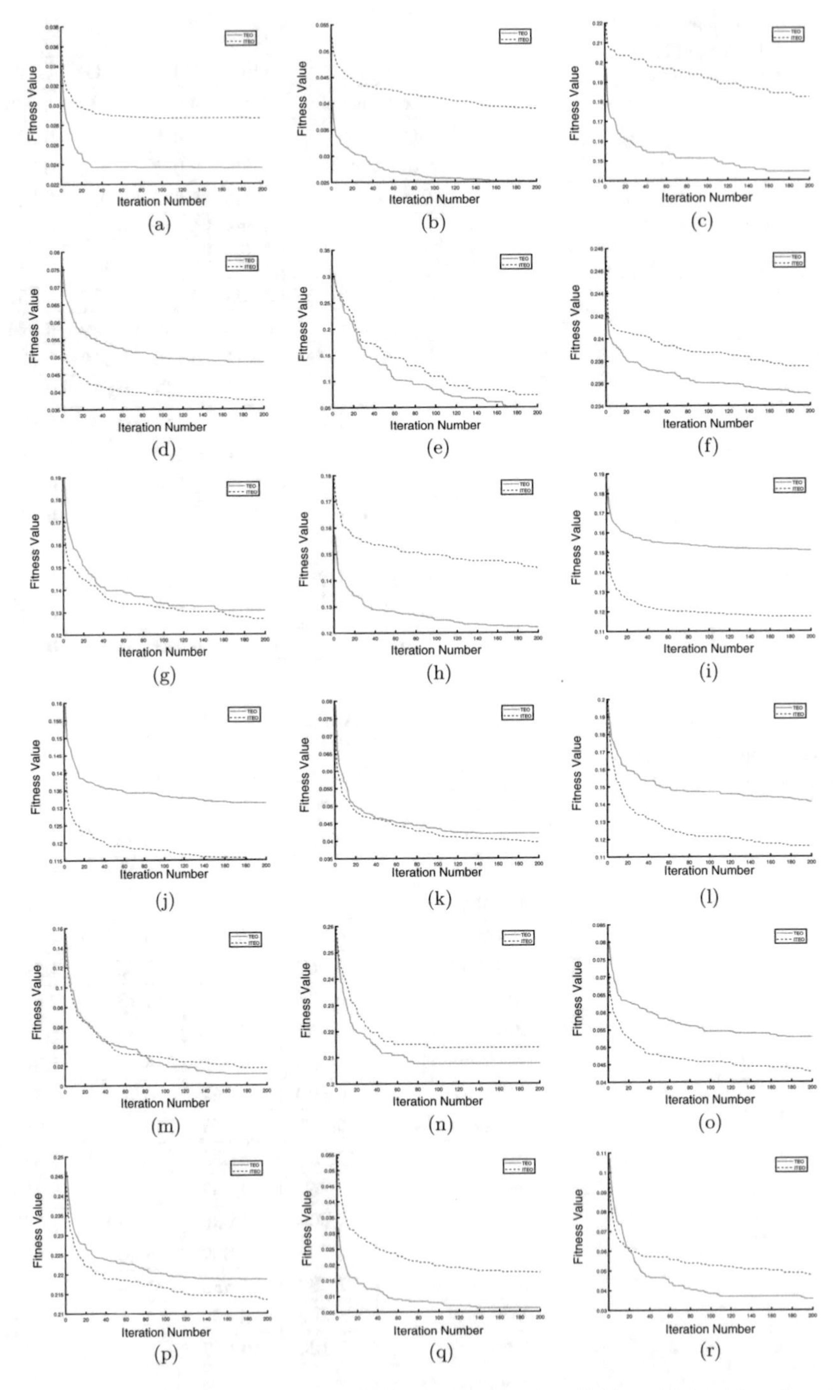

Fig. 4 Convergence curves for TEO and ITEO for all datasets for KNN classifier. (**a**) Breastcancer. (**b**) BreastEW. (**c**) CongressEW. (**d**) Exactly. (**e**) Exactly2. (**f**) HeartEW. (**g**) IonosphereEW. (**h**) KrvskpEW. (**i**) Lymphography. (**j**) M-of-n. (**k**) penglungEW. (**l**) SonarEW. (**m**) SpectEW. (**n**) Tic-tac-toe. (**o**) Vote. (**p**) WaveformEW. (**q**) WineEW. (**r**) Zoo

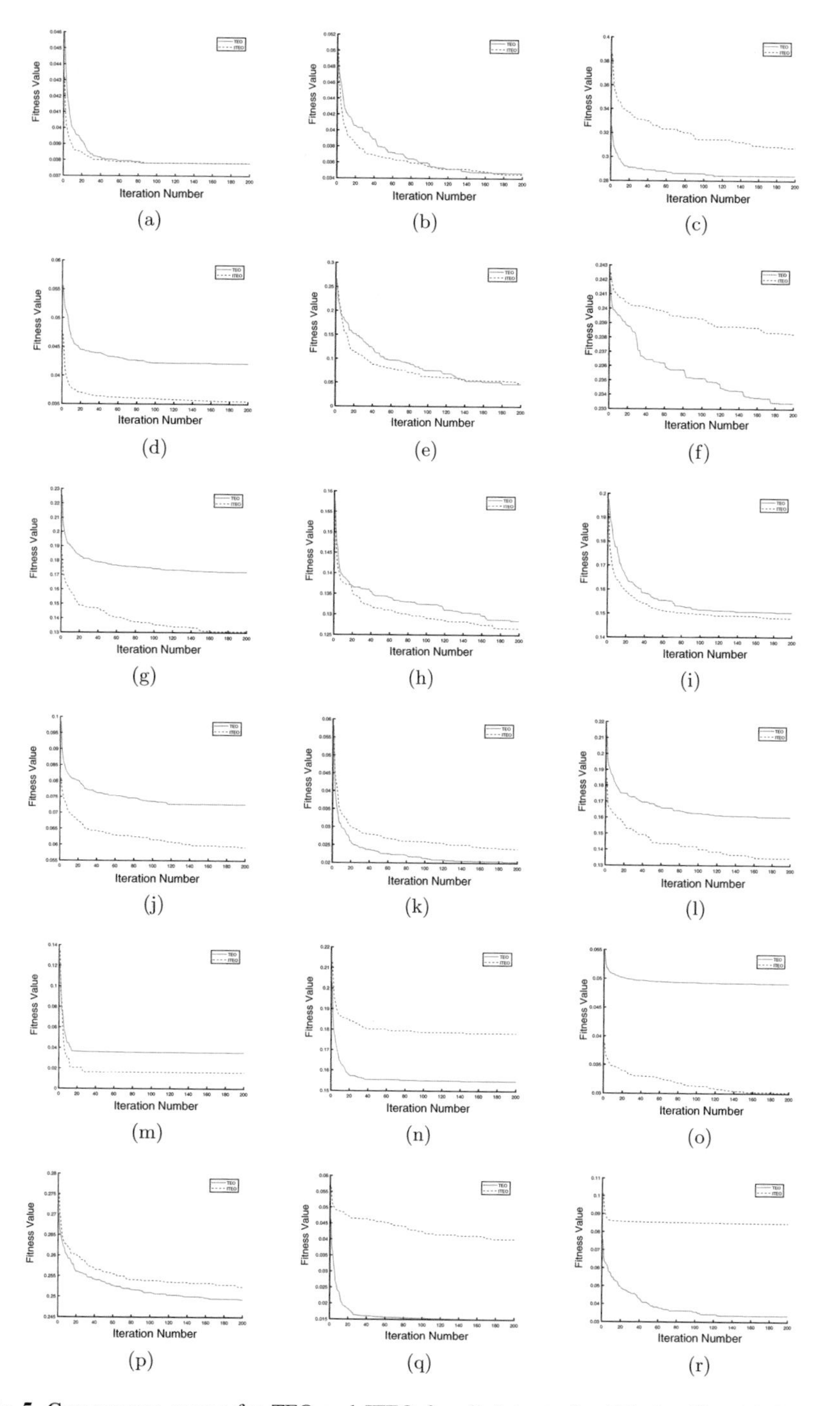

Fig. 5 Convergence curves for TEO and ITEO for all datasets for DT classifier. (**a**) Breast-cancer.(**b**) BreastEW. (**c**) CongressEW. (**d**) Exactly. (**e**) Exactly2. (**f**) HeartEW. (**g**) IonosphereEW. (**h**) KrvskpEW. (**i**) Lymphography. (**j**) M-of-n. (**k**) penglungEW. (**l**) SonarEW. (**m**) SpectEW. (**n**) Tic-tac-toe. (**o**) Vote. (**p**) WaveformEW. (**q**) WineEW. (**r**) Zoo

4.3.1 ITEO Improves Classification Accuracy over GA, PSO, and GWO

Table 8 shows the average classification accuracy result for ITEO and other state-of-the-art well-known feature selection approaches (GA, PSO, and GWO). The following remarks can be made by inspecting the table; ITEO performed with better KNN accuracy than other algorithms in 61.1% of the datasets, while PSO and GWO performed better in 17% of the datasets. When DT is used, ITEO performed with better accuracy than others in 72.2% of the datasets. While GA performed better in 17% of the datasets, GWO in two, and PSO in one dataset, respectively.

The results of the p-values in Table 9 generated from the Wilcoxon test—ITEO acts as a pairwise reference—show that the superiority of ITEO is statistically significant because most of the p-values are less than 0.05 for both KNN and DT classifiers.

4.3.2 ITEO Improves Classification Accuracy over Other Approaches in the Literature

After analyzing the results of ITEO and comparing it with the state-of-the-art approaches, here we are interested to compare it with similar approaches from

Table 8 Comparison between ITEO and the state-of-the-art FS approaches in terms of classification accuracy

	KNN classifier				DT classifier			
Dataset	GWO	PSO	GA	ITEO	GWO	PSO	GA	ITEO
Breastcancer	**0.980**	0.972	0.973	0.980	0.960	0.946	0.964	**0.966**
BreastEW	0.954	0.948	0.953	**0.966**	0.948	0.926	0.958	**0.970**
CongressEW	0.927	0.957	0.940	**0.966**	**0.982**	0.948	0.958	0.968
Exactly	0.731	**0.994**	0.748	0.932	0.752	0.913	0.759	**0.956**
Exactly2	0.758	0.743	0.761	**0.765**	0.759	0.751	0.760	**0.763**
HeartEW	0.853	0.795	0.832	**0.888**	0.809	0.808	0.834	**0.854**
IonosphereEW	**0.893**	0.883	0.876	0.888	0.940	0.927	0.924	**0.946**
KrvskpEW	0.955	**0.965**	0.930	0.965	0.984	**0.987**	0.953	0.983
Lymphography	0.831	0.759	0.815	**0.888**	0.816	0.779	0.825	**0.868**
M-of-n	0.910	**0.993**	0.877	0.988	**1.000**	0.970	0.883	0.990
penglungEW	**0.868**	0.661	0.861	0.821	0.681	0.449	0.643	**0.694**
SonarEW	0.795	0.763	0.853	**0.877**	0.797	0.709	0.802	**0.873**
SpectEW	0.833	0.810	**0.864**	0.859	0.842	0.818	0.852	**0.877**
Tic-tac-toe	0.790	0.783	0.759	**0.795**	0.815	0.832	**0.850**	0.829
Vote	0.940	0.933	0.931	**0.960**	0.932	0.958	0.925	**0.973**
WaveformEW	0.784	0.788	0.761	**0.790**	0.748	0.735	0.739	**0.751**
WineEW	0.980	0.937	0.967	**0.988**	0.952	0.951	**0.964**	**0.964**
Zoo	0.924	0.817	0.930	**0.959**	0.888	0.845	**0.924**	0.918

Table 9 p-Values obtained from the rank-sum test for the results in Table 8

Dataset	KNN classifier				DT classifier			
	GWO	PSO	GA	TEO	GWO	PSO	GA	TEO
Breastcancer	**4.34E−02**	**1.25E−08**	**4.63E−13**	**2.58E−11**	**2.46E−11**	**7.21E−10**	**8.46E−04**	**2.79E−10**
BreastEW	**1.74E−11**	**2.02E−11**	**1.96E−11**	**1.33E−11**	**1.82E−11**	**2.17E−11**	**7.12E−11**	3.70E−01
Exactly	**1.91E−11**	**1.02E−02**	**2.66E−11**	**8.34E−11**	**2.43E−13**	**2.46E−02**	**5.35E−09**	**2.43E−13**
Exactly2	**2.38E−11**	5.76E−02	**4.43E−08**	**1.90E−02**	**7.49E−11**	7.93E−02	**1.23E−10**	3.51E−01
HeartEW	**1.52E−12**	3.73E−01	**1.45E−08**	**6.29E−05**	**2.02E−10**	**8.95E−03**	**4.43E−11**	**2.95E−11**
Lymphography	5.21E−01	**2.68E−11**	**5.91E−11**	**1.13E−12**	**1.91E−12**	**4.47E−07**	**2.70E−09**	**7.25E−04**
M-of-n	**2.36E−11**	**1.75E−05**	**2.02E−02**	**2.58E−11**	**3.91E−06**	8.26E−01	**1.18E−05**	**1.52E−11**
penglungEW	**1.17E−07**	**1.27E−02**	**8.80E−11**	6.97E−02	**1.41E−02**	4.36E−01	**2.79E−10**	**1.47E−05**
SonarEW	**3.46E−08**	**1.33E−09**	**2.40E−09**	**1.53E−08**	**1.22E−03**	**8.34E−07**	**9.22E−08**	**2.95E−08**
SpectEW	**1.36E−10**	3.30E−01	**5.59E−11**	6.49E−02	**1.69E−14**	**1.69E−14**	**4.47E−03**	**1.69E−14**
CongressEW	**2.76E−02**	**3.16E−12**	5.52E−01	**2.59E−12**	**2.78E−10**	**1.22E−11**	**3.07E−09**	**5.05E−06**
IonosphereEW	**2.09E−11**	**2.25E−11**	**2.32E−07**	1.03E−01	**1.57E−10**	**1.94E−11**	**6.06E−10**	**1.14E−11**
KrvskpEW	**1.17E−11**	**1.19E−11**	**1.08E−10**	**8.77E−12**	**9.06E−12**	**1.93E−11**	**2.04E−11**	7.30E−02
Tic-tac-toe	**8.73E−14**	3.44E−01	**1.08E−12**	**1.69E−14**	**1.03E−12**	3.46E−01	2.18E−01	**1.69E−14**
Vote	**1.37E−06**	**1.13E−07**	**1.25E−10**	**1.44E−08**	**1.18E−13**	**1.94E−09**	**3.77E−13**	**1.69E−14**
WaveformEW	5.39E−01	1.81E−01	**2.99E−11**	**2.98E−04**	**1.24E−05**	**5.01E−10**	**1.21E−09**	**9.06E−04**
WineEW	**5.32E−12**	**2.70E−12**	**2.19E−12**	**1.39E−12**	**1.04E−12**	**1.17E−08**	**5.91E−13**	**1.55E−13**
Zoo	**4.33E−11**	**1.35E−11**	**3.63E−11**	**1.90E−05**	**6.41E−12**	**8.68E−12**	**5.11E−12**	**4.46E−13**

Bold values are less than 0.05

Table 10 Comparison between ITEO and other FS approaches from the literature in terms of classification accuracy using KNN classifier

Benchmark	GA1	PSO1	GWO1	GWO2	GA2	PSO2	ITEO
Breastcancer	0.957	0.949	0.976	0.975	0.968	0.967	**0.980**
BreastEW	0.923	0.933	0.924	0.935	0.939	0.933	**0.966**
CongressEW	0.898	0.937	0.935	0.938	0.932	0.928	**0.966**
Exactly	0.822	**0.973**	0.708	0.776	0.674	0.688	0.932
Exactly2	0.677	0.666	0.745	0.750	0.746	0.730	**0.765**
HeartEW	0.732	0.745	0.776	0.776	0.780	0.787	**0.888**
IonosphereEW	0.863	0.876	0.807	0.834	0.814	0.819	**0.888**
KrvskpEW	0.940	0.949	0.944	0.956	0.920	0.941	**0.965**
Lymphography	0.758	0.759	0.744	0.700	0.696	0.744	**0.888**
M-of-n	0.916	**0.996**	0.908	0.963	0.861	0.921	0.988
penglungEW	0.672	**0.879**	0.600	0.584	0.584	0.584	0.821
SonarEW	0.833	0.804	0.731	0.729	0.754	0.737	**0.877**
SpectEW	0.756	0.738	0.820	0.822	0.793	0.822	**0.859**
Tic-tac-toe	0.764	0.750	0.728	0.727	0.719	0.735	**0.795**
Vote	0.808	0.888	0.912	0.920	0.904	0.904	**0.960**
WaveformEW	0.712	0.732	0.786	0.789	0.773	0.762	**0.790**
WineEW	0.947	0.937	0.930	0.920	0.937	0.933	**0.988**
Zoo	0.946	**0.963**	0.879	0.879	0.855	0.861	0.959

the literature. [4, 10] proposed other FS approaches. Since they used only KNN classifier as an evaluator, we used to compare their work with the KNN based ITEO. Table 10 shows the comparison between TEO and GWO [4], PSO [4, 10], and GA [4, 10].

Observing the results in Table 10, ITEO proved its efficiency in solving feature selection problem. Where, ITEO results were the best in twelve out of eighteen datasets (66.7%), while PSO1 was the best in three datasets, GWO2 in two datasets and PSO2 in one dataset.

4.3.3 ITEO Improves Average Fitness Values over GA, PSO, and GWO

ITEO has been compared with other state-of-the-art well-known feature selection approaches (GA, PSO, and GWO) in terms of average fitness values. By inspecting Table 11, for KNN, ITEO outperformed other algorithms in eleven datasets (61.1%), while PSO and GWO each of which was the best in three datasets, finally GA was the best in only one dataset. While for DT, ITEO is better and it outperformed other algorithms in thirteen datasets (72.2%), while GA in two, GWO in two, and PSO in one dataset.

Table 11 Comparison between ITEO and the state-of-the-art FS approaches in terms of fitness values

	KNN classifier				DT classifier			
Dataset	GWO	BPSO	GA	ITEO	GWO	PSO	GA	ITEO
Breastcancer	**0.027**	0.035	0.032	0.029	0.045	0.059	0.040	**0.038**
BreastEW	0.053	0.057	0.052	**0.039**	0.057	0.078	0.047	**0.035**
CongressEW	0.078	0.046	0.062	**0.037**	**0.025**	0.057	0.047	0.035
Exactly	0.275	**0.011**	0.255	0.073	0.251	0.090	0.244	**0.049**
Exactly2	0.242	0.258	0.240	**0.238**	0.241	0.250	0.241	**0.238**
HeartEW	0.155	0.209	0.172	**0.117**	0.196	0.195	0.170	**0.148**
IonosphereEW	**0.112**	0.120	0.128	0.115	0.066	0.078	0.080	**0.059**
KrvskpEW	0.053	**0.040**	0.075	0.040	0.024	**0.021**	0.052	0.024
Lymphography	0.173	0.244	0.188	**0.116**	0.187	0.224	0.178	**0.135**
M-of-n	0.097	**0.011**	0.128	0.017	**0.008**	0.037	0.122	0.016
penglungEW	**0.136**	0.340	0.142	0.182	0.320	0.551	0.358	**0.308**
SonarEW	0.209	0.240	0.150	**0.127**	0.207	0.293	0.201	**0.131**
SpectEW	0.171	0.190	**0.140**	0.144	0.163	0.185	0.151	**0.127**
Tic-tac-toe	0.218	0.223	0.246	**0.214**	0.192	0.174	**0.157**	0.178
Vote	0.067	0.071	0.073	**0.043**	0.072	0.047	0.078	**0.030**
WaveformEW	0.223	0.216	0.242	**0.213**	0.258	0.267	0.264	**0.252**
WineEW	0.026	0.068	0.038	**0.017**	0.054	0.054	0.041	**0.040**
Zoo	0.081	0.187	0.075	**0.048**	0.116	0.159	**0.080**	0.085

4.3.4 ITEO Improves Average Features Reduction Rate over GA, PSO, and GWO

ITEO has been compared with other state-of-the-art well-known feature selection wrapper approaches (GA, PSO, and GWO) in terms of average features reduction rate. The following remarks can be made from Table 12. Firstly, when KNN is used, ITEO is not better than GA, since GA outperformed other algorithms in eight out of eighteen datasets, while ITEO in seven datasets. The remaining three datasets were for PSO and GWO. Secondly, for DT, ITEO acts much better than in KNN, where it outperformed others in twelve datasets. In contrast to GA's performance in KNN, GA was much worse in DT, where it wins only three times.

5 Conclusions

In this paper, a binary version of the recent nature inspired metaheuristic algorithm (Thermal Exchange Optimization) was proposed, and it is applied for the first time in the literature for solving the FS problem. Eighteen well-known benchmark datasets were utilized to assess the performance of the proposed algorithm. Overall, the classification accuracy, number of selected attributes, and the fitness values

Table 12 Comparison between ITEO and the state-of-the-art FS approaches in terms of number of selected features

	KNN classifier				DT classifier			
Dataset	GWO	PSO	GA	ITEO	GWO	PSO	GA	ITEO
Breastcancer	5.97	6.10	**3.90**	7.000	4.70	4.37	3.77	**3.000**
BreastEW	19.93	17.00	**16.07**	16.333	15.70	14.90	15.07	**14.467**
CongressEW	8.37	6.43	**4.83**	6.033	10.00	8.43	7.10	**5.267**
Exactly	9.97	**6.00**	7.40	6.767	7.37	**6.20**	7.30	6.767
Exactly2	**3.27**	4.57	4.07	6.133	**3.63**	5.67	4.13	4.567
HeartEW	11.73	7.93	**6.93**	8.233	7.87	6.20	6.40	**4.567**
IonosphereEW	18.23	14.47	15.20	**13.000**	20.90	17.43	**15.57**	17.033
KrvskpEW	26.80	19.27	19.50	**18.500**	30.33	26.40	**20.20**	23.233
Lymphography	8.87	9.20	**7.63**	8.933	8.43	9.10	8.30	**5.867**
M-of-n	9.97	**6.33**	7.87	6.767	9.23	9.10	7.70	**6.767**
penglungEW	159.80	161.67	151.30	**147.367**	162.20	161.90	155.30	**152.967**
SonarEW	31.90	29.93	29.47	**28.433**	34.97	**28.57**	28.93	29.867
SpectEW	11.63	10.60	11.20	**9.833**	14.03	11.40	10.87	**10.000**
Tic-tac-toe	8.50	7.10	**5.90**	9.000	7.30	7.40	7.17	**7.000**
Vote	11.17	6.60	7.37	**5.800**	8.00	8.00	6.17	**5.600**
WaveformEW	34.90	22.30	**21.37**	22.533	31.97	21.23	**20.77**	21.233
WineEW	7.77	7.60	6.87	**6.433**	6.73	7.47	6.23	**4.933**
Zoo	9.70	8.97	**8.27**	10.067	7.97	8.43	6.60	**5.800**

obtained from running the algorithm for 30 times were reported. Three popular FS methods were used for comparison purpose. The comparative results reveal the robustness and performance of BTEO in solving different FS problems. In this work, we employed one transfer function to convert the continuous version of TEO to binary, as future work, different transfer functions could be used, and the performance of TEO can be analyzed accordingly.

References

1. Aljarah, I., Mafarja, M., Heidari, A. A., Faris, H., Zhang, Y., & Mirjalili, S. (2018). Asynchronous accelerating multi-leader salp chains for feature selection. *Applied Soft Computing, 71*, 964–979.
2. Eberhart, R., & Kennedy, J. (1995). A new optimizer using particle swarm theory. In *Proceedings of the Sixth International Symposium on Micro Machine and Human Science, 1995. MHS'95* (pp. 39–43). Piscataway: IEEE.
3. Emary, E., & Zawbaa, H. M. (2016). Impact of chaos functions on modern swarm optimizers. *PLoS One, 11*(7), e0158738.
4. Emary, E., Zawbaa, H. M., & Hassanien, A. E. (2016). Binary ant lion approaches for feature selection. *Neurocomputing, 213*, 54–65.

5. Faris, H., Mafarja, M. M., Heidari, A. A., Aljarah, I., Ala'M, A. Z., Mirjalili, S., et al. (2018). An efficient binary salp swarm algorithm with crossover scheme for feature selection problems. *Knowledge-Based Systems, 154*, 43–67.
6. Grigull, U. (1984). Newton's temperature scale and the law of cooling. *Heat and Mass Transfer, 18*(4), 195–199.
7. Guyon, I., & Elisseeff, A. (2003). An introduction to variable and feature selection. *Journal of Machine Learning Research, 3*(Mar), 1157–1182.
8. Holland, J. H. (1992). *Adaptation in natural and artificial systems: An introductory analysis with applications to biology, control, and artificial intelligence*. Cambridge: MIT Press.
9. Jović, A., Brkić, K., & Bogunović, N. (2015). A review of feature selection methods with applications. In *38th International Convention on Information and Communication Technology, Electronics and Microelectronics (MIPRO), 2015* (pp. 1200–1205). Piscataway: IEEE.
10. Kashef, S., & Nezamabadi-pour, H. (2015). An advanced ACO algorithm for feature subset selection. *Neurocomputing, 147*, 271–279.
11. Kaveh, A., & Bakhshpoori, T. (2016). Water evaporation optimization: A novel physically inspired optimization algorithm. *Computers & Structures, 167*, 69–85.
12. Kaveh, A., & Dadras, A. (2017). A novel meta-heuristic optimization algorithm: Thermal exchange optimization. *Advances in Engineering Software, 110*, 69–84.
13. Kaveh, A., Dadras, A., & Bakhshpoori, T. (2018). Improved thermal exchange optimization algorithm for optimal design of skeletal structures. *Smart Structures and Systems, 21*, 263–278.
14. Kaveh, A., & Talatahari, S. (2010). A novel heuristic optimization method: Charged system search. *Acta Mechanica, 213*(3), 267–289.
15. Kirkpatrick, S., Gelatt, C. D., Vecchi, M. P., et al. (1983). Optimization by simulated annealing. *Science, 220*(4598), 671–680.
16. Kohavi, R., & John, G. H. (1997). Wrappers for feature subset selection. *Artificial intelligence, 97*(1–2), 273–324.
17. Lichman, M. (2013). UCI machine learning repository. http://archive.ics.uci.edu/ml
18. Liu, H., & Motoda, H. (2012). *Feature selection for knowledge discovery and data mining* (Vol. 454). Berlin: Springer.
19. Mafarja, M., & Abdullah, S. (2013). Investigating memetic algorithm in solving rough set attribute reduction. *International Journal of Computer Applications in Technology, 48*(3), 195–202.
20. Mafarja, M., & Abdullah, S. (2013). Record-to-record travel algorithm for attribute reduction in rough set theory. *Journal of Theoretical and Applied Information Technology, 49*(2), 507–513.
21. Mafarja, M., & Mirjalili, S. (2017). Hybrid whale optimization algorithm with simulated annealing for feature selection. *Neurocomputing, 260*, 302–312.
22. Mafarja, M., & Mirjalili, S. (2017). Whale optimization approaches for wrapper feature selection. *Applied Soft Computing, 62*, 441–453.
23. Mafarja, M., & Mirjalili, S. (2018). Hybrid binary ant lion optimizer with rough set and approximate entropy reducts for feature selection. *Soft Computing, 23*, 6249–6265.
24. Mafarja, M., Aljarah, I., Heidari, A. A., Hammouri, A. I., Faris, H., Ala'M, A. Z., et al. (2017). Evolutionary population dynamics and grasshopper optimization approaches for feature selection problems. *Knowledge-Based Systems, 145*, 25–45.
25. Mafarja, M., Eleyan, D., Abdullah, S., & Mirjalili, S. (2017). S-shaped vs. v-shaped transfer functions for ant lion optimization algorithm in feature selection problem. In *Proceedings of the International Conference on Future Networks and Distributed Systems* (p. 14). New York: ACM.
26. Mafarja, M., Aljarah, I., Heidari, A. A., Faris, H., Fournier-Viger, P., Li, X., et al. (2018). Binary dragonfly optimization for feature selection using time-varying transfer functions. *Knowledge-Based Systems, 161*, 185–204.

27. Mafarja, M., Aljarah, I., Heidari, A. A., Hammouri, A. I., Faris, H., Ala'M, A. Z., et al. (2018). Evolutionary population dynamics and grasshopper optimization approaches for feature selection problems. *Knowledge-Based Systems, 145*, 25–45.
28. Mirjalili, S., & Lewis, A. (2013). S-shaped versus v-shaped transfer functions for binary particle swarm optimization. *Swarm and Evolutionary Computation, 9*, 1–14. https://doi.org/10.1016/j.swevo.2012.09.002, http://www.sciencedirect.com/science/article/pii/S2210650212000648
29. Nagpal, S., Arora, S., Dey, S., et al. (2017). Feature selection using gravitational search algorithm for biomedical data. *Procedia Computer Science, 115*, 258–265.
30. Rashedi, E., & Nezamabadi-pour, H. (2014). Feature subset selection using improved binary gravitational search algorithm. *Journal of Intelligent & Fuzzy Systems, 26*(3), 1211–1221.
31. Rashedi, E., Nezamabadi-Pour, H., & Saryazdi, S. (2009). GSA: A gravitational search algorithm. *Information Sciences, 179*(13), 2232–2248.
32. Rashedi, E., Nezamabadi-Pour, H., & Saryazdi, S. (2010). BGSA: Binary gravitational search algorithm. *Natural Computing, 9*(3), 727–745.
33. Xiang, J., Han, X., Duan, F., Qiang, Y., Xiong, X., Lan, Y., et al. (2015). A novel hybrid system for feature selection based on an improved gravitational search algorithm and k-NN method. *Applied Soft Computing, 31*, 293–307.

Printed in the United States
By Bookmasters